THE BUSINESS OF MOVEMENT

THE BUSINESS OF MOVEMENT

Principles, Patterns, and Productivity

GRAY COOK

with *Jeremy Hall*
and *Matt Cook*

ON TARGET PUBLICATIONS, APTOS, CALIFORNIA

The Business of Movement

Principles, Patterns, and Productivity

Gray Cook

*with Jeremy Hall
and Matt Cook*

Copyright © 2022 Gray Cook
ISBN-13: 978-1-931046-52-7, paperback
ISBN-13: 978-1-931046-47-3, epub

All rights reserved. Printed in the United States of America. No part of this book may be reproduced or transmitted in any form whatsoever without written permission from the author or publisher, with the exception of the inclusions of brief quotations in articles or reviews.

On Target Publications
P. O. Box 1335
Aptos, California 95001 USA
otpbooks.com

Library of Congress Control Number: 2021951970

CONTENTS

FOREWORD	7
INTRODUCTION: Where You Begin Dictates Where You'll End	9
PART ONE—AWARENESS	21
CHAPTER ONE: Principles—Strategies—Tactics	23
CHAPTER TWO: Changing Perception	31
CHAPTER THREE: A Modern Model of Movement	47
CHAPTER FOUR: Refine Your Value—Recognize Your Opportunity	87
PART TWO—OPPORTUNITIES: Identify Your Non-Negotiables	99
CHAPTER FIVE: Own the Process	105
CHAPTER SIX: Master the Functional Movement Systems	109
CHAPTER SEVEN: Understand Your Client	121
CHAPTER EIGHT: Start with Function	135
CHAPTER NINE: Have a Plan for Pain	145
CHAPTER TEN: Master Your Communication. Own Your Accountability	155
CHAPTER ELEVEN: Create an Experience, Instill Awareness	161
CHAPTER TWELVE: Protect the Quality You Find	181
CHAPTER THIRTEEN: Correct the Quality That Doesn't Meet the Standard	191
CHAPTER FOURTEEN: Develop the Quality to Support Adaptation	221
CHAPTER FIFTEEN: Elevate Performance or Empower Independence	241
CHAPTER SIXTEEN: Know Where You're Going	253
PART THREE—EXAMPLES: Turning Pro	263

CHAPTER SEVENTEEN: Measure What Matters — 267

CHAPTER EIGHTEEN: Build Your Community, Change Your Culture — 295

CHAPTER NINETEEN: Build Your Team — 311

CHAPTER TWENTY: Scale Your Business — 327

CHAPTER TWENTY-ONE: Be Transformational, Not Transactional — 341

CHAPTER TWENTY-TWO: Find Your Path — 345

APPENDICES

SYSTEM OVERVIEW — 353

RISKS TO MUSCULOSKELETAL HEALTH — 357

RED/YELLOW/GREEN LIGHT EXERCISES — 361

STANDARD OPERATING PROCEDURE OF MOVEMENT — 363

EXAMPLE PATIENT PROGRESS NOTE — 365

RECOMMENDED READING — 367

CONTRIBUTOR BIOS — 369

INDEX — 371

DEDICATION — 379

FOREWORD

- Are you ready to question your personal and professional actions when movement obstacles are in your way?
- Are you ready to learn and use new tools to see what you're missing in movement?
- Are you ready to change your movement culture?

These may not be easy questions to get behind, but if you work in the movement environment—whether clinician, coach or trainer—you know we as a profession must be better.

In 2003, I published my first book, *Athletic Body in Balance*, forecasting the problems I saw coming in human movement. That same year a (real) author named Michael Lewis wrote a book that fueled my perspective and made me want to build an even better case for overhauling movement. His book was called *Moneyball: The Art of Winning an Unfair Game*.

Baseball at that time had turned into a statistical payroll game. The teams with the biggest payrolls had most of the success and those with the lowest payrolls had the least success. End of story. America's game was nothing but another financial institution that fixed problems with money instead of through human physical and character development, grit, and better competitive strategies.

In this wonderful game's sad evolution, Goliath kept beating David, and it was getting boring to watch…until the Oakland A's changed everything. They focused on the overlooked statistics that truly mattered and changed the culture of the game. To me, Lewis's book wasn't about baseball; it was about becoming significantly more effective using the same resources.

And that was exactly what we were doing with movement.

My partners and our instructors have been teaching and implementing our Functional Movement Systems around the world. We get paid to talk and then answer questions. Some call that education, but our real value is when we get to *ask* the questions.

When we get to audit you, your team, your intakes, your process, and your outcomes, we usually expose unnecessary assumptions, upstream issues, and poor use of basic feedback loops. It's how we mentored each other and it's how we developed the systems that improved our businesses and can improve yours as well.

Good business systematically develops and redevelops a product or service to stay valuable, relevant, and sustainable. The central key to systematic development in business is *measurement* because what gets measured gets done.

Most financial superpowers of the last 40 years seem to agree in word and action that for sustained success, we must first protect the downside.

Reality check: The business of human movement is statistically one of the poorest examples of failed management of a downside. In the past 40 years, we've allowed the physical culture of much of the world to measurably erode while we managed our profit margins, delivering the illusion of rehabilitation, fitness, and sports performance.

On our watch, the physically healthy and fit majority has become the minority. Physical education has no standard of learning, military physical standards have been systematically lowered, and sports have become profit centers that no longer generate life lessons or character development. Under it all lies a health and physical rehabilitation model that amounts to whatever insurance will pay for regardless of outcomes. These trends cannot continue, which is why we're so driven to teach our systems.

There were early adopters who leaned in and helped us become an international brand through their command of the information and their subsequent actions. Many of their stories are in this book. We've learned, through our work and theirs, that we don't rise to the level of our education; we fall to the level of our training.

This book will ask many questions. Those questions are best answered with information, action and reflection because the entirety of the system isn't about proprietary movement patterns. It's about using feedback effectively and efficiently. It's about learning to listen to what movement is telling you before you take action…and having confidence in the response you provide.

Gray Cook

INTRODUCTION

WHERE YOU BEGIN
DICTATES WHERE YOU'LL END

If you're reading this book, you're probably in a profession that touches movement. Whether in rehabilitation, physical education, fitness, athletics, or even high-end performance, you're most likely hoping to understand how to leverage a fresh set of innovative tactics or a new way of thinking to elevate your business. I have no doubt the information contained in these pages will elevate your level of service well above the rest of your competition.

However, what ultimately distinguishes your business has less to do with innovative techniques and tactics, and more to do with the strategies and systems you learn and embed in your practice. Physical culture and the consumer's perspective about movement will soon change—positioning yourself to gain access to a world of new business opportunities requires learning how to better use the practical science at hand.

For 30 years, I've had a front-row seat to the changing perspectives of human movement. It all started with a central question I had as a young physical therapist and strength coach: What's driving movement behavior—form or function? Is your unconscious decision-making process of movement driven by structure and anatomy or function and behavior? It's easy to say "both," but then we need to have a measuring stick for both.

I wrestled with this because whichever end of movement I was on at the time, people were discussing body parts far more than movement patterns. People aimed procedures, products, programs, and services at a particular fraction of movement without recognizing a whole-movement archetype all humans should own. I struggled with the question of "When is it okay to lose these basic patterns?"

We don't have to go back to look at earlier homo sapiens for a whole-movement archetype—it's expressed in every one of us through the developmental sequence of the first 21 months of life.[1] That progression isn't measured in

---

[1] https://cdn.who.int/media/docs/default-source/child-growth/child-growth-standards/indicators/motor-development-milestones/graph--windows-of-achievement-for-six-gross-motor-milestones04ac-44c38d96466498e7633d9d44c7e6.pdf

https://www.cdc.gov/ncbddd/actearly/milestones/index.html

terms of individual parts, but as a sequence of patterns, each building upon one another as we progress from controlling the motion of our heads to rolling, creeping, crawling, kneeling, squatting, standing, and stepping. That sequence of patterns represents the natural movement operating system on which we install and integrate the complex and robust "applications" and movement skills our environments and activities provide.

The patterns of movement become distorted when an adolescent goes through a growth spurt and the musculoskeletal system is thrown out of balance with the nervous system. When people become injured, the expectation is these patterns are lost, at least temporarily. But as we finish rehabilitation or send patients back into their lives—their fitness, hobbies, or sports—why don't we revisit the whole patterns? And what if the activities or lifestyles we're sending them back to were eroding the quality of these fundamental movement patterns all along?

Across healthcare, the assumption was that if range of motion and strength were good, quality movement patterns were possible. Across fitness, the assumption was that simply scaling the difficulty or finding the right progression of an exercise would automatically resolve faulty parts or patterns of movement. Yet, I view movement as the canary in the coal mine—that delicate and sensitive indicator we can watch to tell us if we're in a toxic environment or if our behaviors and lifestyles are working against us.

When my colleagues and I began looking for opportunities to screen movement, we took otherwise fit people who'd passed a pre-participation physical exam and were cleared for sports, and looked for nothing more than the presence or absence of a few fundamental movement patterns. We found that roughly 20 percent of these athletes who "passed" their physical exams had pain on one or more of the seven movement patterns that made up our simple movement screen.

As shocking as that was, many of the remaining 80% demonstrated significant alterations in the quality of these basic movements.

We had to contend with the issue that with no clear physical impairment in the parts of the system, the internal operating system that allows us to run these basic movement "programs" must be dysfunctional. And if that system couldn't consistently and effectively process the basics, what could be gained by trying to install more onto that system? We thought taking the traditional route of programming new or more complex movements without first trying to restore function to the foundational system offered little to gain…and increased the risk of crashing the platform.

Fast forward a couple decades and, unfortunately, the general approach to movement hasn't changed much in health or fitness. If anything, technology has taken us further down the rabbit hole and mesmerized people with the speed and precision of measuring the tiniest details of a body's functions.

More and more, we're missing the whole perspective Aristotle imparted a long time ago: The whole is greater than the sum of its parts.

The quest to understand the human body continues to reduce us to smaller areas of focus, where we find ourselves arguing over which individual factor is more important to enhance health or human performance. Our myopic approach to health, fitness, and performance severs the lines connecting each deconstructed piece and leaves us without a unified system to put someone on the path toward an ideal physical state.

We know that the whole is greater than the sum of its parts, but we so rarely measure and operate accordingly. The challenge my partners and I explored was to objectively measure and communicate what authentic, quality human movement looked like…or better yet, didn't look like. Our shared purpose was to create a common language surrounding movement and to develop tools that could accurately and reliably tell the story of how the body moves. If we could develop a system to establish a qualitative baseline for movement, it could be one more tool to help us manage movement in more economical and sustainable ways.

Functional Movement Systems emerged from trying to hold ourselves to a higher standard in qualifying and quantifying global human movement, and seeing if that standard could survive in hostile environments. We considered athletics, the military, and even some healthcare and fitness environments hostile because none of those environments were or are begging for a revolution. The decision makers rarely want a different perspective that will injure tradition or the current profitability models despite the increased risk that comes with being the last to change.

Functional Movement Systems evolved over the last 20 years from the data and feedback gathered in those environments, despite the fact a lot of the professions tied to health and fitness didn't make or want changes. For you, that's actually good because that's where new opportunities lie, some of which we'll introduce in this book.

The Functional Movement Screen (FMS™) has been deployed as a frontline movement screening tool in elementary school gym classes, personal training studios, professional sports combines, and military bases. The Selective Functional Movement Assessment (SFMA™) has been used as a tool for clinicians to better direct care in eliminating pain caused by dysfunctional movement, with the Y Balance Test (YBT™) serving as a valuable data point on the quality of motor control.

The Fundamental Capacity Screen (FCS™) has allowed us to identify gaps in fitness and movement capacity to direct better exercise and conditioning programming in the same informed, systematic manner as our corrective strategies in the FMS and SFMA. Most recently, we've implemented the Functional

Breathing Screen to inspect the activity we all do 17,000 times a day, but rarely with the quality or intention it deserves.

This book isn't intended to be a course manual on how to perform the Functional Movement Systems. Rather, it connects the philosophy of the Systems with the selection and application of them as part of your standard operating procedures. Even if your experience is with a single screen or assessment, our goal is to allow you to see the connection that binds these tools together. The whole of the Systems offers information when dysfunctional movement is present and can direct your actions, backward toward the root cause of trouble and forward along a path of growth and adaptation.

If the events of a pandemic have shown us anything, it's that people are seeking movement opportunities that offer greater levels of independence as they learn more about rehabilitating themselves and exercising on their own.

Most people can recognize the potential risk of engaging with new physical endeavors when their movement patterns are poor or painful. But without obvious indicators, many of us lack the ability to question the integrity of our movement operating system, and with it the ability to predict the response and adaptation to the stress of exercise or activity.

Because so many of our movement problems operate outside of our conscious awareness or control, they go unexamined and unaddressed until it is too late. We think of movement quality, balance, coordination, and posture as qualities to be trained, but things like sleep deprivation, dehydration, poor nutrition, and psychological stress can affect these qualities just as significantly as a lack of activity. When these largely subconscious movement patterns are gradually lost, you cannot will them back through focus and concentration—you need to recalibrate your behaviors, activities, and lifestyle choices to restore balance to the system.

If you agree that it's not acceptable to lose the fundamental movement signature we all express as we learn to move, you can bring excellent business practices to the opportunities that presents. Delivering new movement information in an accessible and actionable way will allow you to help people grow strong and age gracefully in a more profound and sustainable way by helping to change their lives and their environments.

> *"The first principle is that you must not fool yourself—and you're the easiest person to fool."*
> *—Richard Feynman*

A PATH OF ACTIVE LEARNING

In our journey to improve, we've all heard some version of the 10,000-hour rule—the idea that with a fundamental basis of knowledge, we just need to put in the required time to practice and master our professional skills and abilities. Going to school, learning all the joints, muscles, and nerves and how to influence them…and then practicing is the simple formula to master our craft, right?

If only it were that simple.

We know that isn't how it works, but that's how many of us operate. The fundamentals needed aren't just more knowledge and more skills, but also constant analysis to prevent us from spending 2,000 of those hours doing something that can be counterproductive to development.

It took us the better part of three decades to learn and refine our model of movement. We hope to shorten that window for you.

Working with the human body is more complex than any single system can describe or coordinate, but the Functional Movement Systems are intended to provide a model on which to orient the direction of your practice. The strategies and standard operating procedures are there to systematically identify the weakest link and allow you to capture, clarify, organize, and work on a weakness until it's no longer standing in the way. Applying and reapplying that process to clear the bottlenecks in your professional practice allows you to see more clearly and creates the mental space to be more creative, more innovative, and more present in your work. This is the core of professional development.

In a day and age when we see so many opportunities for mentorship, I prefer to go in another direction. I still prefer the term "apprenticeship" because it's less about the mentor and more about how the student learns to internalize and apply the practice. The mentor provides the apprentice with the instruction on how to use the map and compass, but the responsibility isn't on the mentor to guarantee the apprentice competency. The responsibility is on the apprentice to apply and build on that knowledge on the path to greater mastery. I've always encouraged people to read, study, and learn as much as they can, but everyone needs to go on a personal journey of putting that information into practice before they become a prophet (or worse, a zealot).

Mirroring the steps and actions of successful coaches or clinicians can lead to a similar level of success, but there are no shortcuts or hacks for building both an impactful *and* sustainable business around movement. Shortcuts and instructions don't help when you encounter an environment or a barrier that didn't exist for those who went before you. The tactics and skills they developed may not deliver the change you need or expect in your particular situation. Dead-ends and false starts are inevitable on any journey unless you set out with an understanding of how to make better decisions or to uncover new information when you find yourself in uncharted territory. Failure occurs when there's no means to get back on course toward the destination.

In this book, I hope to communicate how you can take the work we began with the Functional Movement Systems to create your personal GPS to navigate the changing landscape of human movement. I'm confident that what we've developed can offer you the chance to see movement and your own perceptions and behaviors through a new, more complete lens—whether you've been using our tools and systems for some time or if this is new territory for you. Navigating toward success as both a practitioner and a business owner can be a much straighter line when you're armed with both a clearer map and a more accurate compass to inform your decisions. However, the most challenging and necessary step to starting that journey is understanding where you are today and where you ultimately hope to go.

Nailing down where you are and where you hope to be seems like an easy enough exercise, but most of us don't spend the time formalizing those two points because it requires a self-appraisal and establishing our awareness by asking hard questions:

- ▶ Do I have standards to which I hold myself and my work? What are the principles that dictate the way I treat, train, or coach?
- ▶ Why do I do the things I do? Are my professional behaviors guided by objective feedback…or my personal biases?
- ▶ What's the criteria I use to assess my decisions or say a client or patient is better in the short or long term?
- ▶ Am I as consistent as I could be? Am I as effective as I want to be?
- ▶ Am I ready and willing to change?

If you do nothing more than turn these over in your mind and try to answer them honestly and objectively, you'll already be ahead of the game. Many people spend their entire careers operating off of unexamined beliefs or behaviors, going through the motions or blindly following the rest of the herd. You no doubt ask your patients or clients to reflect on their responses to questions similar to these, so you should hold yourself to the same standard.

This isn't an exercise that just happens once. If your goal is to continue to grow and develop, you should be asking yourself these questions every step of the way, whether formally or informally. Holding your beliefs and actions up to critical analysis can be a painful experience—but a bruise to your ego is far less perilous than your beliefs and actions failing to evolve.

As more professionals in healthcare, fitness, and the performance fields used the Movement Systems, our own perspectives evolved as we realized our early work was only scratching the surface of the conversation. The only way to balance the modern, reductive approach to movement was by creating a holistic model that could work alongside it; so we set out to create a new language around whole movement patterns for everyone to stand on the same movement standard footing.

RADICAL TRANSPARENCY + ALGORITHMIC THINKING

The evolution of our work is the direct result of our continued pursuit of radical transparency and algorithmic thinking. I didn't have the words to describe those two principles until I was introduced to them by investor Ray Dalio in both his TED talk and his book *Principles*. Although he presented both terms from a financial and organizational perspective, the principles of both are equally relevant in the context of health and fitness.

Radical transparency seeks measurable truth, communication, and accountability. It requires that we hold the systems, models, and processes we build (and the outcomes they produce) up to a clear standard of measurement to challenge our assumptions and biases and the validity of our work.

Algorithmic thinking introduces the systems that are one of the best vaccinations against confirmation bias—something that's easy to recognize in others and hard to recognize in ourselves. Algorithmic thinking helps us construct systems to *collect* reliable, objective data, and also to *organize* and *use* it in a way to help build better decision-making models and processes.

Embedded in movement, Nature gave us the algorithm for a sustainable, physically vital lifestyle. Developing the tools and systems to decode that formula while removing confirmation bias from our decision-making has allowed us to cross-examine the current perspective on movement to quickly and clearly see opportunities of which our business competition may not be aware.

As Dalio says, sometimes you need to bet against the consensus—especially when you're confident you're right. The consensus is that healthcare makes its profit on procedures and services to help people suffer less from earlier behaviors that would have easily made them suffer more.

Fitness and performance sell products and services, but don't profit if the client becomes independent in the journey. And unfortunately, even physical education—if it's still a class in school—has no standard of learning to install physical competence at that critical stage of life.

Rather than chasing the current idea that we need equipment pulled from a sports science lab or mountains of data pulled from our wearable devices, maybe we should be embracing the opposite concept. The requirements needed to develop and sustain remarkable human performance are simple:

- ▶ An environment that fosters frequent and challenging work with opportunities to move under a variety of conditions

- Opportunities for self-learning
- And the safety to fail

We can create those conditions through authentic, enjoyable physical activities or highly technical and supervised exercise and training, but neither depend on the latest and greatest gear or instruction. The path to greater performance and production begins with a roadmap to change the perceptions, behaviors, and actions around the often-overlooked link between human health and performance: movement.

At Functional Movement Systems, we've had the incredible opportunity to train over 60,000 professionals in our philosophies, who stress-tested our systems around the world. In receiving a tremendous volume of feedback over the years, we discovered our greatest failure was in assuming the theory and practice of the Systems could be easily applied.

Our goal has always been to make sure each student receives the instruction and reinforcement of the screens to be comfortable using them when returning to work, but information overload is a real struggle when trying to fit a foundational education in systems thinking into a continuing education model. For a long time, we showed people how to screen, thinking they'd go back to their home environments, use the standards we designed, and change their practices for the better.

We didn't appreciate that to deliver the Systems in the way we designed them—as standardized but adaptive processes—requires the technical know-how, and also faith in the process and a willingness to be held to a new standard.

There are questions we ask around movement, but sometimes we don't or won't listen to what movement has to say. Adopting a new way of perceiving movement or new behaviors in how we practice can be daunting when it requires a degree of deprogramming from the way we've all been taught. Trying to reconfigure an approach from one of tactically addressing parts to a more strategic and holistic system of improving the qualities of movement entails a heavy dose of humility.

Many people believe dedicating themselves to a system will infringe on their expertise or undermine their authority, when in fact, the humility that comes with trusting a process actually exposes the fact we're all fallible. We all possess biases that can hinder objectivity, and we can all have a bad Tuesday and fall back on comfortable or convenient habits or methods that may not be serving us.

The practitioners who seem to intuitively choose the right action at the right time have often reached a level of mastery from consciously or unconsciously constructing processes that force them to question what they're doing, why they're doing it, and how. Although we all strive to be objective in our assessments and interventions, when we lack tools to measure or quantify the missing pieces of the puzzle, we're prone to allow opinions or biases to fill the gaps in our logic and reasoning. When we then apply our expertise to solve the problem without an objective feedback loop to tell us if we're on the right track, we compound the issue by laying assumptions of what is or isn't working on top of our assumptions of what was wrong.

We've been lucky because many masters of their crafts have left their marks on the Functional Movement Systems. These professionals supported a common-sense approach to the way we think, speak, and act toward movement that champions communication and accountability.

Even if you're just beginning your professional journey or aren't familiar with every nuance of our work, the ability to see movement more clearly and focus your attention and skills on changing it is within reach. It simply demands that you hold yourself to a higher standard in moving beyond individual tools and tactics to construct the processes and systems connecting your decisions and actions to a holistic plan. In pursuit of that, we hope to give you the confidence to grow in an informed and sustainable way through that new standard built around the science of movement.

The book is presented in three sections, each building on the former toward a systematic approach to designing your own blueprint of lasting change for your clients, your practice, and your business. Creating the environment to facilitate those changes requires a flexible system of checks and balances to help you perform a self-appraisal of your strengths and weaknesses, and produce those blinking red lights that tell us, "Stop and look here first."

SYSTEMATICALLY UNCOVERING OPPORTUNITY

Part One will help you ground yourself in the foundational principles underpinning our philosophy and approach and bring awareness to where you stand today. Part Two outlines the processes and insights of implementing the Systems as a strategy to take advantage of opportunities to raise your effectiveness and efficiency. Part Three offers examples from professionals who built successful careers and businesses across the fields of health and human performance by leveraging those strategies to expand their professional impact.

We structured this book in a practical manner to allow you to build on each component of working with clients or patients and ultimately building a business. If you're new to FMS, reading the sections in sequence will help you learn and implement our best practices in a logical order to ensure your success with the process. If you've previously taken one of our courses, there's value in seeing how we knit the Systems together into a more complete and comprehensive process.

It's impossible to implement all of the pieces at once. In fact, some elements may feel more like deprogramming current behaviors or perceptions, which takes time. What we hope to outline is a process for change, built around consistent practice and feedback to keep you on the path of improvement.

But be engaged with the process. Be a healthy skeptic. Challenge things. Prove us wrong. Taking that approach leads to learning, not blindly following our advice or instruction. Just know this in advance: We've tried to break these processes many times ourselves.

> *"It's what you learn after you know it all that counts."*
> **—Harry S. Truman**

By the end of this book, I hope you'll turn this approach to movement into a more responsible business model than most of what the health and fitness industry is selling today. You won't even need to know our tactics to realize how understanding the larger picture can help you spotlight the weak spots in you or your business—especially if you want to be an early adopter.

You're in a service profession, which means you're in this for relationships. Your service isn't a product, and this isn't a quick sale. Even when you won't be the service provider, you'll be an effective and desirable referral if you believe in this model. You don't have to know how to do an FMS or the SFMA—you just need to know your niche and own it.

This book is about challenging perceptions and changing behavior:

- ▶ Changing clients' behaviors around nutrition, sleep, recovery, and activity
- ▶ Changing your professional behaviors around testing and assessment, applying manual or exercise interventions, and designing and teaching lifestyle and training programs
- ▶ Changing our business behaviors around how we communicate with or market ourselves to clients, how we train and educate staff, and how we build a culture of movement to empower and promote health and fitness

If you're familiar with our work, there will be areas applicable more to your particular challenges as a healthcare practitioner, personal trainer, or strength and performance specialist. But before you cherry-pick from one area over another, don't lose sight that the whole is greater than the sum of its parts.

What we may confidently believe is a strength can sometimes go too long without being re-evaluated, exposing cracks only when we finally shed light on it. If it's been a while since you critically appraised your processes, particularly around the movement screens, I can't stress enough the benefit of polishing those neglected areas.

In our seminars, we often talk about creating windows of opportunity to change the awareness of patients and clients to propel them toward their physical goals. We don't just do this through instruction—we make them face their personal screen results. Today marks your own similar window of opportunity. You have the freedom to assess your personal and professional perspectives and behaviors, and gain the awareness and strategies with which you'll achieve your goals.

It took us the better part of 30 years to master our approach, but by putting the years of combined experience contained in these pages into action, you can make a lasting impact and achieve success in a fraction of that time. The Functional Movement Screen spoke volumes to the early adopters in the professional realm through helping them integrate a movement-focused approach. I now hope those perspectives drawn from the Functional Movement Systems will help you create a Version 2.0 of our work that will speak volumes to professionals and the early adopters in the private sector and those engaging in health and fitness pursuits.

Taking a systematic approach may feel like slow going at times, but you'll soon be a step ahead of the people looking to hack the process. It can be challenging to implement the methodology into your daily work—and impossible to incorporate it all at once—but anything sustainable is best won through a little bit of planning, a little bit of thinking, a little bit of action, and sometimes a bit of struggle.

I challenge you to find at least one part of this book that takes you out of your comfort zone. Does it take you out of your comfort zone because you inherently feel it's wrong or does it take you out of your comfort zone because you're unfamiliar with it? Does it take you out of your comfort zone because you believe it won't work or because it runs counter to your behaviors and actions?

There can be no growth without discomfort, and if nothing changes, nothing changes. Putting knowledge into action is essential in our collective journey toward personal and professional mastery; but we can't lose sight of the words of Hall of Fame UCLA basketball coach John Wooden: "Never mistake activity for achievement."

PART ONE: AWARENESS

CHAPTER ONE

PRINCIPLES—STRATEGIES—TACTICS

"As to methods there may be a million and then some, but principles are few. The man who grasps principles can successfully select his own methods. The man who tries methods, ignoring principles, is sure to have trouble."
—**Harrington Emerson**

Thirty years ago, I was sitting in the same place you might be sitting now. Before the birth of Functional Movement Systems and our definition of the term "functional movement," I was practicing as a physical therapist and strength coach in a small town, struggling with consistently solving the challenges of patients and clients. I believed if I had enough time and enough tools at my disposal, I could fix any patient who walked through the door. In my mind, it was just a matter of doing more tests, collecting more data, and gathering more resources (exercises, manual techniques, communication skills, or specialized equipment), and I could then re-engineer that body.

I dedicated my time and effort to gathering and deploying those resources to coach people toward better movement. Yet, often the faulty patterns of movement I wanted to change didn't improve. The additional tactics I had at my disposal weren't producing the level of consistent and predictable change I believed my clients deserved. I slowly realized that how people appeared after I reduced them to discrete components of bones, joints, and soft tissues wasn't indicative of how they looked once they stood up and moved.

The more my partners and I engaged in our early quest to define what we meant by "functional" movement and to develop a tool to measure it, the more imperative it became to establish and reinforce the principles that would need to underlie any system we designed. We didn't set out to disrupt the status quo, but we realized we needed a solid ground to stand on against the scrutiny of people who may not have wanted us to succeed. We led with common truths that should be the building blocks of any philosophy, program, or system that considers physical development or rehabilitation:

- ▶ We cannot develop ourselves or others better than nature.
- ▶ We can develop ourselves and others safer and faster than nature.
- ▶ Proper progression is demonstration of favorable behaviors at one level of development before proceeding to the next.

These aren't really principles—they're the basic concepts of living within an environment. They speak to the natural biological process through which we grow and thrive in the world in which we live. We too often step on nature in our need to control or optimize a situation. The most robust and healthiest people are often those without exercise equipment or a coach or a periodized or planned program; their environments shape them where moderation and self-awareness provide a competitive advantage.

In the words of Albert Einstein, paraphrased: "Everything must be made as simple as possible, but not simpler."

In healthcare, teaching, coaching, and training, we lacked a shared professional *why*, and without that *why* statement, we'd been looking incorrectly at the basics of movement.

The *why* statement behind all we do is encapsulated in the three principles that make up our foundation. They're simple, yet address the core aspects of physical growth development that allow us to deepen our understanding and guide our efforts to identify and correct faulty movement when we find it, regardless of methodology.

It took a long time to gain enough perspective, but as we formulated our strategy for evaluating and correcting movement, we distilled it into three movement principles.

Principle One: First move well, then move often.

Principle One is our natural principle: *First move well, then move often*. We should seek a qualitative minimum before we worry about quantities. If moving well is the standard, moving often is the foreseeable outcome. Even the most complex, high-level problems of world-class athletes are rooted in the basics. The same fundamentals apply for children as they do for high performers, but people lose the narrative. Rather than jumping straight into exercises or performance training and chasing maximums, we must first get back to ensuring we've first met the minimums.

Principle Two: Protect, correct, then develop.

Principle Two is our ethical principle. It directs us to *protect, correct, then develop* movement…in that order. For those with a medical background, it's the guiding principle of the Hippocratic Oath—First, do no harm. Then progress in a direction of independence and sustainability.

Principle Three: Create systems to support your philosophy.

Principle Three is our practical and cultural principle. It tells us to *create systems that enforce our philosophy*. We should always strive to implement standard operating procedures, practice intelligent selection, and match the stress and recovery cycle to the growth and development we desire.

Just like a laboratory experiment, if we deploy a consistent process within a framework of objective checks and balances, we can identify when our choices and actions are producing the desired effect. Without that process, we lean too heavily on the art of coaching or medicine at the expense of objectivity. The standard operating procedures we developed in the Functional Movement Systems create guardrails to keep us on a path pointed toward progress. That process reinforces the fact that no single data point holds all the answers—patterns and behaviors provide more valuable information because they offer a more complete map on which to work.

> *"All the men can see the tactics I use to conquer, but what none can see is the strategy out of which great victory is evolved."*
> —*General Sun Tzu*

THE PATTERNS OF GLOBAL MOVEMENT

Despite my belief in the importance of how the body moves, my early career was so focused on investigating and fixing faulty parts, I wasn't stepping back to appreciate the global picture of movement. Instead of challenging my perspective and asking myself better questions about how seemingly healthy or strong patients could break down or move in dysfunctional ways, I was feeding everyone the same exercise nutrients and expecting the same end result of better movement. Rather than questioning if I missed a component of the big picture, I just applied different tools and techniques when I didn't get predictable responses to my interventions. I made the assumption that my diagnosis was competent and my treatment was incomplete.

Then I flipped the question and my professional trajectory changed forever.

I was always thoughtful in my approach, but I was fixing body parts and assuming movement would change, instead of looking at movement first and then working through body parts to confirm my observations. I was dedicating my time and attention to spreading the seeds to regrow functional movement without first checking the soil to see if it was fertile enough to support and allow that movement to grow.

Those early iterations of the Functional Movement Screen and the Selective Functional Movement Assessment weren't created for anyone outside the four walls of our clinic. My colleagues and I created them because we wanted better tools to screen a baseline level of function and assess painful or dysfunctional movement to allow us to make better, more informed decisions. Our goal was to maximize our own effectiveness by removing our beliefs or feelings from the equation.

Even with all the data available to us today, it's easy to operate professionally off of our biases. Whether or not we're aware of it, our affinity toward a preferred dimension of movement skews our perspectives, and we focus on finding tools to help us support those preferences. We need to appreciate how often our individual agendas lead us to circumvent the natural layers of movement and lose perspective on what each individual needs.

If you're a manual therapist, you probably look for reasons to do mobilizations or soft tissue work as a solution. A corrective exercise specialist will hunt for imbalances and asymmetries to justify a corrective program. A strength coach or trainer will find new ways of identifying where someone needs to be bigger, stronger, or faster. Our biased perception of a problem may be sending us in the wrong direction from the start. Our fixation on finding the best option of *what* to do and *how* to do it keeps us from consistently digging into *why* we encounter some of these problems in the first place.

"*Why?*" is the most important question you can ask yourself because the answer dictates your emotional connection to the professional actions you take. The best education always tells us why, before how or what—even though the hows and whats are the questions we and our clients often pursue. How do I run a faster marathon? What should I do to get my back to stop hurting? What exercise is the best for strengthening _____?

We've been asking random questions for specific problems instead of stepping back and starting with why.

- ▶ Why do some people move poorly, even when they have no measurable pain or dysfunctional parts?
- ▶ Why are some people more durable than others or respond more rapidly when given the same level of stimulus?
- ▶ Why don't certain patients respond as expected to treatments?
- ▶ Why do some exercises or manual techniques work well for some clients and not for others?
- ▶ Why doesn't everyone move well with good form when the faulty parts are "fixed?"

In a field without shared *why* statements, we've been incorrectly looking at the basics of movement, and to a larger scale, health, fitness, and skill. The challenge in dispelling the assumptions we make about movement (and the reason they persist in the first place) is that we've lacked a qualitative standard for what constitutes "normal" or "good" movement across a lifetime. Without a standard measurement of the integrity of movement, we can't engage in productive conversations about how or when to train, develop, or specialize. We haggle over which methods or tactics are superior in achieving an objective when there's no unifying strategy on the best way to get there.

STRATEGY BEFORE TACTICS

The terms "strategy" and "tactics" are used almost interchangeably when the conversation drifts toward achieving some lofty goal. Both are critical aspects of planning and execution, but despite our familiarity with the words, we often fail to appreciate the difference between the two…and even more often, we fail to put them appropriately into action.

To illustrate the difference between strategy and tactics, think of sports. In competition, the goal of either team is to win. In order to achieve that goal, the strategy may be to neutralize the best opposing player to limit the impact on the outcome of the game. Strategy, in its simplest terms, is the plan of action that will get the desired result. Tactics are the individual actions used to support that larger plan.

If the strategy is to neutralize the opponent's best player, we use tactics to disrupt his or her performance. The best tactic will be dependent upon the context of a changing environment, which means there's rarely a single tactic that will suffice. If the strategy is to limit the impact of LeBron James, the tactics may be to double-team him on defense, get him in foul trouble, or play mental games to try to take his focus off the game.

In the world of health and fitness, we don't apply the same perspective to our daily practice. We spend an inordinate amount of time debating tactics without first understanding or articulating a strategy. We fight over which tests are more sensitive or specific for certain diagnoses or skills…which manual therapies work best…which exercises will develop more power, strength, or endurance…which diet will work the fastest to lose fat or gain muscle. All the while, we're assuming all that can be known is already known.

When the focus is on expanding and enhancing a repertoire of tactics, it's challenging to then combine those tactics and work backward into a coherent strategy. We try one methodology until it doesn't work anymore and then move to the next technique, hoping it's more effective than the previous. For example, how often have you attended a weekend seminar and the first thing Monday morning, squeezed a new technique or assessment into your treatment or training plans? How long did it stay a part of your programming?

In a professional environment where we're forced to see more patients or train more clients, the impulse is to add skills or tools looking for greater efficiency. We keep looking for more resources, believing we can find the perfect combination when we'd be better served focusing on our use of the existing resources. Rather than worrying about how efficient we can be, we need to start asking if we're effective in what we're already doing.

You can have all the skills and specialized training in the world, but without a strategic plan, you're effectively throwing your efforts against the wall to see what sticks. Strategy constructs a bridge to direct us from where we are to where we want to be.

STRATEGIES TO TEST AND REINFORCE TACTICS

Many people operate without a strategy because it doesn't come in a template or pre-packaged program. Strategy is built on principles. If your principles are solid, they should hold you to a certain level of integrity and responsibility in your actions. Your principles shouldn't conflict with your strategy, but your strategy should create a framework of feedback loops that force those principles to be tested and confirmed. The two components create a qualitative standard, against which you can test and assess your tactics to find your most effective and efficient methods.

The incredible outcomes or abilities we encounter from master clinicians and coaches aren't just a product of time, experience, and better skills. Their results come from operating under a set of principles and strategies that are tested, refined, and retested over a lifetime into a repeatable, decision-making system.

Bruce Lee may be remembered as a movie star, but his greatest legacy is as a martial arts philosopher. He created a new perspective on martial arts, but he didn't forge it from nothing—he rooted his learning in the principles underlying traditional martial arts. His goal was to develop a more effective fighting style held against the standards of other martial arts. Through his constant practice and self-experimentation of those foundational principles, he created a new strategy based on new principles.

While we marvel at the novel physical and mental training tactics he used to develop the martial art of Jeet Kune Do, beginning with *strategy* allowed him to develop new and more effective *tactics*. If you don't place strategy before tactics, you may have a collection of tools at your disposal, but you'll have no way of comparing or combining those tools into a single, unified process that delivers consistent results.

> *"Adapt what is useful, reject what is useless,*
> *and add what is specifically your own."*
> *— Bruce Lee*

We often talk about the art and science of medicine or coaching. There's a false interpretation of "art" to mean the personal intuition or beliefs we develop through repetition and exposure. Unfortunately, we lean on the art for easy solutions when scenarios become more challenging. However, any complicated endeavor requires technical know-how and precision as well as creativity. But it has to begin from a solid structure of systems.

To expand on an analogy I've heard Mike Boyle use, take the difference between a line cook and a chef. Line cooks go to work every day knowing what the work will be, and largely do it the same way day after day. They may learn a better method to sear a steak or dice a vegetable and their skills and tactics may improve, but much of the mastery stops there. A cook follows a recipe.

Chefs possess the same technical skills, along with a deeper appreciation of the principles of not just how to cook a recipe, but also the chemistry and interactions of different foods. They begin with a vision and strategy for the menu and, based on the available ingredients, can change and adapt to a constantly changing environment as they sample and tweak the approach—a dash of seasoning here, a little extra time on heat there.

The art of cooking doesn't come from randomly choosing ingredients or methods. It comes from understanding the *why* and appreciating the *how,* and then making decisions based on *what* we observe and taste and experience within the parameters of cooking. Creativity and new ideas and methods naturally flow from a wide and deep understanding of fundamental principles. The same idea holds for our work with a human body.

What began as our attempt to create a movement screen to allow clinicians, coaches, and trainers to both appreciate and communicate the foundations of human movement took on that same second life through the Functional Movement Systems. The hope has always been that understanding and using the Systems as they were intended would provide a standard against which to give you permission to be a chef. You've got permission to taste—and you need to taste the changes because adding new tactics or elements without retesting will usually produce a less-than-desirable end result.

CONSTRUCTING MOVEMENT STRATEGIES

Early on, many people believed we intended to create a methodology around corrective exercise. They saw a funny-looking test of seven movements and a bunch of odd exercises to improve those movements…and questioned the value of our philosophy. They believed our approach meant you had to go slow with a client or that you couldn't train people unless they scored perfect on the screens.

Some thought the constraints of the Systems would infringe on the freedom of their practices. That couldn't be further from the reality. Our only demand has been that you have a *why* behind your decisions and an objective process to assess your effectiveness.

Standard operating procedures don't limit excellence in pilots or surgeons—they're actually the foundation of their professional cultures. That's not to say they didn't initially resist SOPs, which is right where we are as movement professionals today. To this day, we don't have a standard intake practice connecting musculoskeletal medicine, rehabilitation, physical education or fitness and sports conditioning.

How is this oversight not a business opportunity?

Methods change; I've been reminding people of that in lectures for at least 20 years. There will always be new ways to work. Show me someone using the same methods today as five years ago, and I'll show you someone whose practice is frozen in amber. But there's a reason that in the age of modern warfare, generals still read *The Art of War*. The strategies it contains still ring true hundreds of years after it was written because *strategies persist*.

Starting with a strategy firmly anchored to a foundation of principles will create a feedback loop to let you know when you're on the right track. There's no dogma other than that.

First, learn how to be effective. Once you're effective, efficiency will develop simply through consistent practice and critical appraisal of your results. Ultimately, you'll find the freedom to adjust and tweak your methods with greater confidence and greater insight by deepening the grooves of your personal experience.

We're in a constant fight both within and across professions between our methodologies of *how*, instead of stepping back and understanding our shared philosophy of *what* and *why*.

Many practitioners want to embrace a similar model of evaluating and correcting movement, but have lacked the ability to know how to read, write, or correct the language of movement. As my colleagues and I continue to work on our unifying strategy around movement, articulating those fundamental principles requires an understanding of the perspective supporting the Functional Movement Systems.

CHAPTER TWO

CHANGING PERCEPTION

Ask yourself these questions:

- What are my incentives in changing my behaviors, beliefs, and processes?
- What are my risks in changing my behaviors, beliefs, and processes?
- Do I want to see new information so I can take it and do my own thing?
- Do I want to see new information so I can find a unique niche quicker than my competition?
- Do I want to see new information so I'll know when I can afford to take the risk in using it, and how much of it I want to incorporate?

At this point, your answers may not be entirely clear and, if anything, those questions may have produced some questions of your own like, "Why should I change? What if what I'm already doing is right? How does that new information fit with what I'm already doing?" Those are all fair questions that will hopefully have clear answers as you move through this book.

The fact you are reading this book means I'll assume you're looking to chart a different path from the norm. You probably perceive that something needs to change in the way you're currently operating and that the path our culture is walking today isn't leading us to a healthier or happier existence. Being self-aware enough to know something needs to change is all anyone needs, but we don't all paddle into the wave of change at the same point. We aren't all willing to challenge our beliefs, actions, or decision-making processes in the way radical transparency demands, which is why the first requirement of self-awareness is to be honest about the relationship between the risks you're willing to take and the opportunities available to you.

Not everyone can be on the leading edge of a new paradigm because not everyone's situation will allow them to tolerate the risks involved—and that's okay! No matter where we fall on the spectrum, there are always opportunities to improve our effectiveness; asking questions about the type of person we are or want to be is the first step toward understanding the best path forward.

Determining *your* path requires a deeper level of self-awareness…and putting ego aside to question the foundation of your knowledge, work, and beliefs.

So, how self-aware are you?

We all have certain areas of ignorance and certain areas where we've lost objectivity. Can you identify those boundaries in your current practice? Where can you identify gaps in your knowledge versus areas where you have a high level of confidence and competence?

Stages of Self-Awareness		
Self-Ignorance	**Self-Observation**	**Self-Absorption**
There are areas in which we'll naturally be ignorant. We don't know what we don't know.	There are areas in which we're qualified for observation and assessment.	There are areas in which we're probably a little too invested and prone to confirmation bias.

The psychological concept called "the Dunning Kruger Effect" states that the more you learn about something, the less likely you are to be as confident as when you first learned it. Initially, we have high confidence that we understand what we're seeing and doing because our ego is attached to what got us to that point. But the deeper we go in understanding and the more objective we force ourselves to be, the less confident we become. If we continue working to comprehend and synthesize the information, we can ultimately regain confidence, although never to the original degree.

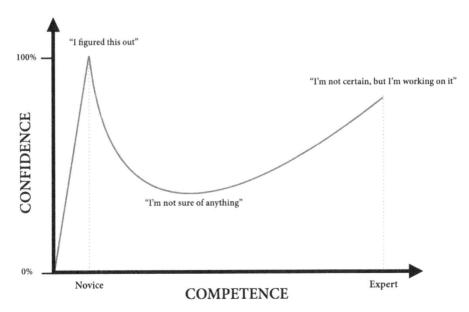

That may seem counterintuitive, but it means that the point where you have the greatest certainty probably needs the most rigorous testing and challenge. I'm not sure where I first heard it, but there's a quote, "The most objective person in the room is the one who knows they are not." If we can apply a process focusing on our decisions and actions through a more objective filter, we can create the transparency to identify the facets of our work that are lacking, that are working, and that need deeper inspection.

My version of the quote about remaining objective is, "The most objective person in the room is the one who knows they are not, *and who creates systems of feedback to manage their own expertise.*" Dissecting where you feel the greatest certainty in your knowledge or ability often exposes the greatest opportunities to accelerate your personal and professional growth.

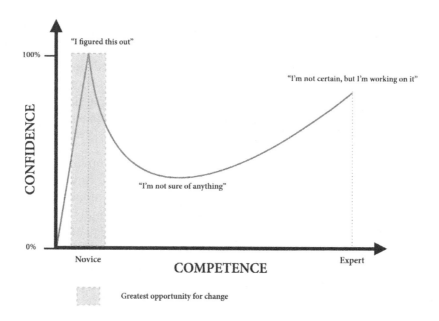

From an early age, I was fascinated by movement. I pursued a career in strength and conditioning and physical therapy because I wanted to learn how my teammates and opponents in sports could perform the same exercises or drills, seeking the same outcome yet would respond so differently. Superior athletic ability, strength, or flexibility didn't always translate into superior movement quality or a greater resistance to injury.

My own experience was one of significant and recurring battles with injuries despite my best efforts in the weightroom. I knew there had to be something that separated those who demonstrated superior physical performance or resilience from everyone else, but I wanted to identify or measure that elusive quality and establish what "normal" human movement should look like.

My years of study made me fully qualified to diagnose and treat musculoskeletal injuries and design programs for patients and athletes to resolve pain and maximize performance. I understood the physical tests of health that told me if someone's heart, breathing, or range of motion could prevent quality movement. I had fitness tests that could give me information on strength, endurance, or power. I could say someone was "tight," "weak," or "slow," but still had no answers why some athletes and clients whose testing showed no concerns ended up with pain and dysfunction.

Anatomy, kinesiology, biomechanics, and physiology seemed clear and concise in supporting the belief that if I knew all the muscles involved in a movement, I should be able to restore and strengthen it. It told me to isolate and measure faulty parts and impairments of structure to relate back to function and movement.

My education in neurology told me that the web of nervous tissue connections meant the whole of the body was always greater than the sum of its parts, but focusing on changing the neurologic system seemed messy, broad, and complex. That inherent fuzziness of the nervous system is why historically, the approach to rehabilitation, fitness, and athletic conditioning is rarely weighted in favor of leveraging neurologic principles, other than instances of a clear neurologic deficit such as a nerve or brain injury.

The components of human movement—locomotion (moving yourself) and manipulation (moving someone or something else)—are fundamental to the health and resilience of the human body. Just as food nourishes the body, movement powers itself to become more robust and complex. Unfortunately, we've been led to believe if we just move more, the benefits of movement will wash backward to correct and restore our bodies to their natural, optimal state. The idea was that if we got stronger or got our cardiovascular system working better, issues of poor health, pain, dysfunction, or impaired production would naturally resolve.

To support that belief, I spent a lot of time and effort drilling deeper into the nuances of how a body works. Today we have more education, professionals, and data in the fields of healthcare and fitness than at any point in history. We've seen science and technology empowering both consumers and professionals with hundreds of ways to measure and micromanage every aspect of physical life.

Yet somehow, with warehouses of data at our disposal, we seem to be moving further from a consensus on what all this information means as we're undoubtedly moving further from the physical robustness of previous generations. We possess the ability to collect measurements to address individual parts with little appreciation for how to piece them back together to establish and maintain physical vitality.

That reductionist approach to health and fitness is leading us down the same misguided route we traveled for nutrition. There, a lack of convenient answers means we fixate on labeling individual nutrients or minerals as "good" or "bad" and building diets around one or two variables instead of starting from a position of first eating whole, natural foods and worrying about optimizing individual nutrients later.

The same flawed logic is working its way into our approach to exercise—debating the most effective exercises or methodologies for some specific problem, and never zooming out and asking if exercise is really the most important component to get someone out of the current condition.

When you impose your professional recommendation on one side of the stress and recovery cycle, you're still responsible for managing both. Whether addressing diet or exercise, we're operating with an unjustified level of confidence that we can simply fit all the pieces together so they add up to the desired result despite mounting evidence of the failure of that approach. Unfortunately, changing our perceptions around the problems and solutions is incredibly difficult when viewed through the lens of our modern physical culture.

A BROKEN MODEL

As a species, we find ourselves on a new path; for the first time in history, our physical culture is making our current and future generations weaker, sicker, and less adaptable to the natural environment.

I believe the purpose of culture is to transfer strategies between generations to help them survive—whether verbally or through song, writing, or art. Physical culture encapsulates those learned perspectives and behaviors we share and integrate across societies that support and develop health and vitality.

> *"The ability to learn faster than your competitors may be the only sustainable competitive advantage."*
> —*Arie de Geus*

The generations that came before us developed a rich physical culture as a by-product of the lives they led, whether it was growing or hunting their food, having to walk and carry that food and belongings, or just being responsible for their independence throughout their lives. Those physical environments and demands were often different day to day, so the behaviors and strategies to navigate the changing environments were constantly being tested and refined.

In biological and organism-to-environment relationships, being self-aware is a competitive advantage because the only *sustainable* competitive advantage is the ability to learn faster. Keeping their bodies and brains tightly connected meant the groups able to collectively learn how to self-regulate and thrive in their environments could pass that knowledge to their offspring, who were able to live longer, develop and refine more advanced skills, and flourish.

Today, that physical culture is broken. We no longer explore the movement opportunities we were formerly required to explore simply to survive. The technical advancements of the last century have altered our lives to such a degree that the rich physical experiences and challenges of our daily environments have deteriorated along with our physical bodies.

Environment creates natural human movement, which is why, regardless of climate, culture, or race, a baby's development for the first 21 months follows the same path as long as she's eating, sleeping, and not in pain or otherwise restricted.

Movement is the expression of the natural feedback loop that readjusts and remanages our perceptions and behaviors to meet a new task, new environment, or new stimulus to which we should be able to adapt. Culture is what takes over and imposes restrictions or allowances that change movement—sometimes for the better and sometimes to our detriment.

Our goal is to provide strategies to help every professional who touches movement. There's value for everyone throughout the book, but we've included icons to highlight areas that are more specific to the needs of clinicians and trainers and coaches.

You will also see QR codes and links offering opportunities for a deeper "whiteboard" discussion of the related material.

Whiteboard	Clinician	Trainers and Coaches
GRAY'S WHITEBOARD	☤	💪

Today, "average" isn't normal. Our bodies are adapting to the engineered conveniences of the 72-degree carpeted comfort zone of life, which has eroded our awareness of our natural physical function and the management strategy to maintain it. We've stopped adapting to the environment and have instead changed the environment to fit our needs. For the most part, this hasn't worked well for the environment…or for us.

https://qrco.de/bcYkbi

Thanks to modern conveniences, we're becoming "zoo humans"—living in less dangerous and less variable environments than what our ancestors encountered. Our movement senses, which allow us to adapt, have become so conditioned to these artificial environments that even the slightest stress that knocks us out of that narrow range of stability elicits the same physical or emotional response as our ancestors would have experienced under the harshest of environmental stresses. Despite our loss of resiliency to even minor disruptions in our environment, our perception of the problem and our response to it may be even more concerning.

To put our current state[2] in a little more context, consider the following:

- 60% of Americans live with a chronic disease.
- 40% of Americans live with two or more chronic diseases.
- 70% of Americans are obese or overweight.
- 50% of Americans report a musculoskeletal condition.
- Less than 5% of Americans participate in 30 minutes of daily activity.
- Yet, 81% believe they're in GOOD or EXCELLENT physical health.

---

2 https://www.cdc.gov/chronicdisease/tools/infographics.htm
40% of Americans live with 2 or more chronic diseases

https://www.cdc.gov/chronicdisease/tools/infographics.htm
70% of Americans are obese or overweight

https://www.niddk.nih.gov/health-information/health-statistics/overweight-obesity
50% of Americans report a musculoskeletal condition

https://www.boneandjointburden.org/docs/BMUS%20Impact%20of%20MSK%20on%20 Americans%20booklet_4th%20Edition%20%282018%29.pdf

https://web.archive.org/web/20200204130347/https://www.hhs.gov/fitness/resource-center/ facts-and-statistics/index.html
Fewer than 5% of Americans participate in 30 minutes of daily activity

How is it that a culture with such advanced medical and health technology at its disposal finds the majority of its population in poor physical condition? Global health expenditures grew to $7.8 trillion in 2017, in addition to the $4.7 trillion spent in the field of wellness—an area that's supposed to be making us more resilient to pain and dysfunction.

The "solutions" to combat our physical decline are often built on complexity and dependence for profit, disconnecting us even further from our bodies and degrading the link between self-awareness and self-learning. We're figuratively and literally paying the price of becoming more reliant on the technologies and industries of health and wellness to manage our physical state for us. While the exploding cost of health and wellness is a more recent development, we haven't been listening to what movement has had to say for the better part of five decades.

EARLY SIGNS OF TROUBLE

Sixty years ago, a study of European and American children showed us that movement was on the decline long before childhood obesity and metabolic disorders came into focus. At the time of the Kraus-Weber study,[3] 57.9% of American children failed a simple postural fitness test that only 8.7% of European children failed. Childhood obesity wasn't on anyone's radar, and despite these kids all looking the same, they were *moving very differently*.

In response to the study, President Dwight Eisenhower established the President's Council on Youth Fitness to create a plan of action for improving the health and fitness of elementary school age children through physical education. Presidents John F. Kennedy and Lyndon Johnson expanded the program to promote health and wellness for high schoolers and adults.

The impetus for the expansion of the program was to address the declining physical function of the general population that was making it difficult to find enough citizens able to meet the minimum fitness standards to serve in the military. Most American adults remember doing sit-ups and shuttle runs in gym class as part of the Presidential Physical Fitness program, but the attempts to use fitness habits and sports skills in physical education to combat the declining function of the population have clearly been in vain.

Case in point: To be considered fit for military service in World War II, six was the minimum number of pull-ups to be performed. Now, five pull-ups is the minimum to be cleared…*as an Army Ranger*. What used to be the minimum requirement to put on a uniform is now enough to qualify you for special ops.[4]

---

3 *https://vault.si.com/vault/1955/08/15/the-report-that-shocked-the-president*

4 *https://www.armyupress.army.mil/Portals/7/combat-studies-institute/csi-books/APRT_Whitfield East.pdf*

The health and fitness fields today are repeating the mistakes of 50 years ago by adopting the same approach to solving our dilemma of declining health and physical function. The current message from physical culture tells us that if we just add exercise, technological solutions, or nutritional supplements to combat our stressful environments, healthier and stronger bodies will naturally manifest. That culture would have us believe our health and fitness fail as the by-product of a harsh and stressful environment without questioning if the health and fitness we possess even reach the world's minimum standards.

Our culture continues to create that false perception as it lowers the bar for everyone to participate in physical activities without providing the tools to determine whether people possess the required capabilities to succeed. By lowering the standards of entry into the military, sports, and fitness activities, we're letting more people sit at a table, eating a meal of a movement nutrient that's too big for their stomachs to handle.

CHASING SOLUTIONS WITHOUT UNDERSTANDING THE PROBLEM

In this modern culture where we're not forced to be active, many people choose to engage in a single activity—be it weight training, yoga, biking, running, or sports—to exercise their way to better health or performance. They don't pursue activities selected for them based on any qualitative measures; they self-select their fitness activities or sports based on what they perceive to be valuable or effective. They assume they're healthy enough to participate without much thought into the quantity of how much to lift or run or play. The idea is usually to just keep adding more reps or miles and maybe a little coaching or instruction—and a relatively straight line of progress will materialize. These fitness activities that are barely stressful enough to cause injuries…cause injuries.

Compounding the issue, fitness often takes on a competitive element, where individual performance is measured against other people in a class or through the social media feed of a fitness celebrity. When fitness becomes a competition that lacks the same selection process for entry as other competitions, the end result is an increased risk of injury rather than a reduction.

A client who wants to be able to perform a kettlebell swing or an Olympic lift will learn just enough before adding sets and reps to iron out mechanics and form, without anyone determining the person could even assume or maintain the basic postures and patterns required to support the movement.

Today's physical culture provides plenty of options for professional health and fitness appraisal, but not for functional self-appraisal. In a world of health, fitness, and coaching professionals, communication between professions either breaks down or is completely absent because there isn't a shared language to clearly link one to the other. A lack of valid, reliable tools that bridge the gap between professions makes it even harder for a personal trainer to identify problems that might not be solved in the gym or for a chiropractor to clearly say when a patient is ready to resume high-intensity training. Information can't flow, and each area ends up myopically addressed.

The combination of an eroded self-awareness coupled with a disconnected model of movement traps people in the endless loop of dependence on the health and fitness machine, searching for solutions and hacks to their problems. We fall into the same traps of constantly hunting for the latest tactics and methods that might help get someone out of pain or get bigger, stronger, and faster in less time. But tactics and hacks without a holistic strategy and system of checks and balances inevitably lead to inconsistent results. We indiscriminately lay complex skilled movements on top of inadequate fitness, questionable function, and poor health, rather than prioritizing the creation of an environment to collect better feedback and promote self-awareness.

Reestablishing a mind-body connection provides perspective of how active or inactive we can be through better self-regulation. To get there professionally, we must reshape the conversation through a shared language of movement and an appreciation for the missing layer of movement that can help our clients and patients reconnect with their own self-awareness and provide the entry point through which we can help them find the right path forward.

We don't need to continue lowering standards—our disciplines can meet the old standards just fine if we *raise* our movement standards and practices. This book is my suggestion for how to do that.

AN INCOMPLETE SYSTEM OF MOVEMENT

Because we're so far removed from a robust, natural movement experience, long-term success in our modern environment requires a more holistic approach to the full expression of our physical growth and adaptation. To successfully deliver on that ideal, we must examine the traditional models of health, fitness, and performance within a modern context. That inspection reveals that we need to redefine our language around the meaning of those words, as well as where our professional responsibility and value lies.

Previous generations had to navigate an uncomfortable world. Historically, people expected discomfort in their daily lives and understood they were ultimately responsible for sustaining their health, albeit with less science to support it. Life was hard enough that they naturally became fit enough to do what they needed to do; survival of the fittest meant that health and fitness were closely correlated.

Our ancestors learned self-management better than we do now out of pure necessity for survival. Those who were more resilient and better able to explore and experience the changing demands of their environments were more likely to discover and refine strategies to adapt and manage themselves than those who were physically unable to cope or thrive. They either learned how to adapt to a physically demanding life, or they didn't last long.

Until the more recent industrialized past, there wasn't a huge distinction between the different dimensions of health, fitness, and performance. Those who demonstrated the highest levels of skilled performance were generally also the healthiest and fittest. In a world without the option to lead a sedentary lifestyle, poor health or inadequate fitness were exposed or exercised through the challenges of a naturally vigorous life.

Levels of Movement	Demonstrated Quantity or Quality	Typical Definition
Health	Vital signs	The absence of disease
Fitness	Capacity (Locomotion and Manipulation)	The ability to meet environmental work demands while maintaining health
Performance (Skill)	Complexity	The ability to accomplish complex tasks or movements for a specific purpose

The three dimensions of health, fitness, and performance and their standard definitions lie on a continuum where each layer naturally supports and develops the next. If one layer is deficient, we expect to find that higher levels of movement are also deficient, as each can only be as strong as the weakest link in the chain. Deficiency at the level of health means fitness will be compromised because physical capacity can't be fully expressed. Deficiency of fitness will impact the consistency and duration of the performance of any skill or activity.

When daily life was a more physically demanding endeavor, there was a relative balance between the three layers required to withstand the environment and function at an acceptable level. Our environments now demand so little effort and we so rarely push the threshold of performance, we can operate for decades with deficient health and fitness. With the slow erosion of bones, joints, and muscular function, injuries ultimately arise from bending over to pick up something from the floor rather than performing a stressful physical feat.

Today we can measure and quantify the qualities of each, but to be meaningful, the terms themselves need to be defined in the context of specific environments, demands, and goals. That's why terms like *healthy, fit,* or *skilled* feel so arbitrary and hard to define, especially as they're currently used.

There are accepted ranges for measurements like blood pressure, heart rate, or vision to declare someone healthy. We have expected measures for many fitness tests based on age, occupation, or sport. We can even biomechanically break down performance to clarify what makes someone more or less skilled. What we consider benchmarks and acceptable ranges of measurement can vary over time or among different groups, but if we aren't accounting for those values on an individual level, we can't stop the overall trend of those numbers, as a species, in the wrong direction.

We're caught in a challenging position of operating on false assumptions. Without first taking the time to examine those physical qualities, we can't confidently identify our greatest need. We can't assume health—we need to look at vital signs. We can't assume fitness or performance—we need to appraise fitness, skill, or activity-specific through appropriate tests. If we cannot confirm that each of those layers is intact (pain-free) and above the required level for the particular environmental or functional demands, we risk the effectiveness of all of our decisions moving forward.

Can Your Testing Confirm Each Layer?

	Pain	**Fail**	**Pass**
Performance	Yes / No	Yes / No	Yes / No
Fitness	Yes / No	Yes / No	Yes / No
Health	Yes / No	Yes / No	Yes / No

EACH LAYER SUPPORTS AND REINFORCES THE OTHERS

One big benefit today is that technological advances have made it easier than ever to measure different physical dimensions. But our growing fixation on individual metrics is leading us to assume that improving one physical aspect will naturally improve the others. That additional data should produce a clearer picture of physical status, but in too many cases, our conversations about how best to maximize health, fitness, or performance focus on developing *more* of a particular physical quality, rather than asking if we possess a minimally acceptable level of each.

Look at many of the highest performers in sports and you'll see the manifestation of the misalignment of health, fitness, and performance. Think of the triathlete who competes in Ironman races and swims 2.4 miles, bikes 112 miles, and runs 26.2 miles in a single day—who also presents with chronic back, hip, or knee pain…or even heart arrhythmia. Consider a powerlifter who can deadlift 500 pounds, but struggles to bend over to tie their shoelaces, or a professional football or basketball player with a 36-inch vertical leap who can't stand on one foot for 30 seconds. If they push their performance measures higher at the expense of their health, can we really say that they are "better?"

Athletes at the pinnacle of performance who are arguably the "fittest" often fail to demonstrate the minimal standards of physical attributes we'd consider healthy for a senior citizen. We could check the boxes and say they meet the benchmarks of performance and fitness, but we have to acknowledge when they're failing in their health. We measure their success by the strengths we observe, rather than the weaknesses that go unreported or unexamined. This should challenge two assumptions we commonly hold:

- Demonstrating elite levels of performance implies every physical quality must be operating optimally
- Improving fitness or performance will naturally improve health as a secondary effect

Health, fitness, and skilled performance depend on one another, but we've been consuming movement information incorrectly for years. Someone with pain or physical limitations can't be functioning at optimal levels, but the message being delivered is that structure—the operation of the parts—always governs function. It says that if we alter the body's structures then function should improve as a byproduct. So with that perspective, we immediately get to work removing pain or tinkering with dysfunctional parts.

Structure does govern function, but function also governs structure. While a lack of physical capacity or structural deficits can absolutely be the drivers of limited function, we have a difficult time reconciling what it means to "function well" because neither consumers nor practitioners are trained to understand movement competency. We have countless tools to tell us when biomechanical, anatomical, or metabolic functions become impaired, but we rarely have the tools to deploy before a problem arises. Identifying behaviors is where the potential for injury or dysfunction can best be addressed, but a shortage of tests specific to function and the behavior of movement has made it hard to support a valid argument.

In orthopedic sports medicine, the structural tests or diagnostic imaging show a sprain, a herniation, or arthritis, and the answer immediately becomes an injection, surgery, or another medical intervention. Even when no apparent injury or damage is identified, we get to work altering the body's structure or chemistry; leaving it up to the miracles of healing or rehabilitation for the physical structure to support a return to activity.

The fitness and performance space falls prey to the same mindset—if someone isn't performing their best, focus attention on some weak or inhibited muscle, or a lacking physical attribute to explain and solve the problem. Sometimes that may be the answer, but I have no doubt that we all know more than a few people who are objectively "fit" and "skilled" who also demonstrate questionable measures of health, dysfunctional patterns of movement, and persistent injuries that aren't resolved through reinforcing the areas where they already have a passing grade.

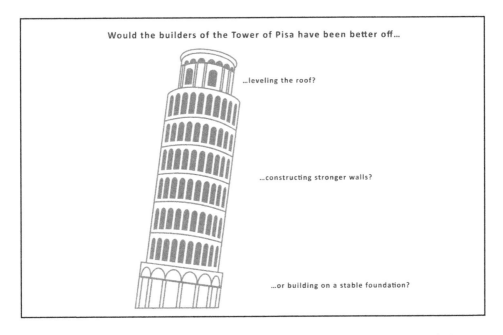

"Move Well, Move Often" is part of our logo because this is the life lesson nature teaches us. We see it in animals and in people who are physically and psychologically the healthiest, which is why I consider this our natural principle. We must protect the beautiful interplay between competency (moving well) and capacity (moving often) because, despite many fitness philosophies, the principle doesn't work in reverse. It's not natural to build capacity on top of incompetence. The quality of the foundation won't naturally improve from building more structure on top.

Looking at movement through the three layers of health, fitness, and performance made sense 100 years ago when we lived with a more authentic physical culture, but we need to reframe the conversation around the world in which we're operating.

Stress and friction are necessary components that can't and shouldn't be avoided in physical growth and adaptation. Likewise, rest and regeneration can't be synthesized. Accelerating advancements in comfort, convenience, and divisions of labor are leaving in their wake specialization and the compartmentalizing of the medical, fitness, and performance realms. The communication and continuity we're losing between professions creates bottlenecks and misaligned solutions for patients and clients, moving us away from a holistic physical culture.

You may not have the skills or knowledge to collect, interpret, and act on all of the relevant information you gather, but improving the effectiveness and the efficiency of your practice lies in finding the connection between them all.

That connection is movement.

Our work at Functional Movement Systems has focused on sharpening the tools for professionals working at different layers of physical growth to quantify and qualify movement under a common, shared language around function. We have an opportunity in defining a new layer within that movement hierarchy—one that provides each of us the same entry point to restoring the natural balance of physical growth and development.

CHAPTER THREE

A MODERN MODEL OF MOVEMENT

- ▶ Where do you fit in the continuum of movement?
- ▶ Is your area of expertise health, fitness, or developing greater performance and skill?

We all have our own branch of knowledge, but viewing the problems of our clients and patients through only our lens of perspective comes at the expense of the larger picture of where movement fits in the framework of being a living, breathing organism.

We need to see movement for what it is—the most distinguishable sign of life. It's a vital sign unto itself.

We're born with mobility and earn stability as we transition from fundamental to functional movements. As those primal and developmental patterns become more refined and complex, general fitness arises from handling and carrying objects, running, and climbing long before specific skills enter into the picture. That understanding of how movement naturally develops to support a child's physical abilities points us to a solution in systematizing that same progression.

Only a few generations ago when the physical demands of life were more varied, we could have more confidently assumed those pursuing skilled activities possessed the movement competency required to safely participate. Exercise was a supplement to daily life—something to help recover from illness or prepare for something that would exceed physical capacities.

Today, treating exercise as the primary solution to our failing health and performance rather than as a restorative or protective tool has led to participation in fitness and sports activities actually becoming a risk factor for injury.[5] Many people without formal exercise as part of their lifestyles could pass a fitness test—and there are just as many people dedicated to exercise who fail to achieve the same standard. That's partly due to the lives we lead, but we also let our biases apply exercise solutions to every problem before we identify where the problem lies.

Food presents a great analogy to this. When we had a diet of whole, natural foods, we didn't have to preface the word *diet* with *healthy* and we didn't have to rely on supplements to cover our nutritional needs. In the Western world when

---

5   https://juniperpublishers.com/jpfmts/pdf/JPFMTS.MS.ID.555562.pdf

trying to explain away heart attacks and our growing waistlines over the past 50 years, we proposed solutions of diets based on a single macronutrient (at different times: fats, carbohydrates, or protein), cholesterol-lowering medications, or health and performance supplements rather than addressing the role of our consumption model. Even as the last decade brought a shift back toward more biologically sensible approaches to what we eat, we still fall prey to marketing and a magic-bullet diet, food, or pill to solve our problems. No matter what the advertisements tell us, popping fish oil capsules and eating a trendy superfood won't move the needle toward better health or performance if we don't identify and address the actual problem.

As more clinicians, trainers, and coaches began to use the FMS, we realized there was a similar disconnect in appreciating where the movement screen fit into a larger approach to health and fitness. I became known as a guy who popularized "functional movement" and "functional exercise," but to me, saying *functional* movement or *functional* exercise is like saying *whole* foods—all natural human movement is functional and all exercise should be in service of growing and developing natural movement. People created mental models where different exercises were labeled as correcting movement or strengthening and conditioning movement, but missed the point that *exercise isn't the goal.*

As long as our health is intact, being active and physical in our lifestyle is the equivalent of eating a diet of whole, natural foods—it should be all that's needed to achieve and maintain a normal level of health and fitness. Exercise should serve as an additive to reinforce or re-establish homeostasis when the system gets knocked out of alignment or when a new environment or activity requires a higher degree of capacity or skill. Whether it's through taking vitamins or engaging in a specific exercise, both are more effective as dosed supplements to restore balance, rather than serving as long-term solutions.

REDEFINING THE LAYERS OF MOVEMENT

The Functional Movement Screen was intended to be a tool to assess when someone's movement required supplementation. When exercise is layered on top of dysfunctional movement or pain, problems are often magnified rather than resolved. We think we can reconstruct movement through exercise when the correct path is to create opportunities that allow natural movement to emerge so we can reinforce that natural movement through exercise and activity. Otherwise, we apply an exercise solution to a movement problem, rather than first finding a movement solution to address the root cause.

The FMS was always intended to function as a measure of movement risk, but with over 20 years of data, we now realize we need to redefine the layers of movement to fit our world as it is today. Quantifying that dimension of risk is more vital than ever, which is why we need to establish a fourth layer of movement: wellness.

Layer of Movement	Demonstrated Quantity or Quality	FMS Definition
Health *(Potential Function)*	Vital signs	Having sufficient structure to support potential function The absence of pain with fundamental and functional movement patterns No medical treatment is required, not possessing a temporary or permanent disability
Wellness *(Demonstrated Function)*	Competency	The ability to be placed in an environment and be able to survive and develop If there's dysfunction, it will be in the lower percentiles of development progress. Those who possess health and function can adapt at an average level or better.
Fitness *(Demonstrated Capacity)*	Capacity	Irreducible physical qualities that aren't sport or activity-specific and are possessed at a young age The ability to do work to match the environment (to be fit for _____) Mapping these qualities can identify roadblocks that may need to be addressed before optimizing specific skill development.
Production *(Demonstrated Skill)*	Complexity	The ability to move in a refined way for a specific purpose The output of efforts (both qualitative and quantitative)

Declaring people "healthy" should mean they have the physical structure and pain-free freedom and control of movement to assume fundamental and functional postures and patterns. When the cycles that sustain life such as respiration, digestion, circulation, and sleep are disrupted, or pain or deficits in mobility, balance, or control are present, we can't connect well with our internal structure. Possessing adequate health should imply the potential for full movement and engagement with the world around us.

Wellness is the ability to be in an environment and be able to survive and develop. It's a projection of health into the future. Wellness considers physical function as well as the psychosocial behaviors we can identify as risk factors that could compromise the ability to engage with the world. The behaviors of fundamental movement patterns and the behaviors that either promote or inhibit the expression of those patterns make up the fundamental software program on which all future movement develops.

In working with wellness, we're trying to determine movement competency—can the person read and write in the language of movement? If people possess adequate health, in wellness, we're looking for an operational problem in the software. We're seeking qualifications and asking questions like, "Are there aspects of the patterns of physical, mental, or emotional behavior presenting a greater risk of failure in the future? Or have those behaviors already led to lost function along the way?"

We can gain a better measurement of fitness once we establish movement competency. The health or fitness fields push a poor definition of fitness; the modern definition is tied to exercise and general guidelines of what it means to be strong, powerful, or possessing endurance. But fitness requires a definition in the context of being a human...literally, does someone's ability match the environment?

Labeling someone as fit should imply "fit for _____." Does this person have the physical capacity to withstand and thrive against the stress of the environment? Fitness develops naturally through exploring and interacting with an environment, which is why children shift from running and playing with friends to participating in organized sports without needing a strength coach or training routine. As long as the foundation of both health and wellness are intact, engaging with activity or exercise in a scaled way allows fitness to evolve to meet the conditions and demands of the environment.

When we can confirm enough health, wellness, and fitness to meet the standard as a functional human being, we arrive at production—the quality and quantity of those unique skills and activities we want to do. Whatever special quality of skill we aspire to perform requires blending the layers of movement into a refined ability to move well for a specific purpose.

PRODUCTION OR PERFORMANCE

There's a reason we value production over performance. Performance asks if we're effective at doing what we want. Production asks if the performance of some skill or activity matches the amount of effort and resources invested to get there—are we as effective *and* as efficient as we could be?

We spend more time at the driving range, circling the track, or working on technique and mechanics, believing that better output is a matter of adding inputs in the time and effort toward the goal. It's those goals that drive us to go to the gym, practice an activity, or change our diets, but our motivation can be so singularly directed that we end up unaware of the qualities needed for support.

If two people are able to achieve the same level of performance, but one person was able to get there by expending 75% of the resources of the other, the one with the reserve is likely to enjoy more sustained success. It's here where we see a breakdown in the old way of thinking, where chasing more fitness and performance ends up costing more without first resolving health or wellness.

The professional tests and interventions that focus on dissecting performance and skill may lead to solutions, but those solutions may be in spite of the client's actual needs. The sports-specific testing and exercises made to mimic the movements of an activity feed people more of the thing they want, without first asking if they possess the ability to digest the plate of movement nutrients they're about to be fed.

Wants versus Needs

Conversations about what people **want** versus what they **need** can be challenging, particularly if they can't understand how those needs connect to their wants. Trying to convince people that you know what's best runs the risk of being received and interpreted as "your opinion isn't as important."

Take the time to lay out the roadmap of what someone needs (backed by evidence and data) with an explanation of how you'll move through the process to get where they want to go.

Take the integrity of a layer of movement away and things start to break down. If we have poor health, we aren't going to move well. If we have dysfunctional movement or behaviors, we won't be able to withstand the stress of building fitness. If we have poor fitness, we can't develop or sustain production of skills. We need to acknowledge that disruptions in health will impair a person long before poor movement, and poor movement patterns will break long before capacity runs out.

And what we really need is to move beyond acknowledgement and actually act in alignment with that natural order.

Professionals across the fields overlook that dimension of wellness because they lack the tools or context to measure function. Even those practitioners who adopt the FMS and appreciate the natural progression and development of movement sometimes struggle to put it into practice in a structured way.

Consider these layers like the parts of a computer. Think of health as the hardware, wellness as the operating system, fitness as the software, and production as the overall output of the system. If you install the latest application on your computer, you'll never unlock the full capabilities of the system with a weak processor or an out-of-date operating system. Even if you upgrade the hardware, an old or buggy operating system will limit the programs you can install and how efficiently they'll run.

Just as with a computer, if we keep looking for problems and solutions in the structure of health or the application of fitness, we'll never be aligned on the right course of action without the connection between the two. Regardless of where your professional practice falls along the continuum of movement, the true value of adopting a movement-focused approach and checking the physical operating system through functional measures comes from providing the most effective entry point to set your clients and patients on the right path.

FUNCTION IS YOUR ENTRY POINT

Function applies to every healthcare, fitness, and performance professional tasked with managing physical potential; function exists within every layer of movement. Function tells us when we're not moving well enough to pursue more complex or demanding aspects of our physical growth or development. Without a systematic approach to first screen function, when clients experience pain or dysfunction, they're presented with only two pathways—health or fitness, both of which often lead to the endless spin-cycle of dependence on healthcare and fitness professionals with no clear path forward.

If we use function as an entry point, we owe it a system of tests to establish a baseline, a minimal level of acceptance at each layer. The FMS filled the gap between fitness and health and allowed us to hold people to their functional problem and provide an environment within which to work before sending them forward into fitness or backward to healthcare.

We developed the SFMA and the FCS as tools to capture and establish minimums of movement competency for the layers of health and fitness. Creating these movement filters allowed us to identify and demonstrate when a foundation of movement was dysfunctional or deficient.

Leading with functional measures forces us to consider risk as the entry point where we ask:

- Is pain present at any level of movement?
- Are we healthy enough to imply wellness?
- Are we well enough to imply fitness?
- Are we fit enough to imply we're performing to an acceptable standard?
- Do we have a system to determine the best path to restore these minimal qualities? And when that minimum is met, is there a system to progress appropriately?

What Does Your Testing Tell You about the Person in Front of You?

	Awareness		
	Pain	**Fail**	**Pass**
Production *(skill or performance-specific testing)*	Yes / No	Yes / No	Yes / No
Fitness *(FCS, strength, power, endurance, agility testing)*	Yes / No	Yes / No	Yes / No
Wellness *(FMS, movement and lifestyle risk factors)*	Yes / No	Yes / No	Yes / No
Health *(SFMA, vital signs)*	Yes / No	Yes / No	Yes / No

Clients come to us with an agenda to improve performance in some aspect of their lives or to find the solution to regain their quality of life. They may realize there's a nutritional component, a rest and recovery component, or a flexibility and strength component that makes them a more complete golfer, runner, or healthier human, but their interest in the other components is only in service to their activity. No one comes to you looking for better movement or asking for a movement screen or a long-term strategy. People want the education or services to get rid of pain or quickly improve their half-marathon time.

But anyone entering athletics or higher-intensity training or activities won't just be as active as they want—they'll be asked to be more active in a structured activity. They'll be asked to learn skills and move their bodies with loads, speeds, and in directions they may not physically be able to tolerate. We can't assume that because people are physically able to swing a golf club or squat with weight they possess the movement competency to sustain an activity. There's no way to know if they possess that ability until you check, and you can't confidently propose a fitness solution if there's a functional problem at play.

As we begin to deconstruct movement, approaching it from the perspective of layers comes from an appreciation of natural development. Engaging with clients first at the level of function points us toward the weakest layer and guides us to the appropriate interventions specific to that person's needs. We need to run through a systems-check like those we have for the first 21 months of life when learning to cover basic postures and patterns.

If a child isn't healthy and can't achieve those foundational patterns of movement, we label this as the lower percentiles of developmental progress, and it's no different for physically mature adults.

But before our conversation on the methods or tactics that promise to address a dimension of physical function, we need to step back and see where our three movement principles merge into a unified strategy of complete physical growth and adaptation.

MOVEMENT PRINCIPLE ONE: FIRST MOVE WELL, THEN MOVE OFTEN

I consider this first principle the "natural principle." Why does this first principle work? Why do we move?

We move because movement affords us opportunity.

Moving "well" allows us to respond appropriately to the environmental signals we receive, to then allow progressive movement learning and growth. Because we're continually exposed to movement opportunities and risk, how well we adapt is dictated by the degree to which we respond to that environmental stress.

From the moment we arrive into the world as newborns, the foundation of movement develops through the same principle we so often cite: Specific Adaptation to Imposed Demand. We need to be able to produce a qualitative physical effort equal to our environment before moving "often" triggers our tissues and patterns to grow and develop in response to the volume and intensity of activity. We improve our software before we improve our hardware.

The exercise paradigm that puts *quantity* before *quality* reverses the first principle and often builds fitness on top of dysfunction—people move often and hope moving well will just happen. It rarely does.

Doing skillful and functional activities can morph a body into a more efficient and effective version of itself, which is why we dedicate so much time and effort to developing muscular hypertrophy, endurance, or strength. We've been conditioned to believe those qualities are the most indicative markers of physical well-being. We fail to equally discuss the fact that the healthiest and highest performers aren't always the strongest, biggest, or best conditioned.

Biology shows us that rather than singular characteristics, patterns and sequences of behavior remain an organism's preferred mode of operation. Undoubtedly, we see the same in those who demonstrate the greatest mastery of the behavior of movement.

DEFINING FUNDAMENTAL MOVEMENT

What does it mean to "move well?" The World Health Organization (WHO) works to develop normal ranges across different ages and population groups for health metrics like heart rate and blood pressure. Doctors use those to determine if a person is "healthy" across a lifetime.

Yet, despite the extensive global research supporting their guidelines, the WHO's agreement on what constitutes "healthy" human movement only extends to 21 months of age.[6] That's because regardless of climate, culture, race, or family situation, as long as a baby is loved during the first two years of life, he or she will generally develop similarly. Infants roll, crawl, climb, kneel, squat, stand, step, walk, and run. Each successive movement requires the foundation of the one before as it grows in sequence, creating a functional blueprint.

These motor milestones from head and neck control and reaching, through the progression of postures and patterns that take a baby from lying flat on its back, to standing, walking, and running are the only agreed-upon metrics of human movement. We can create definitions or measures of what we might consider "good" movements, but those begin to encapsulate measurements of skills or activities that are not uniform across cultures.

As culture and our modern environment expose us to new stimuli, we see more complex movements develop and adapt in response to the feedback loops and perception of the nervous system. Those first two years of life are the staging ground for function, with the basic parts of movement that allow the development of greater and more complex patterns of motion.

---

6 https://www.who.int/docs/default-source/child-growth/child-growth-standards/indicators/motor-development-milestones/who-motor-development-study-windows-of-achievement-for-six-gross-motor-development-milestones.pdf

The infant progression from babies lying on their backs to reaching, rolling, crawling, kneeling, standing, walking, and running isn't something they're taught. Movement is a *behavior*—a response to stimulus from the environment.

The language of movement is developed through perception and repetition; it's experiential.

Our internal feedback loops continue to sample, interpret, and respond to the changing environment and circumstances, making tweaks and adjustments in the short term and gradually, permanent adjustments over the long term. We don't write movement code, at least not consciously—it's biological learning, where patterns of stimulus and response are neurologically and physically mapped through behaviors and actions. Our perception of the environment or task dictates the sequencing and expression of the new program in functional or dysfunctional ways. How the subconscious behaves in response to pain, weakness, or repetitive stress and strain leaves a mark on the body as unique as a fingerprint.

Babies are born with too many physical impairments to be able to walk. They resolve them by doing what they can in a more functional manner…and the impairments soon disappear. The way the software of the nervous system chooses to process sensory input and express it through movement can sometimes be to compensate, avoid, or neglect, whereby movement can alter structure just as easily as structure can alter movement. We need to become better at reading what's written within those patterns if we hope to decipher the language of movement.

Take this example of a shoulder. The shoulder doesn't work independently—it works with the shoulder girdle, which anchors itself on the spine and rib cage. Many things we do with a shoulder aren't directed by an intention of the shoulder; they're directed by an intention of the hand. The way you use your hand influences the way you use your shoulder. Likewise, the way you hold your spine or trunk influences the way you use your shoulder. The shoulder is usually listening to the commands of the hand and responding to the integrity of the spine. The pattern you want to accomplish and the posture you choose to take are both ends of the shoulder movement, the dynamics of which are developed through exploration and experience.

Today, we talk about stabilizing an area of the body with more specific exercises, hoping that adding strength to one region will restore the natural function of another weak or painful area. That's operating off the model that *structure drives function*, which isn't incorrect, but ignores the concept that function also drives structure.

How do babies get their rotator cuffs strong enough to support their body weight? At 3:00 o'clock in the morning when we're not watching, are they working out with a little piece of resistance band? How can kids grow, climb trees, and walk into junior high athletics with no weight training but can still throw a discus or a shot put, jump over hurdles, do push-ups, and run hills?

If they were allowed or encouraged to be active, they likely received a rich sensory experience of running around in the woods, rolling their ankles, skinning their hands, and getting blisters and calluses. Their sensory experience wasn't verbalized. Those abilities to run, climb, or carry naturally develop from repeated exposure to varied and changing environments.

Children explore postures and patterns the same way they grow their bones and develop their muscles. They're driven to do so and, if we don't interfere, they'll do it in a systematic and elegant way. The more varied and challenging the environment they successfully navigate, the more physically robust they typically develop. The signature of function gets left on the structure.

THE DEVELOPMENTAL SOFTWARE OF MOVEMENT

Looking at movement through the lens of a developmental progression, I realized those developmental patterns constitute the basic software of human movement we should all have—the operating system that comes preloaded at birth and grows naturally. We don't want to miss those movement milestones; those milestones are there for a reason. All future movement is built upon those fundamental postures and patterns.

Postures
Lying → prone on elbows → quadruped → sitting → kneeling → standing → single-leg stance

Patterns
Rolling → creeping → crawling → climbing → lunging → squatting → standing → walking → running

When a baby misses a primary movement milestone, limitations or dysfunction will inevitably arise and delay other stages of development because the foundation isn't solid. Although as adults we've mastered far more advanced and complex patterns of motion, these early foundational postures and patterns that should be easily accomplished and re-rendered in adulthood often disappear as our movement exposure shrinks over time.

The human body is built for survival in a world of limited resources, which is why it'll only use valuable resources to adapt or maintain structural change when absolutely necessary.

The formative childhood period allows the software of the nervous system and the hardware of the bones and muscles to discover each other, re-align, and build off one another. Greater movement develops the body, and the developed body has more capacity to take chances and adapt to a more diverse and changing environment. Barring pathology or an environmental constraint, that progressive, self-balancing process naturally develops mobility, stability, and more complex patterns of movement.

We see the same process play out after the early developmental stages when we train a new activity. We'll see our greatest gains in performance in those first four to six weeks of a new activity, but little of that improvement can be attributed to developing stronger physical tissues. We first learn to use our parts in a complementary way and optimize the software application of this new activity. Only when the intensity and frequency of activity exceeds our capacity to respond and recover does the body decide to allocate precious resources toward building greater bone density, reorganizing fascia, and developing stronger muscle tissue and tendons. The trigger for physical adaptation naturally occurs when the quality of function of the body's systems can no longer meet the demands of the environment or activity.

Rebalancing the relationship between the quality and quantity of movement in our lives requires more than just vetting how we use our skills to change the structure and operation of the body's systems. We have to first connect the measurements of what we define as that minimal acceptable quality within each layer of movement.

In business, what gets measured gets done. As we begin the discussion of business development, your next biggest business opportunity might start with the measurements you're not currently taking.

THE FUNCTIONAL MOVEMENT SCREEN—CREATING AWARENESS

In our professional evolution developing a movement-focused strategy, we first needed a tool to help us better qualify and quantify the developmental progression of rolling, crawling, climbing, kneeling, squatting, standing, or standing on one foot because those were the only existing standards.

We were trying to reconcile the abundance of local measurements and interventions with the limited number of global functional tests and interventions. We needed to eliminate the false assumption that correcting those local structural impairments with interventions would ultimately manifest into global improvements in normal, pain-free movement.

Developing that movement tool in our rural Virginia clinic in the 1990s produced the Functional Movement Screen as a tool for sports medicine outreach and pre-participation physicals for 500 local high school athletes. We believed that identifying dysfunctional or painful movements during the physicals could provide the referring doctor more focus on potential problem areas while allowing us, the sports medicine professionals, to suggest alternate ways of exercising or stretching to help correct and prevent problems during preseason training.

It produced immediate effects in the resiliency of the kids we could identify and take action on before they started their sports. However, we wanted to know if we could *detect and measure* dysfunctional movement and better identify the potential risk of injury for those who weren't presenting with obvious pain or limitation. Could we determine who might not be physically prepared to train or compete before they ended up battered and broken?

The Functional Movement Screen came out of that line of questioning to find a way to capture musculoskeletal or movement problems that might present signs of a greater potential risk of injury. At the time, most pre-participation physicals didn't have a movement component…it was just height, weight, some vital signs, and maybe a scoliosis or hernia check.

A screen doesn't answer the question of, "What's the problem?" It simply tells us when there's a need for more investigation. If done well, the same process applied across different scenarios should present patterns. Those patterns present a new opportunity to collect data and refine the larger process. And that larger process helps us more accurately and efficiently detect and monitor areas of concern.

Think of it this way: To determine if you have 20/20 vision, we wouldn't look into your eyes and say, "Wow, you have great vision." We'd observe your behavior of reading an eye chart to get confirmation and then look in your eyes if something seemed off. Using a blood pressure cuff or an eye chart isn't an assessment; it's a screen. It's a tool to evaluate a behavior that might ultimately lead to a deeper evaluation if something falls outside the expected range. A screen is also a way to quickly see if change occurred after an intervention is delivered.

When the internal systems of vision or cardiovascular function become compromised, we have measuring sticks to determine when the behavior of the eyes or heart is dysfunctional or trending in the wrong direction. Those metrics are never stagnant and are affected by a variety of internal and external factors, which is why we recognize their value over a period of time or under different situations. If your blood pressure reading is high at the doctor's office but normal when taken at home, we're more likely to suspect the screen reflects anxiety about the doctor rather than a physical dysfunction. Without a similar screen for movement, movement behaviors either end up completely ignored or investigated only when painful or grossly outside the expected norms.

In scenarios where a screen implies there may be an issue, we need an assessment. An assessment gets personal—peeling back the layers to find the root of movement pattern dysfunction. When blood pressure falls outside the norm, an assessment of additional tests and measures are used to uncover the problem. That's why most assessments have a professional on the other end, offering an expert opinion based on additional screens and tests.

An assessment aims to give a diagnosis at best and at the least, a possible course of action. A valid assessment can uncover the source of a current concern and offer a systematic response to address it. A screen is pass/fail. At its best, a screen can proactively point toward potential trouble on the horizon. Even when problems are present, a screen can help to prioritize which areas require deeper assessment.

When we bring an assessment to a situation that just needs a screen, it becomes easy to break apart and inspect those parts to find a problem that might not exist. Rather than spending time and energy assessing and trying to convince ourselves dysfunction is present, we can quickly deliver a screening tool to tell us if there's something to worry about.

> ### Screens and Assessments
>
> Think of screens like a car. When you take your car for an oil change, the mechanic does a screen as part of a multi-point inspection—checking the fluids, tires, and connection points to spot problems before they cause trouble. The warning lights on the dashboard are *programmed screens,* telling you something isn't right and directing you toward an area outside the normal range. The *specific diagnostic assessment* of a mechanic only comes into play once the signs or symptoms of the car point to trouble.

SCREENING FOR MOVEMENT

While there were accepted proactive screening processes for other areas of physical health, there was nothing like that with movement at the time. If no one in health, fitness, or performance could operate using the same scale or standard of movement outside of saying if someone was injured or in pain, how could we hope to recognize when those basic human movements were changing and leading toward dysfunction?

We wanted to set a qualitative global movement standard and treat it as a new vital sign—one we could objectively measure and monitor. A reliable screening tool could then help us detect when there might be a problem, and also create a feedback loop to check our work.

If that screen could be simple, valid, reproducible, and valuable to the widest range of populations in identifying a minimal accepted level of movement quality, it could provide a common language connecting professionals. We could all recognize movement that fell below the cut of acceptable quality and determine what further investigation and attention was required. If the problem we uncovered wasn't appropriate for our skill set or didn't respond to our interventions, we could communicate more easily when looking for help.

Instead of screening body parts and assuming movement would be normal, we'd screen movements and assume body parts were normal unless the screen told us otherwise. We created a set of rules for a movement screen to:

- Capture movement signs before symptoms
- Capture pattern categories alongside data points
- Create a test nearly anyone in an organization could administer
- Be inexpensive in costs of time, space, and energy
- Filter for minimal acceptable level of movement quality
- Check movement competency before capacity—quality over quantity

The intent was to look at major fundamental patterns to quickly and easily find the biggest dysfunction by testing the individual and not just the problem. The seven movement patterns of the FMS are self-limiting and derived not from specific exercises for specific problems, but from the developmental progressions.

When watching someone squat, lunge, or stand on one foot, instead of jumping to conclusions about parts that look weak or tight, we could appreciate the quality of the larger patterns from both fundamental and functional positions. Then, putting a person into less-complex positions and deconstructing movement into more primitive patterns (think: reaching, rolling, crawling) allowed us to gain better awareness of where that breakdown might be.

STARTING WITH PATTERNS

Starting with patterns made it easy to shift our focus onto faulty parts instead of searching for faulty parts and trying to remember to zoom back out to check patterns. We might be seeing an error in processing and expressing patterns or perhaps a fault in the structure of movement through parts. However, starting wide saved us from spending time hunting for tight muscles or locked-up joints, finding too many (or none), and then having no clear platform from which to work.

This kept our conversations in a productive place, because at that point, debates about needing more fitness or greater skill were irrelevant for someone who couldn't demonstrate the minimums of that developmental ladder. If you have to crawl before you can walk and walk before you can run, why would we assume we could make someone a better runner if we didn't first ensure integrity in walking or crawling?

We often forget or even ignore the question of whether a client or patient can receive and respond to the demands we add. When we encounter a lack of mobility, flexibility, control, balance, or pain, the first action for many of us is to try to solve it with a fitness solution.

The thinking goes that as long as we coach appropriately and scale the exercises as needed, we can accomplish two goals at once: improving movement competency alongside better movement capacity.

The quality of skilled movement can improve with coaching and practice, but at some point, development and adaptation requires pushing our physical limits without a coach there to guide us.

When people can't demonstrate the required control, mobility, or symmetry to perform the developmental patterns of our screens, allowing them to engage with more complex activities will set them up to compensate, substitute…and potentially fail. If the quality of movement is only good when we're controlling the environment, it's telling us that movement is likely to present a consistent barrier to physical adaptation.

Our screens and assessments are designed with the same intention—identifying when the quality threshold of movement isn't being met and is where we need to direct our actions. In those cases, I don't really need to know what the problem is—I just need to know if there *is* a problem. The tests show that somewhere along the line, this person lost functional movement. Hopefully, they'll also identify the movements that could present a risk or a barrier in the pursuit of fitness or new movement skills.

When fitness philosophies ascribe to placing movement capacity (moving often) before competency (moving well), they deny that it's not natural to build capacity on top of incompetence. Those movement problems will only get worse when compounded by frequency. Valuing muscle tissue over the processing of the nervous system leads us to exploit individual body parts while overriding the natural subconscious reflexes protecting the spine, aligning joints, maintaining the center of mass over the base of support, and using advantageous angles and levers.

If we broadly address a problem through exercise without identifying if the internal software can support more complex patterns of movement (and their associated stresses), we're not solving the problem—we *are* the problem.

Good movement keeps impairment at bay, but "moving well before moving often" requires that we define what it means to move well at each layer of physical growth and adaptation.

Our movement tests make up just one set of data points alongside the different objective tests and measures we collect to help paint a more complete picture of movement. We hope to capture more completely that projection of risk and an understanding that the quality of each layer must support the layers above.

Movement Layer	Functional Measures
Production	Skill and Performance-Specific Tests
Fitness	Fundamental Capacity Screen
Wellness	Functional Movement Screen
Health	Selective Functional Movement Assessment

Defining and measuring movement honors our first principle, but there's more to the equation of restoring movement competency than simply placing people in challenging postures or imposing movement obstacles to guide them through a process of self-learning. In the same way "moving more" is incorrectly placed before moving well, our solution to addressing the problems is also often additive—more exercise, more practice, more soft tissue work, more supplemental nutrition, or more gadgets and toys.

Appreciating the impacts the environment, behaviors, and habits can have on movement provides the entry point for our second principle. Just as moving well creates better opportunities for adaptation, removing the negative influences our environments and behaviors can present produces the best conditions and the most effective platform upon which to implement change.

Accomplishing that goal means we need to go back to the foundation of how natural human movement develops. Building on the edge of a person's ability where compensations and mistakes appear is necessary for further development, but an organic solution begins by first asking *what we can take away.*

MOVEMENT PRINCIPLE TWO: PROTECT, CORRECT, DEVELOP

Recognizing there's a problem is the first step to restoring movement. When we find health or wellness metrics that fall below our standard, rather than adding complexity or falling victim to the marketing hype of the latest inventions, we need to first ask, "What can I reduce or remove that's exposing unnecessary risk or impeding the path forward?"

In most cases, the answer comes from our environments and behaviors. Smoking increases the risk of heart disease, cancer, and a host of other issues. Living in an environment with polluted air or water increases the risk of respiratory or systemic disease. In both scenarios, we could add supplements or devices to combat the effects of the harmful behaviors and environmental effects, but removing the source of the problem is a more effective and sustainable solution.

Removing the negative influences and then filling that void with positive activities or environments is the only real solution to promote and develop health, but that isn't always the track we take.

Nature's ability to nurture strong and gracefully aging bodies cannot be bested, but nature isn't concerned about or even aware of our personal or specific development. Nature is big and it can be harsh. It doesn't stop to wait for us to adapt…and sometimes the lessons it teaches aren't survivable.

The natural environment creates exposure, but it's random—some people get too much, others too little. This leads to inconsistent experiences and variable learning, which is why it's so important (and simultaneously difficult) to cultivate environments that help everyone grow and develop to their greatest potential.

We need to gradually scale up an environment that removes obstacles or barriers to learning. Practicing a new skill initially benefits from a quiet, controlled environment of structured drills rather than one that's distracting or variable.

To invoke our second principle, protect before you correct, correct before you develop.

After we've established what it means to move "well" from a qualitative perspective, the second principle is our ethical principle—we'd rather injure your pride than your body.

It's no different than the Hippocratic Oath healthcare practitioners hold to: First, do no harm. Adding a stimulus to effect change should never be the sole excuse to lift more weight, run faster, climb farther, swim harder, or compete in more challenging environments. That thinking again prioritizes *more* before *better,* believing that *more is always better*.

We all fall into the trap of self-selection, particularly around movement. As professionals, we choose a methodology or philosophy based on what aligns most closely with our beliefs or style of coaching or treating.

We see the success we want and don't embrace the slow-growth approach that creates long-term successful development. We're either unable or disinclined to do a self-assessment, and a large part of the problem is the abundance of voices selling specific solutions without the instruction or resources to help us determine for ourselves if it's the right solution for the problem. We follow the advice of trying to hack health or fitness to see the fastest results, and fail nine times out of ten because we haven't looked deeply at the behavioral and environmental factors that introduce risk into our lives.

Before determining the best way for someone to do more of something "good," our first job should be helping identify where they could do less. Recognizing areas of unmanaged risk isn't something most consumers do well, which is why the strongest patients think they need to lift more and the most mobile patients believe they need more yoga. Truly, the greatest value a professional can offer is helping others gain perspective on their personal barriers to success.

MITIGATING + MANAGING RISK

When we talk about risk, we are speaking in terms of a mathematical equation: risk = threat * vulnerability. We can reduce exposure to risk by limiting threats or by reducing our vulnerabilities (and ideally doing both). The reality is that the world is full of external threats that we are not particularly adept at predicting, and we do a poor job of assessing our vulnerabilities to those threats. Many of the negative external forces on our physical growth may be out of our control, but we can absolutely do a better job in identifying, and taking action on, our vulnerabilities.

Our ability to assess real and potential threats and vulnerabilities to our physical growth dictates how well we can respond and adapt. Resilience lies in recognizing those factors that can jeopardize our health, wellness, fitness, or production and taking decisive action to reduce the variables under our control. The greater the integrity of our internal systems and behaviors, the greater our probability of success when it comes time to weather stressful environments or a bad stretch of luck.

Managing our physical risk means identifying those factors that can impair health and function, and then addressing those that are modifiable. The research being done with military personnel by Drs. Phil Plisky and Kyle Kiesel and their team is beginning to point to a collection of risk factors that correlate with changes in movement and an increased incidence of injury.[7] Some factors we can't do much about, but luckily, the majority are modifiable and when addressed can raise the bar of both durability and performance.

IDENTIFIED MOVEMENT RISK FACTORS

Non-Modifiable

- ▶ Age: Older than 26 years
- ▶ Prior history of injury and time lost to that injury

---

[7] *https://journals.sagepub.com/doi/full/10.1177/1941738120902991*

Modifiable

Health and Wellness	Global Function	Fitness
▶ Pain with movement ▶ Perceived recovery ▶ High BMI ▶ Grip strength: asymmetry or below age standards ▶ Reduced physical activity	▶ YBT asymmetries ▶ YBT Composite score below the cutoff ▶ Multiple 1s on the FMS ▶ Ankle dorsiflexion asymmetry	▶ Muscle strength asymmetry ▶ Low cardiovascular fitness (two-mile run)

**See Appendix pages 357–359 for the research and rationale behind these risks.

All of these risk factors can be predictive of injury, but the number of risk factors at play is more critical. The research showed that as an individual's number of risk factors increased, so did the risk of injury.

# of Risk Factors	Odds Ratio[8]	Relative Risk[9]
> 5	1.9–9.6	1.5–2.2
3–4	1.7	1.2–1.4
0–2	0.6–1.2	0.7–1.1

You could argue that many of the modifiable risks are new to us because they're the result of behavioral changes an earlier culture didn't promote. Our lifestyle and movement behaviors have become so physically corrosive that even without an injury, most of us are walking around with four or five of these factors at play. That doesn't mean we're one misplaced step away from an injury, but it does mean many of us are shuffling closer toward that line. Identifying

---

8 The likelihood that an event will occur, as a proportion of the likelihood that an event will not occur. Ratio >1.0 indicates increased occurrence of an event, <1.0 indicates a decreased occurrence of an event. In this example, it represents that an individual with >5 risk factors is between 1.9 and 9.6 times more likely to suffer a future injury.

9 The ratio of the probability of a future event (in this case future injury) occurring in one group (those with X risk factors) compared to another group (those without X risk factors). A ratio of 1 means the future event is just as likely for both groups. In this example, it represents that those with >5 risk factors are 1.5 to 2.2 times more likely to suffer a future injury than those who do not have >5 risk factors.

the factors threatening future function should be the first order of business, and the best first-line action in changing behavior is almost always to look at what can be discontinued.

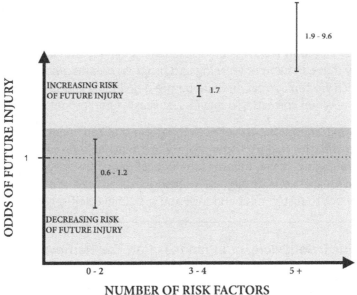

REMOVING NEGATIVES

Something we often speak about in our work at FMS is removing the negatives—eliminating environmental or lifestyle factors contributing to dysfunction. Reducing risk and creating an environment of non-failure is always a better first option because it ensures a more stable environment for recovery, growth, and adaptation.

Protecting a client might mean temporarily avoiding certain activities or types of training that may put the person at greater risk. It could mean holding off strenuous exercise or sports until pain or dysfunctional movement resolve. It can also mean eliminating television for an hour before bed to get a better night's sleep, removing processed foods or drinks, eating smaller portions, or even trying something like intermittent fasting—it's addition by subtraction.

Even in business, rather than buying expensive exercise or rehab equipment or adding services and staff, reducing unnecessary costs or streamlining processes often produces more immediate and sustained benefits. Most industries are built on the concept of complexity for profit, but narrowing your scope and toolkit can make you more resourceful with what you have, and more effective and efficient in your practice. Removing extraneous variables can even illuminate a deficit or deficiency masked by unnecessary layers of interference.

We need to hold fast to the idea that whether in movement or in business, we need to understand our environment, behaviors, and deficits—and remove the factors of each that are compromising the current and future position.

> ### Non-Failure
>
> Don't interpret "an environment of non-failure" as us saying that failure is bad or that we should only let our clients succeed. Removing the negatives or the complexity that can hamper learning and progress creates a better environment in which we can correct an issue before developing a long-term solution. When correcting behaviors, success is paramount.
>
> Removing extraneous inputs reduces the noise that can impact our actions and ensures that the "failure" is temporary and teachable rather than permanent or discouraging. It's no different than developing fitness and skills, where we provide progressions through rich sensory experiences with clear, robust feedback to foster independence and productive self-regulation.

What Activities, Behaviors, or Influences Can You Remove to Reduce Risk and Protect Your Patient/Client/Athlete?[10]

	Awareness	**Protection**
Production	?	-
Fitness	?	-
Wellness	?	-
Health	?	-

? ~ *How would you measure the quality of each layer?*

- ~ *How would you remove negative influences on the quality of each layer?*

Removing negatives is where screens and tests are critical. In our modern world, there are few immediate natural consequences to poor movement quality. Establishing good movement quality and awareness is more important than ever, but it's a hard concept to sell when the signs and symptoms of dysfunction show up later—usually when injury or pain occurs.

---

[10] *You'll see blank or partially completed tables like this throughout this book. We've introduced and included them in this manner to display how we're dissecting the thought process without adding specifics that could misdirect attention. Think of the tools, skills, and tactics available to you that allow you to take action within each box.*

Within a collection of objective data, the movement screens educate those who lack self-awareness, when their confidence and reality don't align. Awareness of movement ability is just as important—if not more important—than the ability itself because it helps us recognize when the risk outweighs the reward.

The people with good self-awareness and who are able to self-regulate can find the opportunity for a teaching moment and transferable activity. Those who aren't aware of the disconnect between the brain and body are those who fail to grow and adapt, and often end up injured. They believe they're getting an A in movement when really, they're getting a D or an F. These are the clients and patients who need a more systematic approach to changing their perceptions and patterns of behavior—an approach of guided self-discovery and learning on the way to physical development.

A PROCESS FOR CHANGE—CORRECT BEFORE YOU DEVELOP

A common misconception of the Functional Movement Systems is that the goal is to use one of our screens to expose a movement problem, and then assign an exercise to correct the problem. That's almost as lackluster as a *Physicians' Desk Reference* for pharmaceuticals—your nose is running; we have these four options. Let's try them one at a time to see which works.

The true goal of the Systems is for both the professional and client to appreciate the critical importance of fundamental movement in sustaining every aspect of life, and how every aspect of life affects movement. That appreciation can then be instilled and integrated through experiential learning, not through talking about it.

Why do we so often insist on coaching movement with verbal cues when movement was first learned before we could follow verbal commands? We don't learn movement through words, pictures, or instruction. If that was the case, children wouldn't be able to get up off the ground until they learned to speak or read. The language of movement isn't communicated verbally; harnessing the internal software of the nervous system to rewire movement patterns means exposing people to a movement, and then fostering an experience that challenges their awareness, perception, and performance at the edge of their ability.

People often use our methods to find dysfunction and then assign a specific functional exercise to help scrub that dysfunction back into function. That's trying to change behavior by inserting another behavior, which isn't nearly as effective as first changing perception.

We try to leverage exposure to the experience. Once we've exposed a movement problem—whether it be through a movement screen or another test—simply describing the problem and giving a supplemental activity to remove it may not be the best investment for a sustainable and independent future.

CORRECTION FLOWS FROM EXPERIENCE

The exposure of the problem and the information to support it isn't nearly as important to the person who needs correction as the experience of the problem itself. Since the words of movement in the body are written *in feel,* not in words or pictures, there needs to be an experience where someone acknowledges, "Oh, I *do* lose my balance on my right foot," or "Wow, I didn't realize how tight it was on that side."

That's a more relevant experience for lay people than the numeric value of a movement screen or the way we describe a movement pattern. They know how they *feel.* They may call it tightness or weakness or wobbliness—and it's important to let them articulate it in their own vocabulary because we can relate our measurement and observation to what they're feeling. We can provide the context so they can see the connections more clearly.

Creating that physical awareness helps realign their perception to their reality. The real essence of what we're doing is engaging the neurological system in a scalable way, which is our most efficient feedback loop. Of all the systems in the body, the neurological system is the most sensitive and most responsive to both correct and incorrect elements.

"Correcting" movement comes from feeding someone a movement experience in a non-threatening, low-risk environment. Positive adaptation follows multiple positive responses, and if we can provide feedback that magnifies the obstacles or barriers and provides an achievable learning path, we should see a measurable response. It may not resolve the issue, but more often than not, people who go through that experience are empowered by seeing how change can happen quickly.

Most people who can't touch their toes think they never will or that they'll need a month of yoga classes or soft-tissue work before they can. We can take many of those people through a toe-touch movement progression and, with guidance, they realize, "I don't have tight hamstrings. When I bent forward, I was sending a signal to make my hamstrings do something that wasn't the most advantageous for that movement, but it may have been necessary for my current state. I have to compensate in one place because my body is using a strategy of bracing or tightening to protect myself or to maintain stability."

That kind of experience is vital because if we can engineer a positive movement experience both at a subjective level for them and an objective level for us, we can both appreciate what happened in a common way. People call that a corrective strategy or a functional progression, but they don't measure it against a functional baseline. I don't think the world sees what we do in the Systems as a way to measure if a particular endeavor is working, but that's exactly what they're intended to do.

That's the thing we've always valued—it's much more than exposing a problem and exercising the demons out of it. Taking someone through a movement experience like we do through a movement progression, and then seeing, feeling, and measuring a change leads toward a corrective path that goes beyond a collection of exercises.

I've always tried to communicate that process of creating awareness through actions, but I've never communicated it well enough to say we're not just revealing a dysfunctional movement and then applying exercise—we're uncovering and engaging with that dysfunction to create a learning experience.

What Activities, Behaviors, or Influences Can You Add to Correct and Restore Movement? What Can You Deliver to Improve and Sustain Positive Adaptation?

	Awareness	Protection	Correction	Development
Production	?	-	+	=
Fitness	?	-	+	=
Wellness	?	-	+	=
Health	?	-	+	=

? ~ How would you measure the quality of each layer?

- ~ How would you remove negative influences on the quality of each layer?

+ ~ How would you improve the quality of each layer?

= ~ How would you enhance and sustain homeostasis/balance in each layer?

If that experience changes movement in a way we can measure and value, that experience can then be converted into a reproducible, scalable exercise. Selecting an exercise through that criteria neurologically strengthens that pattern so we can continue to progress and add layers until we're satisfied it can support greater and more complex movement. Reaping the full physical benefits that come from developing greater fitness and production in a particular lift or activity doesn't come from better exercise selection and coaching—it comes from guiding people through a journey of self-discovery whereby they gain awareness and control.

We suggest exercises we've found to be effective in resetting the body into more complete movement, but we don't want people to be "doing" exercises; we want them to be engaging in activities. Functional movement in the clinic or gym is meaningless if it doesn't translate into the real world. Regardless of the exercises or methods we use, we hold ourselves to a movement standard and assess if our interventions are able to sustain long-term movement development.

We first need to become aware of whether we can quantify or qualify if the layers of movement meet the required standards. Then, taking the proper steps in protection, correction, and development honors our restoring and maintaining a minimal accepted level of movement quality before pursuing more movement quantity.

Following that stepwise progression helps sustain competency and independence in our fundamental movements on the way to greater physical adaptation. Effectively putting that movement process into action requires a system of feedback to tell us if and when to apply the appropriate tactics throughout the process.

Applying our first two movement principles requires a third—to implement standard operating procedures that unify our approach to the dimensions of physical growth and development.

> If you believe in Principle One, honor it with Principle Two.
>
> To take action on Principle Two, implement Principle Three.

MOVEMENT PRINCIPLE THREE: CREATE SYSTEMS THAT TEST AND ENFORCE YOUR PHILOSOPHY

> *"Don't let your schooling get in the way of your education."*
> *—Mark Twain*

The third movement principle is our practical principle. We believe we can develop movement faster and safer than nature, but when it comes time for us to combine our strategy and tactics, we're too often inconsistent, questionably effective, and often unevolved. The solutions we use are prescriptive without basing that prescription on a meaningful objective measure. Are we basing our decisions on pain? Strength standards? What the patient reports as "better?"

How do we hit the target when we don't know where we're aiming?

We see the greatest practitioners in the fields of health, fitness, and performance achieving incredible outcomes more rapidly than the rest of us. We assume following their path and learning to harness their techniques is the recipe for our own success.

Starting with a focus on tactics is the equivalent of learning all the survival and camping tips you need to hike the Appalachian Trail without ever learning how to use a map or compass. A map provides some context on where you are relative to where you want to go. Knowing how to periodically use a compass keeps you pointed toward the right heading, rather than searching for anything that looks like an indicator you're on the right track.

The best performers are so consistently efficient and effective because they use a better map, and they know what tools can help them navigate their choices. Every one of them has a systematic process to generate objective feedback that they allow to wash back over their work and prevent their egos or assumptions from going unchecked.

If the best practitioners try a new technique or tactic that proves counterproductive, they don't stay on the wrong path for long. They also don't let fear of looking like a failure get in their way—they know how to quickly correct their course and get back on track. Operating with a consistent strategy creates a filter to see opportunities for faster feedback and simpler decision-making. The rest of us spend more time debating which fork in the road to take rather than learning to use better filters to align our data and actions and find the straightest route from Point A to Point B.

A PLATFORM FOR SELF-EXPERIMENTATION

The original goal of the Functional Movement Screen was to look at fundamental movement patterns and establish a baseline. We believed that if the structural anatomy fell within average limits, the ability to perform the functional patterns should also be at least average. If people performed below average, their software—the neuromuscular performance—must not be as effective as their hardware. If they had average hardware with exceptional ability, the software of their physical awareness, processing, and skill had all been elevated beyond the sum of the structural components. They were more resourceful with the same physical resources as other comparable people.

Once we established the screen, we presented it anywhere we could. We spoke about the screen at different local, regional, and national conferences to get the information out. The more people we could convince to deploy the screen, the better we could see and question the construct and find what worked and what didn't so we could establish a movement baseline across different groups and environments.

We wanted to know: How do different people from different environments move? Do we see consistent problems? Which patterns are most important? And…is this tool valuable for its intended purpose?

Although this all seemed like a logical, non-threatening perspective on what constitutes "functional" human movement, we knew this perspective was likely to meet resistance. The implication that we'd all been professionally misguided and were operating in a less-than-optimal way could give rise to negative emotions. But rather than saying the old way was wrong, we were simply asking people to give the process a fair shake, and then give feedback on if they were seeing what we were seeing.

Like any good experiment, we asked everyone to follow the same process and report back on what worked and what didn't so we could collectively hold to a standard measurement. We didn't initially talk a lot about exercise because we didn't have an exercise agenda—we didn't even fully understand what the movement screen told us. We already had a lot of corrective exercises based on our unique functional evaluation, but how we laid things out continued to evolve as we collected more input from the field. Those 10 years of in-the-trenches work provided a lot of mistakes and false starts, but also a lot of feedback and empirical evidence from the early adopters.

Luckily, early in this process, professional sports teams started using the movement screen. The great thing about professional sports is that professional strength coaches, athletic trainers, or athletes don't initially rely exclusively on research. They can't wait on research because being ahead of the consensus is their competitive advantage.

The Soviet sports complex was built on that principle—start from a scientific hypothesis, apply a logical intervention, see which coaches and athletes excel with specific techniques or methods, and then allow the research to uncover or confirm what was occurring. The Soviets were way ahead of the Silicon Valley idea of failing fast—try a variation of an original idea, measure its effect, and then move on if there's no measurable impact.

If we waited for the research to overwhelmingly confirm something to be superior, every profession would come to a standstill. How many studies have you read that don't end in "more research is needed?" But think of this: The first research study on the Functional Movement Screen didn't come out until 2007—10 years after we first introduced the screen.

The early-adopting professional teams weren't doing the movement screen because research said to do it—they were doing the movement screen because they saw benefits in using it. That's when we knew those first seven tests told us something.

Fortunately for us, today there's much more positive research on the movement screen than negative, and the biggest victory to come out of the research so far is that the screen is a reliable way to look at movement.[11]

---

11 Cuchna, J. W., Hoch, M. C., & Hoch, J. M. (2016). The interrater and intrarater reliability of the functional movement screen: A systematic review with meta-analysis. Physical Therapy in Sport, 19, 57-65. doi:10.1016/j.ptsp.2015.12.002

Having scientific support behind what you do is vital, but don't close your eyes to what's been learned by practical application. If you hope to be at the top of your profession, at some point, your sleeves need to go up, your hands need to get dirty, and you need to risk the embarrassment of making a mistake where you're the only one to blame.

A PROBLEM OF APPLICATION

In those early days, we personally made more than enough poor assumptions and mistakes. Initially, we believed all movement patterns were represented in the overhead deep squat; we assumed the deep squat could either be the fundamental starting point or the tip of the iceberg of the movement patterns. Many of us put a lot of value in fixing the deep squat, thinking it would wash backward across the movement screen, enlightening the other more primitive, less complex, or fundamental patterns.

Boy, were we wrong.

The same thing happened with the push-up. Unlike the leg raise, shoulder mobility, and rotary stability tests, the push-up is a high-threshold movement that doesn't quarter or cut the body in half to enable a left-right comparison. It asks, "Can you zip up your skin suit and accomplish this movement before getting on your feet?"

Failing this test could explain why people had problems on their feet or when training with loads, and we were forced to reassess our processes when we realized our testing and approach allowed people to slip through the cracks and end up stuck with a poor push-up and compromised movement.

We acknowledged this movement hierarchy, but even we didn't follow it at the beginning. We were trying to hack someone to a better deep squat or push-up, hoping it would clear everything below it, when really the developmental progression was there to inform us we had a pre-built progression. We should honor it not by weighing each test democratically, but by making sure we read that first line on the eye chart.

Honoring that system meant the first line for us became the active straight leg raise, and the second line was shoulder mobility. We needed to re-establish that developmentally, the extremities move in a symmetrical and at least average fashion before we progress into different levels of core control on our way to moving upright.

Early on we made errors in our tactics, and we saw other people making those same mistakes. We tried to eliminate biases in our screening process, to allow movement to speak—but ultimately, once people left our clinic or one of our presentations and went back to their gym or clinic, the same scenario of operating off of false assumptions reared its head.

The biggest challenge was that many people who saw inconsistent results were deploying what we designed as a systematic, stepwise process in non-systematic ways.

One of the more common mistakes was the "buffet approach" to the movement screen. Many people, out of convenience or preference, chose to do some tests and skip others…and still proceeded with the confidence they were accurately screening something. The screen is built to look at the way each of these individual movement tests play with the others—they're creating a gradient of movement to look for a theme. Going back to the analogy of an eye chart, if we arbitrarily pick a small or large line on the eye chart or delete lines without a scaled approach to shrinking letters, we won't get an accurate picture of visual competency.

People who perform the parts of the screen they believe are more important than the rest and then take their programming cues or ideas from it are embarking on a journey ill-prepared. Too many people assume that modifying the screen toward a particular sport or activity or using a piece of the screen is as good as the full standard screen, but it's not. That's using a tool in a different manner than it was designed instead of using that tool appropriately in as many environments as possible to discover if it renders better information to take better action, and then moving forward.

Many coaches and trainers were more interested in manipulating the measuring stick of the screens to fit a niche because they see the generalized postures and patterns within the screen as nonspecific to the demands of their sports. When people need to sprint 100 meters or throw a baseball 90 miles per hour, what value is there in lying on their backs and raising a leg up and down?

A GLOBAL PERSPECTIVE ON SCREENING

When you screen without confirmation bias and with as much reliability and objectivity as possible, you see distributions that tell you the movement needs of a group, and where an individual falls within the group. The value lies in seeing the democratic distribution of these movement patterns in a particular environment with specific populations so you can take the most appropriate action.

Certain people and environments demand higher standards than others. A professional basketball player has a higher movement standard than a weekend golfer, but those higher standards belong on the other side of the movement screen, not in place of it. Baseball players take the same eye test your grandmother does to get a driver's license, but the expectation is that their "normals" won't be the same.

The tests aren't as valuable in comparing the movement scores of a factory worker to an Olympian—the importance is comparing workers to other workers, and athletes to other athletes. People can achieve amazing things with a normal movement score—without it being exceptional—but there are few scenarios where people in a higher-performing, more physically demanding environment are able to do well with lower movement scores than their peers. Distinguishing those whose baseline function is a barrier to physical adaptation allows you to deploy your resources and effort where they're most needed.

The movement screens offer a multi-stage filter scaled and strategized like the neurodevelopmental progression. If dysfunction or a deficit in one of the lower patterns catches something, we assume the lower pattern is a fundamental domino that needs to be flipped over before confronting the next. If we take the right action, the ripple effect of human behavior will occur, and we need to be there with the same scale to measure what changed, what didn't change, and then use the information to progress. The whole point is *Test—Take Action—Retest,* but many people take the first two steps and never objectively employ the third.

Incorrectly using the screening tools, incorrectly sampling the environment and then deciding to act based on incorrect assumptions is unlikely to produce the desired effect. Staying true to the system of movement and working on the weak links until they meet a minimal qualitative standard may sound like a slow process, but it actually streamlines our decision-making into yes or no propositions. Instead of trying to shortcut or speed up the process only to hit a dead-end of our own creation, that algorithmic model often results in more rapid gains simply because we're less likely to stray too far off course.

The multi-layer filter generated by our principles of movement and the Functional Movement Systems allows us to assess and respond more quickly and course correct more efficiently. Time is a limited resource; instead of waiting for a sustained plateau in progress to indicate when it's time to adjust, we can constantly sample the output and tweak the input in an objective, scalable way. Every decision or intervention should pass through the Systems at some level and demonstrate a positive change. Otherwise, we have to ask if our time and effort is better spent elsewhere.

In a world engineered to protect us from many of the natural barriers and challenges that shape our physical growth and adaptation, the negative feedback telling us when we're off course is usually slow to emerge. Even if you're individually leaving an imprint on movement, our Western model forces us into silos of health, fitness, and performance, and we still leave too many parts of movement behavior mismanaged or unmanaged, and other parts over-managed.

Now is the time to go beyond a systematic approach of our technical skills and professional decisions toward an even larger system—one that weaves together our professions and responsibilities in service of every patient, client, or athlete.

Think of this thought process as the most basic example of how to implement a standard operating procedure for your work:

- How can I screen or measure _____?
  - Perform screen or measurement
- What action can I take to change _____?
  - Take desired action
  - Rescreen or remeasure
- Did I see a change?
  - Yes
    - Proceed if the change was positive; try a different action if the change was negative
  - No
    - Did I measure it right?
    - Did I deliver my tactic/technique right?
    - Do I need more time to see change?

https://qrco.de/bcYnIQ

THE 4X4 MOVEMENT MATRIX

People think of processes or systems as restrictive—something reduced to a recipe or script that hinders creativity or flexibility. In reality, good processes and systems are built with just enough structure that they facilitate greater freedom. They're intended to first provide protection by setting up guardrails and checks on your work, and second, to confirm the effectiveness of your actions. Following a recipe might not produce the best version of a dish, but it will help prevent you from making the worst. As you get better at identifying the things that matter, you can experiment and test the boundaries with greater confidence in the quality of the end product.

When well designed, systems create a safe environment to work and expand our field of vision and attention.

> *"Freedom is what everyone wants—to be able to act and live with freedom. But the only way to get to a place of freedom is through discipline."*
> *—Jocko Willink*

For us, "system" implies a body of work set up to check itself when we follow the instructions. When performed appropriately, an eye chart and a blood pressure cuff function much the same regardless of the environment in which they're used. That's where we wanted to start the movement conversation. The Functional Movement Systems provided a set of standard operating procedures to use when boots are on the ground in an environment—whether that environment is a clinic, a training room, a weightroom, or the practice field.

Just as with a pilot's preflight check, standard operating procedures are intended to reduce risk, improve performance, and minimize variation and miscommunication through a checklist approach. We didn't ask people to unflinchingly follow our dogma, but the number of professionals who engaged with the movement screens and our corrective strategies on a critical level allowed us to establish the standard operating procedures we use to collect information, devise an intervention, and then measure the result. Starting and ending a task or action with that checklist of confirmation ensures that problems are identified early, errors stay small, and significant decisions have a trail of breadcrumbs to follow back in times of trouble.

We're not just looking for a positive change we can reinforce, but also appreciating negative side effects. That constant measuring and sampling of the response to our protective, corrective, and developmental strategies keeps us from misapplying our efforts and discovering too late that we made the wrong decision. It keeps us from putting fitness on top of dysfunction or applying a fitness solution to a medical problem. It simultaneously informs us in healthcare that the job of removing risk is not done just because symptoms are managed.

If we can measure a positive change with no negative side effects, it sets up the program. Taking an individual response and turning it into an adaptation is built on the repetition of measured, favorable, and positive responses—you'll get the adaptation you need and the tissues will grow with no insult to the neurological system along the way. If we can't measure a positive response to an intervention, or the intervention actually diminishes quality, it wouldn't be fruitful to base an entire program or an assumption of adaptation on that path.

I want every movement professional to be able to work in unison, guiding people through the layers of physical growth and adaptation. The Functional Movement Systems provides a shared perception and language of movement to bridge the gap in professional communication. Now, this simple 4x4 grid can provide the same map for each of us to navigate our own way and ultimately find each other.

What Actions Are You Taking in Each Layer of Physical Growth and Adaptation?

		→ **Physical Adaptation** →			
		Awareness	Protection	Correction	Development
↑ *Physical Growth* ↑	Production	?	-	+	=
	Fitness	?	-	+	=
	Wellness	?	-	+	=
	Health	?	-	+	=

? ~ How can you measure the quality of each layer?

- ~ How can you remove negative influences on the quality of each layer?

+ ~ How can you improve the quality of each layer?

= ~ How can you enhance and sustain homeostasis/balance in each layer?

The vertical orientation of the table represents the dimensions of your physical growth, and the horizontal orientation is your progression of adaptation to your environment. The structure is in this order because addressing the components of each box supports the next.

The 4x4 framework appraises the dimensions of physical growth that may be dysfunctional or deficient for an individual, and it also allows us to identify the best actions to take in restoring the natural balance of each.

Within this framework, we have the opportunity to drop every patient, client, or athlete we work with onto a grid to gain immediate clarity into their needs.

This system is not a list of rules, but rather 16 sets of decisions that proceed in a particular order. Each box holds an endless supply of tactics and tools that can be deployed to create change—therein lies the opportunity for creativity, experimentation, and innovation in your work.

As long as we respect the progression of growing and adapting to our environments and hold ourselves to a consistent, objective set of standards in appraising the impact, the effectiveness and efficiency of the process only grows stronger as time and experience offer better inputs to feed into the system.

I can't tell you exactly what to do or which direction to go because everyone begins the journey at a different starting point, with a different set of resources, a different base of knowledge, and different goals. Whether you're mapping a client or yourself onto the grid, everyone will have a different level of needs to be addressed. What I can provide are better instructions on how to read the map and select the best tools to determine when your decisions and actions are leading you off track.

Whether you're the first or last person to adopt a new way of thinking or working, starting with a personal inventory and identifying your own areas of greatest need are necessary to successfully change yourself before you worry about your business.

> Dissecting the layers of human anatomy can be a daunting and intimidating task, but the appreciation of the human movement miracle only grows with the dissection of each layer. This movement matrix creates the same opportunities of finely slicing the layers that profoundly affect human movement. In either case, going beneath the surface is the first step to awareness, understanding, and the ability to reconstruct a more complete model of our physical selves.

What Information Do I Need?	What Actions Can I Take?
Awareness—can we measure those qualities that will confirm this person currently meets the most basic standard of health, wellness, fitness, and production to meet their needs?	**Health**—vital signs, SFMA **Wellness**—functional risk factors, FMS **Fitness**—FCS, 1RM, VO_2 max, etc. **Production**—skill or performance-specific testing
Protection—is this person engaging (or not engaging) in behaviors that will sustain the health, wellness, fitness, and production he or she already has?	**Health**—stopping negative lifestyle behaviors (smoking, eating junk food) **Wellness**—avoiding new environments or activities that may expose the person to failure or injury **Fitness**—removing painful exercises or activities **Production**—removing or modifying skills or tasks with a high likelihood of failure
Correction—is this person engaging (or not engaging) in behaviors that will help correct dysfunction or deficiencies that may be present or appear later?	**Health**—improving hydration, sleep, mental or emotional balance and removing pain **Wellness**—addressing modifiable risk factors and reinforce function **Fitness**—corrective activity and exercise to restore capacity **Production**—retraining activity-specific skills
Development—is this person engaging in behaviors that will reinforce and expand the quality or quantity of each layer of movement?	**Health**—daily walking, eating healthy **Wellness**—maintaining mobility and function through whole-body activity **Fitness**—training functional capacity **Production**—teaching and practicing skill

A PERSONAL APPRAISAL OF MOVEMENT

The business of movement must begin on a personal level because we should be able to cross-examine our personal lives as we would our professional lives. If you're a critical consumer of your service, you should believe in what you do. You can sell a car you wouldn't drive, but I'm not sure you should be part of a service you wouldn't consume. Those are different because service is a continual, evolving relationship, while selling a product is a finite transaction. When the sale is complete, the product may be guaranteed, but the relationship isn't.

Think of your professional growth and adaptation as you would your physical growth and adaptation. Ask yourself these questions as you move across each layer of growth:

- ▶ Am I healthy/well/fit/producing at the level I want?
- ▶ How am I aware if I'm healthy/well/fit/performing? How am I measuring each?
- ▶ How am I protecting the health/wellness/fitness/production I already have?
- ▶ How am I correcting the problems in health/wellness/fitness/production?
- ▶ How am I maintaining or developing my health/wellness/fitness/production for the future?

The 4x4 grid builds from health awareness as the first problem you can have because if you're not aware of how to identify and measure the qualities needed to be a balanced, stable human organism, there's no way to confidently make objective decisions with more advanced levels of growth and development. Being able to shade in the boxes in each row means you should be able to provide examples of behaviors and actions you're taking to measure and address each layer of growth from the bottom up.

Try to plot yourself on this grid in an objective way, and you'll find it even easier to use to plot your patients, clients, or athletes. We've offered our definitions of what each dimension represents, but even superficially ask yourself:

- ▶ Are you aware of where you are or what you need in each layer of growth?
- ▶ Do you have ways to measure or quantify your competency in each?
- ▶ Once you know your status in a particular dimension of growth, are there behaviors or barriers you can remove to protect your current position?
- ▶ Are there behaviors or resources to add to correct the limitations you identified and measured?
- ▶ Have you done enough to sustain and develop this new baseline before you focus on the next level of growth?

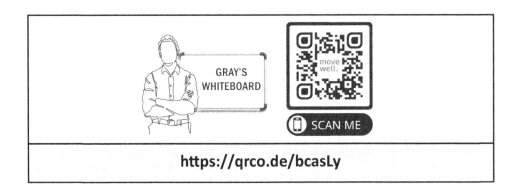

https://qrco.de/bcasLy

Where Are Your Opportunities?

		→ Physical Adaptation →			
		Awareness	Protection	Correction	Development
↑ *Physical Growth* ↑	Production	✓	-	+	✓
	Fitness	?	-	✓	✓
	Wellness	?	✓	+	=
	Health	✓	✓	✓	=

? ~ What can you be doing to measure the quality of each layer?

- ~ What can you be doing to remove negative influences on the quality of each layer?

+ ~ What can you be doing to improve the quality of each layer?

= ~ What can you be doing to enhance and sustain homeostasis/balance in each layer?

Any unshaded boxes where you lack a clear "Yes" to those questions represent areas of uncertainty where you've just found opportunities. If you fail to measure quality in that first box of Awareness, any other actions to Protect, Correct, or Develop a layer of movement are potentially incomplete (and likely out of alignment with what is needed). You may be an athlete, working to develop greater fitness and production, but if you can't first provide objective evidence that your wellness and fitness are adequate or at least being maintained, you can't be confident the action you are taking is in service of what you really need.

Right now, *perspective* is the goal. If you plotted your personal problem and can now see yourself in a different way...that's the point. Don't worry about solving it right now. The real objective is to see if you can solve problems with a fresh perspective while using the resources you have before trying to overhaul what you're already doing.

If you can do this in your personal life, you can ask the same questions about where you are as a professional. Where are you in your profession today? Where do you want to be in 10 years?

I've always attempted to make my processes as simple as possible, which is why I feel these 16 grid boxes can adequately capture and support the strategies and tactics required to build resilient human beings.

When I initially wrote my core movement principles, I started with 10 before I realized they could be reduced to three. I could probably think of more boxes to address growth and development, but not fewer. Any fewer than these core components and we miss something critical in the recipe. It's my application of Principles One to Principle Three, demanding quality first and quantity second on our system of movement.

How early or how deeply you pursue these layers of growth and adaptation comes back to how willing you are to challenge your current approach. The risk-to-reward ratio we're each willing to take is unique and, to be honest, there aren't many people willing to be early adopters in every category—myself included. In 99% of my life, I'm a middle adopter. In my lifestyle, my exercise, and my training, I want to use tried and tested tools with at least a solid proof of concept, but I'm willing to take on risks in finding better ways to wellness.

I want to drive a safe and dependable vehicle in every other aspect of my life, but with movement and finding the weakest links in human patterns and behaviors, I love being a test pilot.

CHAPTER FOUR

DEFINE YOUR VALUE— RECOGNIZE YOUR OPPORTUNITY

- Is there a need in your community for health, function, fitness, or production?
- Can you fill that need?
- With your skills and knowledge, can you provide something better than what's available?
- What are your areas of weakness and areas of strength?

Most often, the question we get at the end of our courses is, "How do I implement this?" Our response is, "Where are your opportunities?"

When I returned to my small town in Virginia to start a practice, I wasn't in an academic environment or trying to compete in a major market. The health and fitness options were limited, so I had to wear a lot of hats to meet the needs of the community in those early days. I had a background in strength and conditioning in addition to my physical therapy training, so I could provide my knowledge and perspective in that regard, but I wasn't a strength coach. My medical training allowed me to perform health screening for children and adults with poor eating habits, high blood pressure, and mental and emotional challenges, but I wasn't a nutritionist or a medical doctor.

I could have taken full advantage of any of those opportunities, but I never lost sight of my greatest opportunity and value: restoring movement health and making people aware of options enabling a more physically productive lifestyle.

As you envision your ideal business, your skills likely support one or two particular layers of movement. But with so many people unknowingly walking around with deficits in health or wellness, it's rare that you'll get to work with someone who needs only your specific set of skills. That is why screening is so important regardless of your expertise—you may be the first line of defense in identifying the risk factors at play for these clients and patients.

I have no doubt you can see opportunities in your business to address every layer of movement, but think about where your greatest opportunity lies. What your community, tribe, or team needs and your particular strengths play a tremendous role in where and how you should direct your focus.

THE SPECIALIST

Some professionals go the route of specialization to set themselves apart, refining their skills or businesses and going deep into a specific area or segment of the population. This might mean a manual therapy practice offering structural integration or acupuncture, or something like a training environment catered to working with outdoor athletes or tennis players.

There are plenty of examples of successful professionals who built their businesses on being the experts in one area, but specializing requires a strategy for what happens when the person who comes to see you has needs outside that specialty. If you're a manual therapist and what your client needs won't be solved solely by your hands, what do you do? If you fashion yourself as a "Corrective Exercise Specialist," but you screen someone and don't find significant dysfunction…technically, you're out of work.

The benefit of becoming a specialist is the depth of knowledge and skill you have to offer, but that narrow focus may limit your abilities with people who have multiple areas of concern. Even though it's not exclusive to specialists, the risk of losing objectivity is also higher when looking at every problem through a single lens. If all you have are highly specialized tools or methods, you risk turning every problem into something that needs what you have to offer. However, with a broader strategy, you can position your contributions within a sustainable framework that still supports your specific goals.

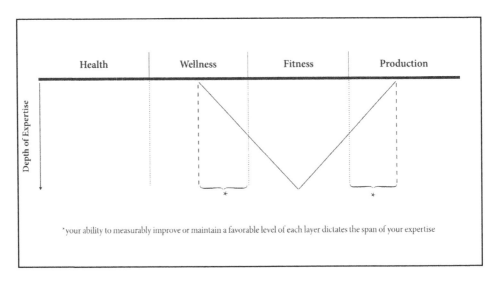

THE GENERALIST

The other path many professionals choose is the route of the generalist. Being able to provide complete care for clients is often the motivation for generalists, which is why you can usually identify them by the number of certification initials after their names.

More professionals are getting multiple certifications or expanding the scope of their practices into lifestyle coaching or a hybrid of physical therapist, chiropractor, and strength coach, all in the name of providing a holistic solution. This can be great for continuity of care and concierge-level service for some clients, but in our experience, professionals who try to be everything to everyone inevitably sacrifice their effectiveness in the process.

You should absolutely expose yourself to varied training and try to provide comprehensive services, but you can only wear so many hats. While there are some double- and triple-threat professionals, being exceptional in multiple dimensions is rare. Your brain possesses a finite storage capacity; the broader your knowledge, the harder it is to keep expanding its depth. Whereas a specialist's deep knowledge is typically effective within a narrow range, a generalist can often only maintain general competency across that wide range—diluting the effectiveness in all of them.

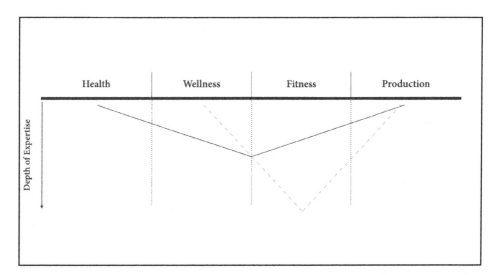

Defining the category of physical growth where your respective service fits offers plenty of breadth for professional development. There may be scenarios where your environment demands going wide to fill additional roles, particularly if there are no other options for your clients to receive guidance. In those instances, offering even superficial direction will be better than none. But even though there's value in offering services across the span of health, wellness, fitness, and production, that's not where the greatest opportunities lie.

Professional growth requires communication and accountability at the forefront. Being comfortable acknowledging our strengths and weaknesses allows us to ask ourselves honestly, "Am I really good enough to be all of these things? Is it important to fill all the roles someone needs? Or should I become the best clinician, trainer, or coach I can be and acknowledge when it's time to pass the baton to a professional who can best meet my client's other needs?"

The real differentiation between your level of service and everyone else's lies not in your ability in a single layer of movement, but in your ability to look backward and forward through the other layers to identify those opportunities where you can measure and act. Regardless of your expertise, a strategy that helps you recognize the weakest link is the key to success because wherever you stand on the continuum, you're responsible for upstream awareness and downstream results.

OPPORTUNITY LIES AT THE INTERSECTIONS

We all appreciate the synergy created when the members of a team enhance one another's skills. If your goal is to raise the performance of your professional service, it's critical to find peers to complement your skills. This can protect you from the specialist's trap by leaning on others whose expertise is complementary to your own. You can mitigate your weaknesses with the added benefit of creating a collective knowledge that's both deep and wide.

That's why so many environments try to replicate the professional sports model. Constructing a team of doctors, athletic trainers, physical therapists, chiropractors, nutritionists, massage therapists, strength coaches, and sports psychologists allows everyone to wrap their collective arms around the athletes from every angle of health and production. The team can be in your employ or in your referral network, but you must all be connected on strategy. Your 4x4 matrix will facilitate this communication and accountability.

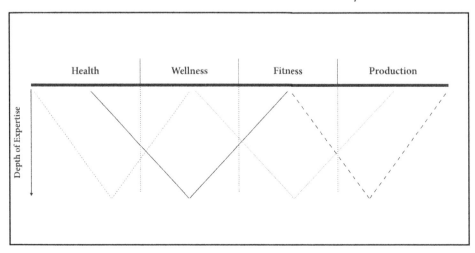

When done well, the results can be incredible. Blended environments of orthopedic surgeons with in-house rehabilitation and sports training, gyms with an attached physical therapist or chiropractor, or yoga and Pilates studios that also offer massage or acupuncture can thrive with a similar approach. The benefits to having multiple specialists working together is clear: keeping everything in house creates a closed loop where regardless of the client's condition, someone can provide value. The financial benefits of a single business that can meet those needs are obvious. Instead of having to refer someone out when a patient is released or when an athlete gets injured, people become lifelong clients as they shift among the team.

Not everyone has the luxury, resources, or desire to create an everything-under-one-roof model. It's great if you hire a team of practitioners who can do their jobs effectively, but that also creates more plates you need to simultaneously keep spinning for the survival of your business. You might not want the responsibility of managing a large team or facility, or tackling the logistics of different schedules and payments—and that's fine.

The good news is that more isn't always better. You can be successful as a generalist or a specialist as long as you don't operate in a silo.

> Regardless of our respective knowledge base, if we're concerned about the best interests of patients and clients, it's in our best interests to know where the value of our skills stop and someone else's begins.

KNOW WHERE YOUR GREATEST VALUE LIES

You need to decide whether it's in your best interest to be a specialized expert and general tactician or a general expert and specialized tactician. If you're an orthopedic surgeon, you're a specialized expert in health, and you should be able to deliver general tactics and advice to help direct a patient in other layers of movement. If you're a therapist or strength and conditioning coach, you need a wider range of expertise to be effective, but you'd better possess specific tactics in your core area of focus to differentiate yourself.

My clinic's expertise is in getting people out of pain and restoring function on the way to fitness and production, whatever physical task, vocation, or sport that may be. We need to know enough about nutrition or medical diagnoses to counsel patients on lifestyle choices and to recognize when they need to work with a nutritionist or a medical doctor. We need to know enough about Olympic lifting or the demands of a particular sport to know when someone can safely return to training or participation, and also when we need to allow a personal trainer or coach to do what they do best.

The strength coaches and personal trainers we work with recognize when pain or dysfunction won't be corrected through better fitness or coaching. They don't think twice about referring back to us when appropriate. Even though pain, fitness, and production command much of the attention, our focus on function provides the feedback loops we require. It's that approach that makes us successful—by maximizing our effectiveness and nailing those transitions and handoffs from one professional to the next.

For every chunk of knowledge you add across the layers of movement, you'll inevitably have to sacrifice some of the depth in your area of expertise, and vice versa. Your business can often be leaner, more effective, and more sustainable by deciding where you can make the greatest impact, and then cultivating a multidisciplinary team in your community. Your work may not be responsible for covering each box in the 4x4 grid, but every box matters. You either need to have tactics to improve those areas, or you need to know someone else who does.

The greatest opportunity for every movement professional lies in what we choose to do in those transitional periods of a patient's or client's journey between the layers of movement. We can't always prevent injury or dysfunction, but we can prevent poor lifestyle, bad rehab, and lousy training strategies from creating unnecessary pain, injury, and disability.

HEALTHCARE: DISCHARGE TO WELLNESS ON THE WAY TO FITNESS

If you work in the healthcare space, using the model of movement offers opportunities to accelerate rehabilitation, and to logically confront and correct the medical model that forces us to discharge people with unresolved risk factors. Using the Systems won't help your business on the frontend—that's about getting referrals and networking and creating contracts. Using the SFMA as part of your clinical evaluation can improve the effectiveness and efficiency of your treatments, but it won't help you on the backend either, because it only tells you the patient can move without pain.

When we only deal with the diagnosis an insurance company gives us permission to work on, we're not dealing with the holistic care of the patient. Even though most of us in healthcare view ourselves as specialists, we really operate as general practitioners. This means the active lifestyle of our patients is ultimately our responsibility. When pain or disease is resolved through a course of treatment, we may confidently say their health is now in order, but their function may not be.

This is where many health professionals miss their biggest opportunity.

If you're discharging people from medical care who can't check that box of wellness, they'll likely end up right back in your exam room after returning to their previous behaviors. Dysfunction needs to be handled and patients need the awareness of what that means because otherwise they're leaving your care with unaddressed risk factors. It's in gaining expertise and a strategy in the measurement and interventions of those risk-generating behaviors where we can restore the behavioral health that defines wellness and future function.

Implementing an exit screen at discharge alongside better education and better movement behaviors is the greatest business opportunity in health and rehabilitation. That exit allows you to sell your services again—repackaged not in a diagnosis or reimbursement model, but in a functional-fitness model. That alone won't drive more patients through your door, but the patients leaving will understand what they now need from you is different from what you just provided.

Where's Your Greatest Opportunity as a Medical Professional?

	Awareness	Protection	Correction	Development
Production	?	-	+	=
Fitness	?	-	+	=
Wellness	?	-	+	=
Health	?	-	+	=

Dark to light = Greater to lower opportunity

> How relevant are you in each of these categories?
>
> Do you have the skill set to be an expert in that category?
>
> Do you have a way to provide value in those areas that may be outside your scope?

The beautiful thing is that the same language, the same strategies, and the same equipment used in rehab can transition people back into independence or whatever degree of support is needed to restore their physical function. In that transition, patients regain function, but they're not fit and they're also not being rehabbed. Many of those people have so many risk factors and dysfunctional behaviors to be managed that they might be six months away from the fitness they imagine for themselves.

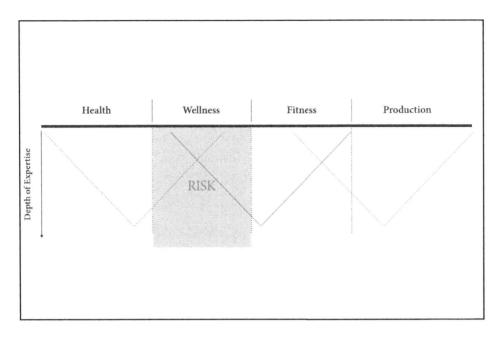

If you work in healthcare, you must know how to foster better health and how to support wellness and resolve risk factors. If you can deliver value in fitness or production, that's an even greater advantage, particularly if you can offer a long-term incentive of sustainable development.

On the other side of that opportunity, the greatest impact for a trainer or coach is in identifying and prioritizing those same risk factors for the people showing up at their gyms and training facilities.

Being a responsible professional in fitness and production requires learning to exercise restraint from the start because lower body fat, muscle hypertrophy, or a better vertical leap can be built much more easily on a firm foundation, having addressed those risk factors that will ultimately hamper progress.

FITNESS:
ENSURE WELLNESS TO POWER GREATER FITNESS AND PRODUCTION

If you work in fitness, your value lies in developing physical capacity, but the best thing for your business is knowing more about improving production and wellness. You can become a better fitness professional when you know how to convert wellness clients into fitness clients by reducing risk factors, and when you can restyle clients seeking greater production into fitness clients when their physical capacity is limiting their skill.

Where's Your Greatest Opportunity as a Fitness Professional?

	Awareness	Protection	Correction	Development
Production	?	-	+	=
Fitness	?	-	+	=
Wellness	?	-	+	=
Health	?	-	+	=

Dark to light = Greater to lower opportunity

If there's one common pattern we've seen among successful health and fitness professionals, it's in treating those patients and clients pursuing fitness and production with more integrity. The unrecognized opportunity for most professionals is in capitalizing on that exit from rehab and the entry into fitness and in the transition from general fitness to high-performance training—realizing that taking the same actions but wearing two hats can accomplish the same goal.

For health professionals, there's more cheese left on the cracker at discharge than commonly thought. Insurance won't pay for it (yet), but patients are often willing to pay to solidify their wellness and fitness if they understand how the strategy supports their long-term resilience.

For fitness and performance professionals, identifying risk factors and dysfunction standing in the way and delivering a solution at that first encounter can establish your value to clients before they ever lose a single pound or set a new personal record. Taking the steps to first establish the integrity of more fundamental layers of movement ensures that clients' efforts go toward pursuing greater production rather than scaling obstacles in their way.

We see many professionals blending their businesses because they intuitively sense the opportunity in these gaps, but then fail to put it into practice with systematic strategy. We either see a big training facility with a little chiropractic or therapy office, or we see a big PT office with a wellness program they simply tolerate. It's either a fitness concept that's so poorly regulated that it requires an in-house sports medicine presence, or a wellness program meant to keep people tethered to the clinic until they ultimately need more rehab. Neither is correcting the underlying problem: that few people are ready for fitness without regulation.

You picked up this book for greater success in health, fitness, or performance, but I hope you put it down realizing that how you address wellness impacts everything you do. Your competitive advantage isn't in the billboard you hang or the number of credentials after your name—the advantage lies in the processes and feedback you can internally embrace that move you into a new area of influence while your competitors keep fighting over the same patch of territory.

That's how we'll reshape the current culture of the profession, by creating more effective and efficient systems that allow us to protect, correct, and develop the right things, for the right individual, at the right time. You'll do this:

- ▶ By demonstrating that your outcomes are consistently better
- ▶ By delivering your particular skills within a model of movement that first ensures the integrity of health and wellness in service of greater fitness
- ▶ By applying those same skills to establish more robust fitness to elevate and sustain production

But we can't take you from a philosophical reshaping of your practice and your business to a profitable metric unless you're willing to do what we've done. You need to hold yourself to a new standard.

PART TWO: OPPORTUNITIES

IDENTIFY YOUR NON-NEGOTIABLES

- What are the core values of your work?
- What are the behaviors you value so much that will always be done… no matter what?
- What do you refuse to compromise in your business and your work with clients?
- Are your professional behaviors supporting your professional goals?

Before diving into the second part of this book and the practical strategies for implementing the Systems, take some time to do a personal appraisal. People fail to achieve the goals they set for themselves by underestimating the demands and pressures that arise as the pace of life and work steadily climbs. Challenging or confusing situations arise and the first impulse is to take the path of least resistance—to compromise. There's a time and place when it's better to follow the advice of Bruce Lee to "be like water" and adapt to continue moving forward, but without a guiding philosophy, you run the risk of responding reactively rather than intentionally to external pressure.

Your values and principles shape that guiding philosophy and, in turn, define your non-negotiables. Non-negotiables are those points on which you're unwilling to compromise in your personal and professional life. They are the actions that, no matter what, will always be done. They are those behaviors you will or won't accept from others—and more importantly, what you will and won't accept from yourself.

Non-negotiables make it easier to vet opportunities because it makes part of your world more predictable and consistent. If your non-negotiable is to dedicate the first 30 minutes of every morning to quiet meditation or exercise, the decision to get out of bed or hit the snooze button is less difficult. If your non-negotiable is to avoid eating meat or processed foods, your shopping list and grocery trips end up being more efficient.

You're already operating with a collection of non-negotiables subconsciously governing your behavior and directing the decisions you make, the people you hire and associate with, and the way you treat or train clients—you just might not realize it. The problem is that some of those non-negotiables may not be promoting behaviors that are moving you and your clients toward your collective goals.

And if your non-negotiables aren't reflected by those who you hire or work with, you probably won't be making progress toward your business goals.

Dr. Jason Hulme, a chiropractor in Hendersonville, TN, has a list of non-negotiables that define his practice. Some follow the standards of healthcare, but the others shape the direction and impact of his practice. They dictate the level of care every patient who sets foot in his clinic should receive. His non-negotiables are:

- Always treat from the SFMA.
- Demonstrate improvement in measures of pain, functional outcomes, and disability.
- Exceed a patient's measurable goals.
- Exceed the expectations of the referring providers and athletic trainers.
- Restore functional movement at discharge through the FMS.
- Empower patients to embrace self-selected fitness.

These non-negotiables don't just apply to Dr. Hulme; his entire staff operates along the same standards. These non-negotiables align the clinic during challenging periods or when it comes time to set the expectations for new members of the team.

When faced with declining insurance reimbursement or the challenge of managing a rapidly expanding schedule of clients and responsibilities, compromising a non-negotiable by shaving off some level of service, or worse, allowing a lack of passion to slowly plague the practice isn't an option. If those non-negotiables are truly non-negotiable, the responsibility is to stay true to the values and find new or different ways to remain profitable and continue to grow.

Not sure what those might be for you? Think of it in these terms: What core values of your practice or business would you be willing to put on the wall for every customer to see and hold you accountable?

> ### Non-Negotiables for Clients
>
> Strength coach Mike Perry, who runs Skill of Strength in Massachusetts, has created a list of non-negotiables for working with older adults who come to his facility. Because he believes his role is to maximize functional independence for these clients regardless of their goals for training, he makes sure the overall program always:
>
> - Promotes their ability to get from the floor to standing without using their upper body
> - Improves lower body strength
> - Increases grip strength
> - Improves foot speed
> - Maintains the deep squat range of motion and control

MANAGE YOUR MINIMUMS

So what are the non-negotiables in your work that you could put on display? Hopefully those non-negotiables align with your professional goals. Non-negotiables make up the DNA of a successful practice because rather than saying what you could do more of, they demand that you outline what you can't afford to do less of. They capture the essence of your minimal standards.

The Talent Code (Daniel Coyle) and *Talent is Overrated* (Geoff Colvin) are two books that share a common thread about the way we develop perspective and the way we practice. If you look around, you won't find many people posting their minimums at the gym or on the internet. You'll find them posting their maximums in the weightroom or the biggest victories in their businesses, but you won't hear about the lost opportunities or defeats.

But the talented and successful are just as clear on their minimums and make that a part of their identities because when our minimums also represent our areas of weakness, leaving them unaddressed will never allow us to achieve our maximum potential.

When we work with professional sports teams, we ask them which athletes are available, performing, contributing, and demonstrating an above-average level of durability. That's typically a small percentage of the team, but if you measured the strength, agility, BMI, movement, sleep, or diet of those athletes, you'll often find they're not the best on the team in any of those metrics. They're more productive than everyone else because they're the best at *not failing*. That strategy of non-failure means their focus isn't on being superlative in one area to cover up failure in another, but to make sure their weakest quality is still good enough to succeed.

The best coaches have an excellent perspective of athletes' maximums and minimums because combined, they help identify problems and potentials. It's the seasoned coach or the wise mentor who quickly appraises both strengths and weaknesses and delegates training time to remove or at least hit the essential threshold of the weakest links. That wisdom continues when they measure and monitor the trajectory of those qualities to confirm the effectiveness of their work.

When you're on the path alone, those minimums can often be unknown entities. People seek our professional advice because they believe we possess the knowledge to help them identify what's robbing them of their true potential, but we rarely turn the lens back on ourselves.

We see it all the time in our seminars when intelligent and fit people are surprised with their less-than-optimal screen results. It's always uncomfortable to challenge our own perceptions, but with the right tools to provide an honest self-appraisal, we can uncover the behaviors preventing us from achieving the success we seek.

YOUR PRINCIPLES SET THE STANDARD

Our three movement principles form the core non-negotiables of Functional Movement Systems because there's a common *why* statement found in them. Something has been lost in movement, health, and fitness that we're passionate about reinstalling, and there's an ethical way to do that. Demanding quality over quantity (move well before you move often) and pursuing change through an ethical framework of *Protect, Correct, and Develop* is the only way to operate within our current culture and professions if we want to stay on the right side of the conversation.

We won our street cred by getting the best sports medicine professionals on the planet to recognize we have to evaluate, measure, and interact with movement in a different way. They all had to move beyond the point of discomfort when, inevitably, the data and the feedback pointed a finger back at them and asked the same question we had to answer, "Are you making the impact you believe you are?"

Your willingness to adjust the way you test, treat, train, and educate will ultimately dictate your success. We only ask of you what we asked of them: Don't cherry-pick. Learn how to navigate that system with what you have today, and then add to it. Owning the process will allow you to understand how to ultimately build and program your innovations within that framework and take what we've built to another level.

Don't start with a success strategy and think of all the things you can layer on to maximize what you're already doing. Begin with a strategy to first protect yourself from failure. Identify the weak links in your business and your craft. If you can identify those areas where you fall below the cut, raising them to a higher professional standard will put you on steady ground.

It can be an intimidating and humbling path to follow, but it's the most complete form of training and education you can achieve because once you raise your floor, it makes it a whole lot easier to reach a new ceiling.

OPPORTUNITIES FOR CHANGE

For added guidance along the path, we'll present a sampling of steps to help adopt the practical and professional strategies of the Movement Systems. After each practical strategy, there will be questions to challenge your perception of your areas of weakness, action steps to facilitate behavioral change, and opportunities to reflect and collect feedback to ensure you're on the right track. This process of questioning, taking action, and reflecting on the outcome is essential if you want to improve your skills as a clinician, trainer, or coach.

Your success in translating this philosophical approach into a practical application for you and your business requires more than just following the instructions. We ask that you trust the process ahead, but that you also actively engage with it. Moving toward mastery in your profession is only possible when you treat each and every decision as an opportunity to run a mini experiment. Filter your work through that 4x4 matrix and see what comes out the other side, and I guarantee you'll ultimately find opportunities to assess and refine your perceptions, skills, and abilities into something powerful and uniquely your own.

In the words of the Greek poet Archilochus, "We don't rise to the level of our expectations; we fall to the level of our training."

CHAPTER FIVE

OWN THE PROCESS

If your career lasts long enough, you'll inevitably hit what Dr. Hulme calls a "split." A split is a point of complexity that challenges your expectations and the status quo of how you're operating. If you're growing and successful, you'll hit multiple splits that force you to adapt over the course of your career.

In our minds, we expect our business growth and our passion for what we do should increase in an even, linear fashion over the course of our working life. In reality, businesses can grow while our ways of practicing largely stay the same until at some point, things feel different. You start thinking, "This doesn't feel comfortable anymore. I'm not getting the same level of fulfillment. I can't put my energy where it needs to be. The economics are getting challenging, and I'm not sure if I'm moving in the wrong direction or if I need to change my tactics to continue to grow."

If you're a business owner, no doubt you've already felt the friction at different times, slowing your progress and fabricating many of those thoughts. But you can feel that same pressure building as an employee, trying to carve out success in a niche on your own within a larger practice, or maybe as a manager, tasked with the growth and expansion of someone else's business. You may not feel the friction to your progress yet, but it comes for us all, and without a strategy to keep yourself centered, you're staring down an uneven journey ahead.

Providing business strategies on how to run things more effectively or efficiently are irrelevant if what you're creating and selling isn't producing consistent and meaningful results. The best marketing or business plans won't make you more successful than your competition if the perception of how good you are doesn't match the reality. What will separate you from 80% of your competition is producing consistent results that exceed the expectations of your clients and patients.

In the four layers of movement, we've tried to craft a strategy to help you identify where you are and what you need to create those results. Your setting or the people you work with may dictate how deeply you need to engage with each layer of movement, but appreciating how each layer complements the others allows you to ask better questions covering the hows and whys of your decisions. When you move from just following instructions to making calculated decisions, you move from being a cook to a chef—as long as you know how to use the right tools to sample and taste the results of the decisions you make.

The skill that develops from that sampling is the skill of *pattern recognition*. The greatest strength coaches, clinicians, and trainers might not be the most innovative, but they're able to recognize the signature of deficits or dysfunction more quickly and direct their coaching or care more effectively. They strategically manage non-failure all the way to success, by standardizing the process of learning and their operating procedures.

Following a process provides the consistent repetitions that allow them to fine-tune their tactics. The value in adopting that approach, particularly early in a career, is to establish patterns of behavior around how you deliver those inputs and how you respond to the outputs. That's how to achieve a level of mastery where outcomes seem to flow systematically and effortlessly.

A QUESTION OF BEHAVIOR

When a successful career in health, fitness, or athletics means more people and more demands on our time, too many clinicians and business owners slowly succumb to the weight of reacting and responding, minute to minute and day to day. We all start each day with a finite amount of decision-making power—and without systems and processes to produce faster and more effective decisions, we're more likely to deplete our mental resources before we make it halfway through the day. It doesn't take much from that point to spiral into a steady succession of reacting with ingrained behaviors to the challenges of the day instead of responding with intention or proactively setting up processes to stay ahead of whatever new hurdles arise.

The habits we have are there because the repetition of routine tasks or coping methods ingrains them into our subconscious, allowing us to divert our attention elsewhere. The problem develops when the strongest habits or behaviors are so embedded that we become largely unaware of their presence—not so different from the dysfunctional movement patterns we're often trying to change.

When we fall into the cycle of reacting to our environments, we become blind that our behaviors are driving the car. We can usually rationalize why we chose to act in a particular way, but changing behavior isn't done through logic—or people wouldn't struggle with quitting smoking or biting their fingernails.

Sometimes behaviors serve us, but often we serve them. Initiating change first requires looking critically at yourself to recognize which behaviors are moving you forward and which are holding you back.

The greatest barrier to making the changes necessary to develop your practice and business won't come from your clients, your time constraints, or mastering the screens. It'll come from reshaping your own behaviors and habits and possibly your perceptions of how you've been practicing. I hope the first portion of the book either shifted or reinforced your recognition of the value of taking a movement-centric approach to your work, but it still takes conscious, consistent practice to change.

We began this book with *Awareness,* because we wanted you to take a serious look at your strengths, weaknesses, behaviors, and goals. Once you have those baselines and can see your gaps on the 4x4 grid, a practical appraisal is the first step in building a better business—by identifying those parts of your work where you have an opportunity to become more effective. When you have a strategy to tackle your weaknesses, adding effective business strategies provides that extra bump that can elevate your efficiency and grow your reach and impact.

Forming a Professional Strategy

As you move through the practical appraisal, each chapter encompasses a single strategy and begins with a few key questions. These are questions to ask yourself to gain insight into your own perceptions and behaviors. When you find one that's difficult to answer, you may have found an area in which you can act. If you encounter one where you don't have an answer at all, you've uncovered a facet of your practice that may have gone unexamined, buried behind previously installed beliefs, assumptions, or behaviors.

The power of the Functional Movement Systems are the feedback loops to consistently sample your outcomes and measure your impact. The tests, screens, and assessments act as a compass to point you toward better movement quality and more precise musculoskeletal risk management; the strategies can help you construct that map to where you want to go. After you review each strategy, you can immediately start to put it into practice by repeating three simple steps along the way:

- ▶ Ask questions to gauge your own perceptions—gather baseline data.
- ▶ Take action to create new behavioral patterns—find and remove bottlenecks to progress.
- ▶ Seek opportunities to gather data and feedback to gauge if things are changing—reflect on the degree of change.

The tactics you employ or the path you take are up to you, but I have one piece of advice: *Put each strategy into practice first.*

Don't worry about telling people about it, marketing it, or factoring in how much to charge for it. Create and own each step of the process of how you interact with every client who comes through your door.

Build a system that's repeatable and effective and *then* worry about where your business grows from there.

OPPORTUNITIES FOR CHANGE

Perceptions

- What do you believe is most important to the current success of your professional practice?
- What do you believe is the greatest value you provide to your clients?
- Looking at the 4x4 Matrix, which areas do you see as weaknesses or gaps in your practice?
  - What steps are you taking to prevent failure in those areas?

Actions

- Write down five personal and five professional goals.
  - Include short-term (six months or less) and long-term goals (one year or more)
- Write down five personal and five professional non-negotiable behaviors you currently follow.
- Compare those two lists. Are your behaviors supporting your goals?
  - If they aren't, do you want to change your goals or do you want to change your behaviors?

Reflections

- At the beginning and end of each day, run a quick mental review of your non-negotiables. Are you consistently demonstrating those behaviors and actions?
- Learn what your successful friends, team members, or mentors see as their non-negotiables. Can you find trends or consistent behaviors?
- Consider putting the Three Principles in practice in your personal life and professional life: Well before Often; Protect, Correct, Develop; Create Your Systems.

  Would that fundamentally change your day-to-day life?

CHAPTER SIX

MASTER THE FUNCTIONAL MOVEMENT SYSTEMS

- ▶ Where do the tests, screens, and assessments fit in your examination?
- ▶ What process have you used to establish consistency in your testing?
- ▶ What data are you collecting from clients that directs your actions? What data is the most valuable in that regard?
- ▶ What kind of feedback are you using to keep yourself accountable to consistent improvement?

Before you worry about how to integrate the Systems into your current practice, how to interpret the scores, or what correctives or interventions to use for a particular patient, you need to master your process. If you're like most people who take our weekend or live virtual courses, you probably get excited and show up first thing Monday morning and dive head-long into screening every person who wanders into the clinic or gym.

That's a challenge because the screens don't seamlessly layer into the workflows most people have in place. You're no doubt working in a time-constrained environment. Trying to drop the screens into a rushing river of initial evaluations, treating, training, and paperwork can ultimately feel more like someone handed you an anchor instead of a life raft. Sacrificing the efficiency of your current process by struggling through the mechanics of the FMS or FCS or the breakouts in the SFMA is the number one reason people fail to put them into long-term practice.

Prioritizing training time over training integrity produces less integrity over time. This is another way of saying move well before you move often, but you can just as easily substitute the word *training* for *learning* or *practice*. If we don't first ensure the quality of our practices, just practicing more will lead us to compromise the constitution of our skills. This is why Army snipers don't practice their shooting on the battlefield and why football kickers don't learn how to kick in front of 50,000 fans. Those are extreme examples, but they illuminate the point that learning the skills of screening and correcting movement in an environment demanding your attention or with stakes at play won't provide the cleanest feedback to hone your ability.

You need to learn the chords before you can play a song. Elicit time from friends, family, or generous people who have no stakes in the outcome of your screens or assessments. You're under no obligation to correct what you find until you're first reliable, consistent, effective, and confident in the process.

People get so focused on the corrective piece, that they don't spend the time to get proficient at screening. Better pattern recognition first comes from collecting more consistent and reliable data, which allows you to train your eyes to see normal versus abnormal. When you can confidently categorize movement or behavior that "passes" or "fails" the standard, you can more clearly detect the nuances or changes you expect to see.

For the movement screens, we recommend picking a number of screens to perform each week or in a month—make it your goal to do 20 screens in the first 20 days. The objective is to be consistent in the language you use and the set-up and execution of testing each individual pattern.

Drill it—get tighter with your words and the sequence of testing until executing the screen is as automatic as taking a blood pressure reading.

You'll make mistakes. You're going to grade movements too generously or too stringently. Your brain will interpret the scores on the page and create a personal narrative of why this person is moving this way. That's all part of the learning process. Working through it with people who aren't paying you takes your ego and anxiety out of the equation.

The screens are designed for the user, not just the subject. People who perform the screens consistently for at least eight weeks tell us they see movement clearer. They have direction for their actions within 10 minutes of meeting someone, and additional testing is cleaner and simpler as it narrows the funnel toward whatever corrective strategy or intervention they choose. Ingraining the screens or assessment into your normal workflow allows you to gain almost immediate feedback on your tactics and strategies.

Once you feel confident in your delivery of the screen, use it on clients or patients with whom you have an established relationship.

The first screen you do on people provides a baseline that tells you who they are and what they've been working on…or not working on. The second screen reflects what *you've* worked on—and if movement hasn't changed or it's gotten worse, that's on you. It may seem like a harsh place to be, but that's the kind of feedback loop you need to save yourself from chasing unproductive paths.

Before starting someone on an exercise path, that feedback lets you know when the movement nutrient you're feeding them is what they need. It doesn't mean they need to put down their fitness or activity—just the fitness and activity that's counterproductive.

By the time you feel confident in effectively delivering the screens with your friends, family, and established clients, embedding screens firmly into your professional practice is easy.

DON'T BREAK APART THE TOOLS

Deconstructing the screens or assessments and applying only parts based on an area of interest is one of the most common application problems we see. People gravitate toward screening only the top three patterns of the FMS—the overhead squat, inline lunge, hurdle step—or the jumping movements with the FCS because those look like the exercises they want to train. They then proceed on a particular path with an overconfidence that they have a full picture of the movements.

But with complex movement, the brain can cover up certain pieces through subtle compensation that might not be apparent on the surface. The screens are built as they are and tested in a particular sequence to try to construct a complete picture of an individual's movement capabilities moving from simple to complex. That progressive order illuminates the weakest link in the chain potentially impacting the quality of those higher-level patterns.

If someone trains Olympic lifts and you only screen the overhead squat, the compensations or limitations seen with the movement are left open to interpretation. Is that person rounding the upper back and letting the head fall because of thoracic spine stiffness? Or is it from weakness of the spinal or scapular stabilizers? Is it to help maintain the center of gravity because of poor hip or ankle mobility?

Coaches see an overhead squat they don't like and tell people to foam roll their upper back or stretch their hips or calves or shoulders, and then hop under the bar. They take one data point and dispense a solution based on an untested assumption. They place efficiency over effectiveness.

The truth is, without looking at how each of these individual movement tests play together, the odds of choosing the correct strategy go down, as does the speed in finding a sustainable solution.

For that faulty overhead squat—what relations exist between patterns? Could it be dysfunction or limited mobility at the hips? Test the active straight leg raise and if that's good, then it's not likely. Could it be tight or unstable shoulders? If we find dysfunction or restriction at the shoulder, we can work on it, recheck the shoulder, and recheck the squat.

Did better shoulder mobility change the quality of the squat? If it did, we now have a direction to drive our actions because our feedback loop tells us the shoulder is at least one driving factor.

We could do these individual tests to try to work backward, deconstructing an overhead squat, or we could do one screen of all the movements and discover the level where dysfunction may be impacting multiple patterns.

Staying true to the tests means everyone deserves at least that initial complete screen to provide a global picture. If a client has a particular pattern that seems to resist change or needs regular checking, you can probably get away with rescreening that single pattern from session to session. But if that pattern begins to change for the worse, returning to a screen of all of the movements can sometimes uncover negative changes creeping in elsewhere.

The screens are just like any other test—once you start deleting components or delivering them in an inconsistent manner, the quality and reliability of the results will suffer. And if you can't deliver them with consistency, you can't confidently say you have the complete picture of your client's movement.

CREATE SYSTEMS OF FEEDBACK

The best way to accelerate your learning of a new skill—particularly the skill of screening movement—is to collect and use real-time feedback. We all have the tendency to do more of what we're good at, rather than focusing on areas we may need to change.

Clinicians want to get on with treatment. Trainers and coaches want to get on with programming. But the best marksmen aim more and shoot less, and expert craftsmen measure twice and cut once. Whether by choice or just complacency, if we aren't consistently monitoring and measuring the actions we take, it becomes hard to install and trust a process.

Screens are intended to tell us when we need to perform a deeper assessment, which is why screens themselves are a type of feedback. A screen tells us if we need to do more testing of the individual parts. Once we deploy a solution, the screen should tell us if we made a successful change. That provides a better judgment on what the person needs and which methods are having the desired effect.

The easiest, albeit most humbling, feedback tool for mastering your testing ability is to capture your process on video or simple audio recordings. Just like perfecting a golf swing or a jump shot, repetition with feedback connects what you're doing with what you're feeling and experiencing.

Recording both your instruction and your test subjects in your early screening practice serves multiple purposes:

1. Listening to your language can improve clarity and timing of instruction—where can you be more clear or consistent?

2. Reviewing how your client moved on video takes away the burden of splitting your attention between what you're doing in the moment and grading the movement.

3. Your clients can accelerate their awareness by aligning what they experienced with a visual of how they performed.

4. You now have a record of their baseline movement on which to measure change after you've carried out your treatment or corrective—demonstrating value for your client (more on the value of video on page 158).

Finding opportunities for feedback to challenge your perception and your processes is what the Functional Movement Systems are all about. Otherwise, it's too easy to slide back into old, comfortable patterns and behaviors without something—or someone—to challenge your perspective and protect you from complacency or bias.

FIND AN ACCOUNTABILITY PARTNER

Finding someone to embark on the journey with you is another valuable but often underutilized source of feedback. It's underutilized because we struggle... and no one wants to look bad in front of a friend or peer. Initially, you won't do it well and your ego will take a hit—but there are thousands of other people who have walked that path.

Early in the process of learning the Systems, it's easy to succumb to discouragement or self-doubt, and it's even easier without somebody to hold you accountable. Every difficulty or seemingly insurmountable barrier you encounter has most likely been tackled by those who came before you.

Our proudest achievement is bringing people together under the umbrella of movement, where groups of professionals can come together to talk and stay accountable and grow their practices. If you made a connection at a course you attended, you have a buddy to support the process. If you can find a coworker or peer who's also exploring the screens and is willing to be a supportive, collaborative learner, you can combine your efforts.

If you don't have a coworker or peer also learning the Systems, the Functional Movement website provides a direct connection to a network of certified professionals you can contact and learn from and with. If there are other trained professionals in your local area, make contact. Looking at like-minded folks as competition rather than comrades is a short-sighted approach and a perspective that's likely to slow your mastery.

> ### Don't Sacrifice Your Strategy for New Tactics
>
> In the first clinic I ran, we had a two-week grace period after attending an educational course or seminar that offered an interesting new tool. If one person of the team went to an educational course that seemed like it had value, we'd commit to inserting the new learnings outside of our normal standard operating procedures for the next two weeks.
>
> We didn't lower the level of care we provided—we leaned in. Instead of cherry-picking when we did or didn't use it, we'd use it in any scenario where it should provide value and would then reflect on what was retained and what was interesting.
>
> It changed what we did, but not what we measured—it changed the tactic, but not the strategy. If the new information helped us in our decision-making or interventions, we would insert it into our process.

The ideal scenario is for everyone in your facility or clinic to be exposed to the same tests and processes because if everyone is operating from the same set of instructions, the outcome should look the same. When the outcome depends on the person using the tool, there's a clear opportunity for everyone to come together and find where things are breaking down. If that can happen in an environment of honest and open collaboration where everyone is working to elevate one another, criticism or input will accelerate the learning process and the impact of the entire team.

HAVE A PLAN WHEN SCREENING GROUPS

Consistently capturing reliable and accurate information from the screens takes time and repetition, but how to screen groups is probably the most common question we get from people learning to screen for the first time. We're all pressed for time and resources, which is why group screening is so desirable, even though we can't stress enough the importance of fully developing your screening process on an individual level before trying to deliver it at scale.

We've screened large groups in professional, collegiate, and youth sports, school gym classes, fire academies, the military, and large utility companies. Each setting presents its own set of challenges, but rarely do they afford the opportunity for one tester to do a single screen on a single person.

If you have an entire high school sports team or a military company that needs to be screened, performing individual screens is always better, but also requires a commitment of time and resources you probably don't have. Working with groups will always require some trade-off between the ideal way to do something and how to do it within the restrictions and limitations of the real world. With that trade-off, there's likely to be some erosion of the quality of your data.

To screen a group, you don't have to be a mathematician, but you do need to think about logistics in how you deploy those resources. What's the time frame? How many people will you test? How many testing kits do you have? How many people will you have to assist you? Are those assistants qualified to deliver the screens; can they record the scores or will they provide a supporting role?

When we screen groups, our primary goal isn't to find a perfect movement screen. The goal is to establish a baseline level of risk by finding people above the cut of the lowest acceptable FMS score. This is what screening and then training a group or a team is all about—to leave no one behind.

Mike Contreras, Division Chief of the Orange County Fire Authority and founder of FMS Health, screened hundreds of firefighters and utility workers and then prioritized the scoring of the test to simplify his decision-making. If a 2 on the FMS is the lowest acceptable score (good enough), his priority was to identify those with pain (0) or dysfunction (1) and trust that his programming would grow and support the development of those who scored a 2 or a 3.

For those who scored a zero, that pattern needed to be protected from unnecessary strain and the person referred to the right medical professional. For those who scored a 1, a deeper assessment was needed to determine the root of dysfunction and the activities that would need to be modified while correcting the pattern. Using the screens to compress the focus and attention onto that small subset meant that his resources could be brought to bear on those who needed the most help.[12]

We've seen plenty of examples of creative ways to screen groups, but there's no single solution to group screening, other than whatever solution provides the most reliable data with the resources at your disposal. Rather than becoming paralyzed trying to dream up the perfect solution, put the process in motion. Once you get over that initial hump, you'll find better and less upsetting ways to accomplish your goal.

MAP YOUR PATH

Becoming comfortable with the mechanics of the screens and assessments is the biggest hurdle in adopting the Movement Systems. That comfort only comes from consistent reinforcement. Those who show up on day one after one of our courses and successfully put everything into practice are few and far between. The path to success entails consistent practice, in a reduced stress environment,

---

[12] We'll further discuss training groups beginning on page 232.

with real-time feedback to help internalize the process. Once the mental burden of the testing procedure falls away, you can reapply cognitive power and expand your perspective to hone your effectiveness.

If you find a new process, don't stop doing what you're doing, but hold yourself to using this new tool or activity a consistent number of times each week. It'll initially take longer and force you through growing pains, but that approach always yields superior information. With time, it allows you to look back at your previous model and make more purposeful decisions. You can identify the unnecessary components and avoid the unfruitful endeavors limiting your effectiveness and hampering your efficiency.

Not performing a functional appraisal at the front end of your work with a client is the biggest mistake to avoid. Without establishing the value up front, it's much harder to reinforce it later, during those transitions to higher-level activity. Even with people now becoming more functionally minded, we still see professionals who miss opportunities because they worry about how it will be received or don't appreciate the perspective they can provide in connecting the layers of movement.

Don't worry about what people think—worry about the results you get. Foster the awareness of your clients to their bodies and the connection between their movements and their behaviors. This requires putting your own ego aside and recognizing that most people don't care if you look at their neck or shoulder when they're there for knee pain or when you perform an FMS when they just want to train. You'll find that even though it may take some effort and repetition for *you* to get comfortable, your clients probably trust you.

Don't perform the screens on everyone right out of the gate, as that's likely to disrupt your workflow. Don't immediately overhaul the way you're practicing either. First strive for consistency and effectiveness in the mechanics of screening (your words, setup, and scoring), and then strive for efficiency. Once you're consistent in your performance and feel confident in your ability, add the screens in a way that fits in the flow of your normal work, and then gradually experiment with developing your overall process.

As you'll see, regardless of your role or profession, we recommend using the FMS as your point of entry. The FMS will always point you in the correct direction of health, wellness, or fitness, and will create opportunities to gather deeper layers of information to navigate the most effective path forward.

The list that follows isn't exhaustive, but it should provide guidance on the natural opportunities where you can begin to build the screens into your normal practice with the lowest risk.

FMS

Trainers and Coaches:

- Use it for existing clients coming back to training or sports from injury.
- Use it for existing clients coming back from vacation or a break in training.
- Use it before initiating a training plan or before moving into a new training phase such as in-season or off-season, conditioning or competition.

Clinicians:

- Use it for patients during a reevaluation.
- Use it for patients with chronic or recurrent injuries.
- Use it for patients at discharge.

SFMA

Clinicians:

- Use the top-tier movements for a reevaluation.
- Use the top tier on patients with a non-specific or unclear diagnosis.
- Use the top tier as part of your standard exam on all new patients.

Trainers and Coaches:

- Although the SFMA is a tool for medical professionals, the top-tier movements can be used by anyone as a quick assessment of a client or athlete's readiness before training or activity (see page 286).

> You should screen *all* the top-tier movements of the SFMA, but it's initially better to focus on a single dysfunctional pattern to work on. Both effectiveness and efficiency suffer when we try to do too much at once.

FCS

Trainers and Coaches:

- Use it before a phase change or before adding high-intensity exercise in the training plan.
- Use it for clients whose goals are to participate in any activity involving running, jumping, impact, lifting, agility, swinging, throwing, striking, and similar activities.

Clinicians:

- Use it as part of your return-to-play testing for patients returning to sports.

OPPORTUNITIES FOR CHANGE

Perceptions

- What's the value of the data you're currently collecting?
  - Are there components of your testing that could be removed?
- What do you believe is the greatest barrier to implementing the screens?
- How will you know when your screening has become both effective and efficient?

Actions

- Pick a number of screens to perform each week or try for at least one or two per day. Try 20 full screens in 20 days where you'll screen friends, family, and coworkers.
- Script your screen, and save your explanations for later. Streamline your comments to the essential language and directions and discuss a hypothesis only once additional testing confirms what you saw.
- Keep a record or spreadsheet of client's scores to track and show change (and your progress) over time.

Reflection

- Film or record yourself and your client while screening—are you effective in your instruction and feedback for your client (i.e., are you tight on your language)?

- Time yourself when testing to gauge changes in your efficiency. Are your speed and efficiency improving?

- Don't just practice your screening—try to explain the screens to your subjects. Can they articulate their findings or begin to self-screen and score themselves?

CHAPTER SEVEN

UNDERSTAND YOUR CLIENT

- What do you know about your clients?
- What do you believe are the greatest needs of your clients and their greatest barrier to success?
- What do they believe is their greatest need and their greatest barrier?
- What data are you collecting at each layer of the 4x4 to support your belief?

Many of the questions we asked in Part One were about you. Now it's time for questions about your clients—or rather, what you know about your clients. When a new personal training client or medical patient sits across from you, what do you want to know about that person? Probably something like:

- past medical history
- training or injury history
- occupation
- day-to-day activities
- goals for starting a training program or coming in for treatment

A complete profile of their history, goals, behaviors, and motivations would probably take hours to complete, but the typical history-taking process for most professionals lasts just long enough to get the bare minimum of information before diving into an evaluation or training program.

But what's the goal of our questioning? What if that minimal level of information doesn't provide the data that would best serve us in choosing which tests or measures to use? Do you ask what they believe is their greatest weakness or deficit, or what they believe is the reason they find themselves in their current condition? Is there some aspect of their life that represents the domino that, once knocked over, could set in motion a chain reaction of benefits?

A holistic approach to health and wellness doesn't mean just giving advice or interventions to address the physical, psychosocial, and emotional dimensions of clients. The profession shows us time and again that most people won't change their behavior just by hearing what to do or being told what's "right" or "wrong."

The knowledge of anatomy and exercise physiology, biomechanics, training, rehab science, or nutrition tells us what's going on to some extent, but if we incorporate a psychosocial model when we look at a behavior, we must also consider what's being perceived. If perception drives behavior, we need to look beyond just labeling behaviors as being "good" and "bad," and acknowledge them as *responses to a stimulus*.

Rather than just trying to teach away bad behaviors and reinforce good behaviors, we must find the input, people's perception of that input, and if they're even aware of the stimulus-response loops that drive their actions.

A complete physical reconnaissance requires a collection of hard, objective data, and it also requires a collection of people's impressions and perceptions of their lifestyles and their movement. The answers they provide don't simply supply a list of motivational talking points—they provide an opportunity to improve self-awareness of their personal movement journey.

THE LIFESTYLE SURVEY

No doubt you have standard intake paperwork for new clients that covers a history of their activities or injuries, but rarely in that intake do we capture specific lifestyle behaviors. However, leading with a lifestyle screen or questionnaire can help us understand movement problems in a deeper way.

We know that things like sleep, hydration, and nutrition can impact the quality of tissue and movement. A lack of sleep and dehydration can impair mobility, balance, strength, and endurance, which means finding and following the right exercise path for someone with chronically poor sleep or hydration habits may still not be enough to overcome that deficit for long. These are all areas that can be measured and managed, but people's opinions about sleep, hydration, or nutrition also provide valuable action items.

Many lifestyle choices are behaviors—they're outputs. The opinions or projections of clients about their behaviors before the data collection of the behavior itself is an often-overlooked management key, but it's a good one because it helps understand the inputs.

People want a hard number about sleep, hydration, nutrition, and movement, but we don't capture their perception before we get their behavior captured. How can we try to control behavior by suggesting alternative behaviors without first recognizing if their perceptions are actually guiding their behaviors in non-fruitful ways?

There's an effective way to restore and develop movement when the soil is ready to plant that seed, but it's easy to assume methods and systems are broken without realizing the seeds we're planting are being dropped on dry, depleted ground. We wonder why we don't see the changes we expect to see—it's because we rely on tactics and tools to force movement to grow naturally in an unnatural environment.

Capturing a view of a client's life outside the four walls of the clinic or gym and the readiness to engage with your rehabilitation or training program is as important, if not more important, than the actions you're planning to take.

Discovering if they believe they're functional before we prove if they are (or aren't) is the first piece of getting people out of their own way in a functional movement model. Taking that approach creates a teaching moment—and the chance for us to tailor and stack education at the individual level. A questionnaire or some version of a lifestyle survey is beneficial alongside a movement sample because it can offer a snapshot of an individual's impressions or perceptions about movement.[13]

SCREENING MOVEMENT PERCEPTION

As a part of our practice with the movement screen, we show new patients or clients faceless silhouettes of someone moving through the movement screen from a starting posture through a particular pattern. While they sit in a chair we ask, "Could you do this movement?" They'll answer yes or no, to which we follow up with, "If you could, would it hurt? If you think you can, do you think you'll be perfect, average, or below average?" The answers are purely subjective, but they uncover people's impression of their personal movement thumbprint.

Then we ask, "Should somebody your gender and age with average health and fitness be able to do this?" Now we can gauge what they think they should be able to do and their expectations of movement across the board.

It allows people to tell us what they think and how they feel about movement, both personally and on a larger scale against everyone who could be in their health and fitness peer group. If we get those pieces of information before we screen or even see them move, we gain an idea of their movement awareness.

Do they believe this is a normal, representative movement, that they can do it, and if they can or can't, do they think it will cause pain? We're checking their

---

13 See "Opportunities for Change," page 132 for an example.

confidence-reality ratio. We'd like to think that ratio is 1:1, but it never is—most people's confidence in their ability doesn't align with their reality. Once we do a movement screen, we discover if they overshot or over-forecast their movement ability…or if they undershot.

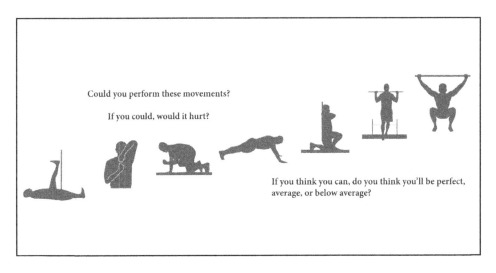

Even if they don't understand the vocabulary or meaning of a movement screen, those whose confidence is too high are effectively telling us that, "I think I'm a far better movement image than I actually am." Many of these people can easily get into risky situations, not just because they're moving poorly, but because they ambitiously tackle environments that a more physically self-aware person might avoid.

TACTIC—Screen The "Good" Side First

If you suspect people are skeptical of the value of the movement screen or their movement confidence exceeds their reality, try testing their stronger or more functional side first on the bilateral tests. By leading with their more functional side, you can then create an experience where they're more likely to perceive the difference on the opposite, more dysfunctional side.

It can serve as an opportunity to challenge their awareness of movement and gauge their perception of what they believe is causing the issue. The more complete a picture you have of their perception, the better you can address their behaviors.

What if they think they move far worse than our objective scale says? Those people often avoid physical challenges or experiences that could easily make them more self-aware and more robust. Having low movement self-esteem can keep people from becoming better even if they possess good quality movement, whereas those with high movement self-esteem that's unsupported by objectivity can put themselves at risk in environments in which they have no business performing. The same goes if they believe they're sleeping enough, drinking enough water, eating the right foods, or engaging in the right activities when they aren't.

A lack of self-awareness is as big a risk factor as poor movement. We regularly work in highly athletic and hard-charging environments, with college and professional athletes, police, firefighters, and the military. We've seen people who do below average on a movement screen survive a lot of physical work and activity with demonstrated durability. When we see amazing physical capacity and athletic feats from those with lower-than-average movement screens and poor behavioral patterns, we can only explain it as them being self-aware of the things they can and can't do. That means movement isn't the only variable—movement awareness plays a tremendous role as well.

People can get injured who have a great movement screen and poor movement awareness with a ton of risk factors in other behaviors, or they can have a low movement screen but be self-aware and able to avoid or compensate in a constructive way so as not to put themselves at risk.

I've tried to reconcile this in my teaching, realizing we don't just fix movement by adding supplements of movement to people's lives. We first must use our objective scale to gauge their confidence-to-reality ratio and make sure they gain that awareness of when they have more or less movement ability than they think.

Most people need to personally experience this before you'll get the latitude to say, "Let's see if we can work on developing a path to change this and reclaim what was lost."

Understanding where our perceptions are misinformed is a catalyst for change. This is more than simply providing a lifestyle or movement instruction sheet; this means showing them where their perceptions of "average" and their forecasts of their own ability aren't realistically represented.

That's a valuable gauge because perception drives behavior in both lifestyle and movement. The closer we get to screens that allow those opportunities to be collected before we start sampling the true behaviors will give us a better leverage point to see where the problem is and how to deal with it.

THE KEY QUESTIONS TO ASK YOUR CLIENTS

A lifestyle questionnaire can show clients' perceptions before they set foot in your clinic or gym, but a time will come to have an honest conversation to peel back the layers. The value in this portion of the intake process starts with beginning to identify the underlying cause of their problems, and moves into the weak links and barriers in the perceptions or behaviors that can ultimately hinder progress.

You can execute the best manual and exercise interventions known to man, but if your client is living off junk food and sleeping four hours a night, no change will stick. You need to dig deeper into lifestyle cues…or your clients will be doing correctives forever. This lifestyle portion is also an opportunity to direct your questioning to the high-value information to align the objectives and expectations to build rapport moving forward.

Strength coach Eric D'Agati of ONE Human Performance has a handful of questions he asks of every person who comes to work with him. He calls these his "key questions." There's nothing remarkable about the questions, but each is delivered with consistency and intention. If the wording of the following questions isn't how you'd ask your clients, think about what you'd say instead. Ponder the potential answers and what your follow-up might be. Eric is able to design specific and effective programs clients are invested in because managing people through these initial questions helps them buy into everything that comes afterward. This is great advice across all the populations we work with—patients, clients, and athletes.

What is it you're looking to accomplish? Why is that important to you?

We all ask this of clients, but how often do we receive more than a surface-level response? We need to get to the layer beyond "I'm here to lose weight" or "Because my back hurts." The answers we receive are generic because there's often pain attached to the actual, deeper answer. A loss of self-esteem or an inability to participate in activities with family and friends may not be something people share when you meet them, but if we don't engage in an open conversation and explore at least a couple of layers of the *why* under their goals, we can't gain actionable information.

These two questions can lead us to the root of the problem, and if done well, can also tap into their true motivations and meaningful goals that will keep them engaged. Some people's "stronger" may just mean being able to lift and carry their kids. If we don't get to the *why,* we're more prone to put our own lens on what's important to them—and it's often wrong.

How will you know when we reach that goal?

What metrics do you use to determine when a patient has achieved a goal? Is it based on functional outcome scores on a piece of paper, a certain FMS score, or a performance metric? You should have an answer because you'll need to operate off the same scorecard as your clients if you want them to appreciate your value.

You may think your clients are doing great because their movement scores are improving or their strength is going up, but if they can't carry their daughter on their shoulders around Disneyworld without pain, all of your objective measures don't matter. Almost no one comes to see you to improve their movement or to lose a certain number of pounds. People often have quantitative goals, like losing a specific amount of weight or reaching some performance standard, but they're more than likely also seeking a qualitative goal. That qualitative goal is usually the driver behind seeking professional assistance in the first place, and if all you're talking about are quantitative measurements, they may not fully appreciate your impact.

Capturing a client's perspective on what the ultimate goal looks and feels like, and then aligning it with your objective indicators of progress can honor both the qualitative and the quantitative as you guide them along.

During training or exercise, are we building up or breaking down?

You probably just read that question believing the answer is such common sense that asking it is a waste of time. Although you'll encounter more people today who can appreciate the basic physiologic principle, this qualifies as a key question because in balancing stress and recovery, changes in one necessitate off-setting changes in the other.

This question provides an opportunity to have a conversation about taking ownership of those lifestyle behaviors from your questionnaire that may sabotage progress. When people understand that training and exercise break down the body's tissues, you can help them appreciate that the other 23 hours a day are when that seed of exercise can grow. It creates an easier entry point to discuss recovery, nutrition, or the daily activities they may need to simply move better.

Once we establish that the greatest training or rehab program in the world can't combat a poor diet, minimal sleep, or 13 hours a day of sitting, we can ask,

"Are you willing to take the steps needed to change those behaviors?" They need to understand they're in control of their own success if they take ownership in the process.

Only when we're ready to accept ownership can we ask ourselves, "Is something wrong or am I doing something wrong?" This can be hard to accept, but it's a healthier setup than looking at problems as a product of a faulty system.

How will you know if I've done my job and how will you know if we've had a great training session?

Do you know how most clients judge the value of a training session? Nearly always, they say some combination of: It was hard; I sweat a lot; I was sore afterward. D'Agati often tells his clients if that's their goal, he doesn't even need to charge them—they can come to his house and do manual labor in his yard. They'll sweat a lot; it'll be hard, and they'll probably be sore afterward. He just doesn't know if they'll be any better at what they want to do or that they'll be any closer to their goals.

It's frustrating, but the general public—and actually, a lot of professionals—confuse "hard" and "effective." Resetting expectations for clients (and sometimes ourselves) can be the most challenging, which is why this question is so valuable during the first visit.

We need to set a higher standard for what people expect from each training session and let them know that sweat and soreness are by-products of training, not goals. Knowing that for some clients that's a challenging mental shift, Eric tells his clients his goal for them is to walk away from each session doing something today they couldn't do yesterday, or having learned something that will allow them to do it in the future.

Setting expectations before touching a weight can help clients value the process and not just the sensation of training.

How broad and deep is your history in training and exercise? What have you had success with in the past, and how did you know it was successful? Is there anything that didn't work, and how did you know?

Training age and experience play a huge part in the planning and progression of your work, and also provides insight into the physical stresses that might cause pain or dysfunction. Even still, the greatest benefit of these questions may be getting buy-in from your clients. You want to know what they positively or negatively respond to not just from a physiological, but also a psychological perspective.

If they feel their concerns or input are being heard and incorporated into the larger plan, you'll earn their trust. Simultaneously, if you believe a particular intervention or approach is likely to be of benefit but they believe the opposite, you have an opportunity for education or compromise on a course of action that can move you both forward. The customer isn't always right, but the customer should feel heard—and clear and simple testing provides the transparency and objectivity most people can appreciate.

What do you see as your biggest obstacle or obstacles you'll have to overcome to achieve your goals? What does your physical lifestyle look like outside of our time together?

Again, this question comes back to understanding their perception. Do they see their biggest obstacle the same as you do? Creating long-term behavioral change is hard, and challenges will always arise whether from work, family, or time commitments. Identifying barriers to success in advance and formulating strategies to remove obstacles and stay ahead of potential roadblocks can at least provide a roadmap to get back on track.

Creating treatment or training programs would be so much easier if we could just recreate the Soviet sports model of total control on when and how people train, eat, and sleep. Unfortunately (or fortunately, depending on how you look at it), that model doesn't exist for most of us. We think we can prepare a path that's smooth and straight by controlling the variables, without acknowledging that we can't control everything that matters.

Designing detailed periodized programs is a good mental exercise, but in practice, those often hold up for a week or two before an extended work trip or an injury playing a pick-up basketball game knocks people off course. As well as we can, we need to understand where the bumps and distractions are most likely to appear so we can build in the space to adapt. Designing a flexible long-term plan that fosters growth and development requires that we work alongside our clients to provide the map and compass to navigate the obstacles in their way.

Questions about Injuries

For the fitness professional or coach, asking questions about injuries often only happens when pain shows up during testing or training. That can be partly because many clients don't even recall a past injury or surgery until they struggle to perform a movement or experience pain or limitation. Many fitness and performance professionals lack the rehabilitation knowledge to actively address those areas that fall under the jurisdiction of medical professionals, but diving a little deeper into a medical history can provide valuable background on dysfunctional or painful patterns of movement.

To establish a strong working relationship with your training clients, identify previous injuries, how they occurred, what treatments were used, and whether an injury is still an issue. The answers can inform your choices on how best to proceed and knowing when to refer out to a trusted medical professional. Helping solve underlying dysfunction establishes you as a valuable resource, not just another trainer or coach.

> ### TACTIC—Hold Your Prognosis (Jason Hulme)
>
> On a first visit to the facility, once we've gone through the history and exam, we'll quickly get deep into goals. We'll lay out the whole narrative by explaining that it's crucial for two things to happen during this first visit.
>
> Number one: At the end of this, I should be able to tell your story as well as or better than you.
>
> Number two: When we're finished, it's crucial to talk about where you want to go and what you'll do. I need to know if the corrections you're going home with will help me get some pattern recognition of how quickly we'll be able to help you get better.
>
> I make no hard prognosis or determinations of how long it will take until I have these data points. If I send them home with a couple of correctives and they come back and it looks like I didn't give them anything…well, that's a different person than if I sent them home with a couple of correctives, a positive change stuck like crazy and the movement patterns are already clearer.

READINESS

Those questions boil down to the one question that dictates our decisions on a path forward: "Is this person ready for the work?"

By capturing the patient's behaviors and perceptions around movement, sleep, hydration, exercise, diet, or stress, we can match that lifestyle survey with a lifestyle screen. We can identify where certain behaviors are misaligned in a positive movement environment and find those metrics to provide us with feedback as change is made. It's getting easier to collect metrics like heart rate variability, sleep duration and quality, pH levels of bodily fluids, patterns of breathing, or the quality of movement—really, any area that can identify the state of a body's nervous system and its ability to respond and adapt to the input received.

When we see behaviors or representations of stress degrading movement, we should first challenge lifestyle, not movement patterns—but that doesn't mean we can't exercise that day. By being prescriptive with simple changes to lifestyle and basic awareness of how to assess and manipulate movement, breathing, and relaxation, we can begin to shift the nervous system back into a better sympathetic-parasympathetic balance.

When people respond well to their environment, they can work regularly on consistency and adaptation. The Movement Systems are valuable tools to direct us to biomechanically safe patterns scaled for what people need beyond just delivering the right exercise.

For example, when I work with Ironman triathletes or professional basketball players who get incredibly fatigued doing corrective work, it's not because I'm challenging their metabolic system in any way—it's often because their sympathetic system isn't allowing them to efficiently accomplish a task. Asking them to extend their hip or retract their shoulders may be the right biomechanical thing to do, but it can also be a sympathetic movement trigger if we don't teach them how to breathe through that posture or position themselves to downregulate their system.

Laying the right exercise on the wrong state of readiness might only leave someone slightly better off than before. Removing peripheral triggers of stress or learning how to better manage those unhelpful behaviors can uncover unbelievable real estate of movement to help people reshape themselves.

If we don't first account for those sympathetic triggers, people will struggle with something as fundamental as standing on one foot…and not know why. They'll learn to avoid balancing behaviors because we showed them how bad they were instead of giving them a way to get organized for daily success.

If I review a survey and then support it with a screen, the only thing I may tell people is to drink more water or get an extra hour or two of sleep, and they'll come back and demonstrate a host of positive responses the next visit. They'll still have a tight hip flexor or a stiff neck, but now they're more likely to respond to what I can provide because I regulated the system to better accept my input.

Your initial intake is about more than just learning why your clients or patients are there to see you. By the end of your review of their paperwork and their answers to your questions, you should have a 360-degree picture of the level of awareness of their abilities and deficits. Your decision on the first action to take should be based on the most limiting factor you uncover. Sometimes that's something you can lay your hands on, and sometimes it's in the hands of your client.

Before the real work can begin, you need to find common ground to stand on where you and your clients agree about where they've been, where they want to go, and what barriers may be standing in their way. Without that understanding, you've put yourself at a disadvantage in choosing the right path forward.

OPPORTUNITIES FOR CHANGE

Perceptions

- Where's the perception-to-reality gap the greatest for your client? Movement? Diet? Sleep? Exercise? Expectations?
- Which lifestyle behaviors aren't supporting your client's goals or your work? Can you take action there?
- What objective measures are you using to connect lifestyle behaviors with markers of progress?

Actions

- Create an intake form that captures basic lifestyle and history information at the very least. What are some of the areas of risk that could stand in the way of progress?
  - Injury history (time, severity, duration) and perceived recovery
  - Activity level (type, frequency, volume)
  - Hydration (how many glasses of water a day)
  - Sleep (how many hours a night)
  - Stress (perception of work/life stress)
  - The goals and expectations for working with you
- Ask the clients what they perceive to be their biggest barriers—and be prepared to provide evidence why their perception is aligned or misaligned.
- Pick one or two health behaviors to address - consult on those you feel qualified and provide a professional resource for the areas where your skills or knowledge are inadequate.

Reflections

- Look for trends in the answers—if every one of your patients or clients says sleep is an obstacle, level up your skills on good sleep education and behavioral modification.
- Pick a time to reassess those behaviors along with your client's perceptions.
  - Does your client perceive an improvement in health, fitness, or production?
  - Can you measure that improvement?
  - If modifying lifestyle doesn't lead to changes in movement, does the person need more time or does the problem lie elsewhere?

CHAPTER EIGHT

START WITH FUNCTION

- Are there any clients or patients who wouldn't benefit from a movement appraisal?
- How do you prioritize the weakness that needs to be addressed?
- What interventions are you performing to promote function?

Perceptions and behaviors offer an initial list of areas that may need attention, but even if the intake paperwork passes inspection and someone tells us there's no pain or restrictions, we still need the body to tell us the truth. Filtering our observations through more global tools and screens allows us to more clearly capture signs and symptoms that can often reveal upstream influences within the layers of movement.

Prioritizing a screen then directs our focus to more relevant local tests where we can test our subjective opinions against the data we collect for a complete representation of the client. Then we can proceed with a plan more likely to succeed by identifying those people who may seem to be doing everything *right,* but aren't able to tap into their movement potential.

Wellness, and the function it captures, is the untapped entry point to a movement-focused approach. It's the safest place to stand and is a natural entry point to pursue greater fitness or determine when health needs a deeper assessment, which is why I like to think of the FMS as the hub of the wheel of movement.

The FMS isn't a health thing or a fitness thing—it's an "everyone" thing because its target is risk. It's a test to tell us if someone meets the minimal human movement requirements. Passing or failing that minimal standard points us toward the likelihood of future failure and what additional information we need to gather to support a plan of action.

FUNCTION TELLS US WHICH WAY TO PROCEED

Everything we do through the FMS (as well as the SFMA and the FCS) are attempts to make movement binary. The algorithm of our decision-making demands that we pose those questions with as close to a Yes/No or A/B answer as we can, to direct us to the next step in our process. We expect physicians, pilots, teachers, referees, and umpires to operate in that manner, but when we get deep into managing patients or clients, too many professionals lean on what they "feel" is the problem or answer. The purpose of anchoring the process to screens is to more confidently identify when to proceed, when to proceed with caution, or when to stop and move backward for a deeper investigation.

	Awareness (?)	Protect (-)	Correct (+)	Develop (=)
Production				
Fitness				
Wellness	FMS			
Health				

Identify Risk First

CONFIRM AND ESTABLISH HEALTH AND WELLNESS FIRST

Regardless of the primary level of movement you work with, beginning with wellness and function allows us to ask better questions and find better tools for faster feedback. We end up with a more effective path by avoiding unnecessary detours, and also a more efficient path as we strip away additional tests that won't provide relevant information.

For example, when clients don't "pass" their paperwork or intake because they report pain or other red flags of concern, we have enough information to determine that wellness is compromised, and health needs to take priority. Diving into an FMS likely won't provide relevant data because the number one goal of the screen is to identify pain and risk, and we already have that information. The correct path is to move backward and screen vital signs and protect them until we can assess movement health with the SFMA and more specific tests and assessments to identify where we can further protect them or correct the problem source. Sometimes we have to focus on the markers of recovery before creating opportunities for stress.

Conversely, if someone reports positive lifestyle behaviors and can demonstrate the mobility and control to "pass" an FMS, is it necessary to measure the range of motion of the involved joints or the muscle strength of individual muscles? Maybe not.

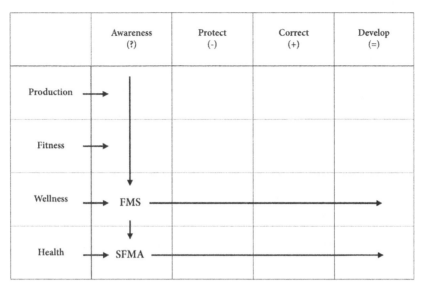

Identify Risk First

If our collection of wellness data points toward a low risk of future dysfunction, rather than collecting even more data that may be redundant, we can move forward into screening fitness with the FCS to chart our course of action.

Effective solutions to unclear problems come from systematic processes that provide reliable feedback. Once a failed screen alerts you to a potential problem, you can dive deeper and act on the root cause of pain or dysfunction before running everything back through the same filtering process to confirm if you were correct in your hypothesis and your interventions.

Depending on your expertise and training, you may only make use of a single layer of that movement algorithm, but the branches that can develop ensure every box is being checked and acted on appropriately by you or a trusted peer.

Quantifying the Layers of Movement

	Awareness (?)	Protect (-)	Correct (+)	Develop (=)
Production	Movement Performance			→
Fitness	Movement Capacity Deficiencies			→
Wellness	Movement Risk Factors			→
Health	Movement Vital Signs			→

LET THE SCREEN GUIDE YOU—DON'T FIXATE ON IT

The movement screens are built to *detect failure, not predict success.* The only way to appraise success is through competition in a realistic scenario—but everyone doesn't deserve to compete right away. We want to predict risk so that clients know when not to put their body on the line. Once people pass the cut and have as good of movement as the successful people who came before them, they can compete, get bruised, build calluses, collect that experience, and then come back to see if they met the level of success they wanted or if we need to continue working on another weak link.

People use a screen or assessment to try to predict both success and failure, *but it can't do both.* Natural selection selects non-failures, not necessarily successes…and so does the FMS.

Our scoring system might be the most debated aspect of the Movement Systems in general, and the FMS in particular. We set our scoring to highlight those presentations of movement with an increased risk of failure in more complex movement.

0 = pain with a movement

1 = an inability to complete the movement

2 = an ability to complete the movement with compensation or substitution

3 = an ability to complete the movement without compensation or substitution

Our early work using the FMS in professional sports told us that athletes whose total score on the seven movements fell below a 14 had a greater likelihood to sustain a time-loss injury.[14] Many people took that number and ran with it, focusing solely on the total score and saying if you scored lower than 14 you'd get hurt, and if you were greater than 14, you were bulletproof.

If you do poorly on the screen, we can say you have a greater chance of failure than similar people who don't fail the screen, but most people failed to appreciate that people can score an 18 and have a pattern that's a 0, placing them arguably at a greater risk of injury than someone with a 14 who scored all 2s. The total scores can help when comparing across groups, but the real practical value of the screens is in telling us which patterns present with pain (0s), dysfunction (1s), or asymmetries.

Scoring a 3 on a particular pattern or scoring a perfect 21 doesn't imply "perfection" but rather that the problem is unlikely to be functional in origin. It simply means a demonstration of the required qualities of mobility and control to not fail in performing the functional pattern. If patterns aren't problematic or painful, moving on to general fitness testing will tell us more about the resilience of those patterns under stress.

Many people who get high scores on the FMS are actually hypermobile, which can be the kiss of death if strength and stability aren't adequate in extreme environments, like MMA, gymnastics, or the NFL.

A 2 means performing the pattern with an imperfection. It's something that can be remedied by simple adjustments in programming, lifestyle, or environment. A 0 or a 1 means there's a barrier, be it physical or environmental, that's restricting the expression of fundamental movement that needs protection and further investigation.

The world is debating the line between a 2 and a 3, while we're debating the line between 0s and 1s and 1s and 2s.

Think of the scores in a slightly different context:

- 0 = organism problem—a physical barrier to movement
- 1 = often an environmental problem—an inadequate physical or behavioral response to the demands of the environment
- 2 = rarely an organism problem and can often be remedied or maintained by simple adjustments in the training program, lifestyle, or environment

---

14 Kiesel, K., Plisky, P. J. & Voight, M. L. *Can Serious Injury in Professional Football be Predicted by a Preseason Functional Movement Screen? N. Am. J. Sports Phys. Ther.* 2, 147–158 (2007).

Kiesel, K. B., Butler, R. J. & Plisky, P. J. *Prediction of injury by limited and asymmetrical fundamental movement patterns in american football players. J. Sport Rehabil.* 23, 88–94 (2014).

- 3 = no limitation from the functional baseline—movement is intact but requires capacity testing to determine durability in more demanding environments

These values let us know what movements to avoid or address in the short term, and what movements are safe to train and develop.

About 20% of those who go through an FMS experience pain with at least one movement pattern.[15] That presents us with a physical deficit or dysfunction that needs to be addressed through a health intervention because the response to exercise will be unpredictable and, at best, inconsistent.

If people score a 1 on the screen, they can't perform under the most basic demands of the environment in which they find themselves. That may be due to a deficit in motor control or a mobility issue, but we can't coach them into better mobility or better intrinsic body control. Good coaches intuitively don't put those people under additional stress—they protect their clients and athletes from the demands of the environment or address the physical limitations before demanding more from the pattern.

Once someone can demonstrate a 2 or a 3 on a pattern, you should feel comfortable in allowing them to engage in structured training or activity. Those who score a 2 can see their movement quality improve as a by-product of intelligent program design or lifestyle adjustments.

However expansive your corrective exercise knowledge might be, when people score all 2s and 3s, your time is better spent elsewhere. Those clients don't need corrective exercises as much as they need a thoughtful movement-focused program that builds the required movement capacity and skill to succeed in the environment they want to perform.

SIMPLIFY YOUR APPROACH

As you practice your screening and data collection, look at the entire profile of your subjects and try to appreciate the implications of the scores for each individual pattern.

Keep your focus narrow and your priorities clear:

- Identify your 0s (pain)—Protect.
- Identify your 1s (dysfunction)—Protect against potential harm, correct dysfunction.

---

15 Teyhen, D. S. et al. What Risk Factors Are Associated With Musculoskeletal Injury in US Army Rangers? A Prospective Prognostic Study. Clin. Orthop. Relat. Res. 473, 2948–2958 (2015).

Teyhen, D. S. et al. Identification of Risk Factors Prospectively Associated With Musculoskeletal Injury in a Warrior Athlete Population. Sports Health 1941738120902991 (2020).

Lehr, M. E. et al. Field-expedient screening and injury risk algorithm categories as predictors of noncontact lower extremity injury. Scand. J. Med. Sci. Sports 23, e225–32 (2013).

- Identify your asymmetrical patterns—Restore balance to the ASLR, shoulder mobility, rotary stability, inline lunge, and hurdle step.

- Identify your 2s—Proceed with an eye on correction through development.

Operating from these four priorities and taking the appropriate actions to address them can immediately make you more effective. Whether you're a clinician, a trainer, or a coach, people seek your expertise because they believe you possess the skills to help them improve their physical condition. No one comes to your clinic or gym asking for better movement or a better FMS score—improving scores on the movement screens can be your primary strategy, but not your primary goal.

In the words of strength coach Dan John, "Keep the goal, the goal." Help people safely and successfully pursue their desired fitness or skilled activities and empower them to sustain health and vitality. To connect your movement strategy to your client's desired outcome, you need to get agreement and buy-in on the weak links you believe stand in the way, and the actions that will carry you both toward success.

Avoid the three biggest mistakes of the FMS, SFMA, and FCS

- Don't try to convert movement dysfunction into a singular anatomical problem until you investigate further.

- Don't obsess over imperfections you see on each test—use them to prioritize pain, significant or fundamental movement limitations, or asymmetries.

- Don't attempt to link corrective solutions to movement problems before you collect all of the data on a global and local scale.

PROVIDE CONTEXT

It's inevitable to have expectations when getting analyzed, including our movement behaviors. Pains, problems, and desires are the driving forces behind most people seeking a deeper assessment. For those who overestimate their movement competency or who perform poorly on the screens, putting the results in perspective can be the difference in their coming back to work with you...or not.

Your clients need to understand that a low movement screen doesn't imply they're destined to get an injury or that they can't successfully perform their desired activity. It simply implies that their gaps in movement will make it more challenging to perform at the level of people with better movement quality. It's not that they can't get there, but at the lower end of the distribution, they'll need more resources—time, energy, money, or expertise—to get where others get with ease. People don't need a perfect movement screen if they want to be a Hall of Fame athlete, but it's going to require even more effort and support if they don't hit the basic movement thresholds.

If we know there are things we can't do, we don't let ourselves get into those situations. We head them off early and never get put in those positions or scenarios. We've seen that demonstrated time and again, primarily in our work with the fire services.

Firefighters need to perform under the most randomized stresses; the people who handle that better and longer have their physical abilities and physical awareness in check. It's not that they're superior at everything, but they know their limitations and don't go where they know they can't until it's demonstrated they can.

Your clients need to understand you don't need them to be perfect. They can live a long, happy life with an average movement screen—for context, the average FMS score in the NFL is between 14 and 15. But if those same clients are hoping to compete or excel in some physical endeavor, they might need an NFL-level health and performance staff at their disposal to achieve those goals.

A good movement screen doesn't mean people are ready to take on the world, just as a poor movement screen doesn't mean they need to be wrapped in bubble wrap. The results identify the weakest links in movement and point to a physical development path focused on working on that weak link first.

For some people, that means a few corrective movements built into a training program. For others, it means temporarily avoiding certain exercises or activities and charting a conservative course forward. And for some, it means completely revamping their physical lifestyle.

We never argued that the better someone's score on the FMS, the greater their injury insurance. Injuries or dysfunction in the neuromusculoskeletal system are multifactorial and complex. The environments we navigate and adapt to are varied and ever-changing—there's no single, best screen or test to provide a full picture of resilience. Any movement screening should exist as one component of a more comprehensive system of screening and testing to identify the number and magnitude of risk factors for each person. This protects you from making decisions based on the findings of a single isolated test.

If we can't prevent injury, let's ask ourselves, "Can we prevent poor rehabilitation? Can we prevent poor pre-participation physicals? Can we prevent people from engaging in activities or environments where they have a higher likelihood of failure? Can we design better programs and teach better strategies that help clients identify and manage their weak links independently?"

Yes, we can.

Let your clients know the movement screens aren't indicative of them as people or as athletes—the screens are simply decision-making tools. Communicating how the screens are informing your actions and why those actions are important in mapping out a movement strategy provides the transparency to visualize the path ahead.

OPPORTUNITIES FOR CHANGE

Perceptions

- ▶ How do you form your hypothesis for the source of dysfunctional or painful movement?
    - ▶ Does the person have a health problem, a functional problem, a fitness problem, a skill problem?
- ▶ What's your priority to work on? Where do you go from there?
- ▶ How are you communicating your findings and your plan? Does your client understand the connection between the screens and their goals?

Actions

- ▶ Ask patients/clients/athletes for feedback from screening—what did they feel? What do they believe was best or worst? Why do they think a movement was challenging? This provides the information to align perception to reality.
- ▶ Find patterns with 0s and 1s—prioritize your initial work by addressing the most fundamental dysfunctional pattern and then progressing.
- ▶ Have a go-to tactic—what's your first action when you encounter a particular dysfunctional movement? What about an abnormal vital sign? Or pain?

Feedback

- ***Clinicians***: Screen your patients at discharge. How many of your patients present with movement as a risk factor based on the FMS score?

- ***Trainers and Coaches:*** Screen every new patient. How many of your fitness or performance clients present with pain or dysfunctional movement when they come to work with you?

- Look for trends in the screens—does an entire sports team present with poor shoulder mobility? Does someone demonstrate systemic levels of dysfunction? What could be the root cause of such extensive dysfunction?

CHAPTER NINE

HAVE A PLAN FOR PAIN

- ▶ Are your clients in pain because they're moving poorly, or are they moving poorly because they're in pain? How do you know?

- ▶ How will you change your approach for a client who presents with pain?

- ▶ When people report pain, will you still train them?

- ▶ Have you built a trusted referral network?

Pain is complex. The mechanisms at play are more involved than just a few irritated pain fibers or a weak muscle somewhere causing poor mechanics and stress. In the presence of pain, information being relayed between the brain and the body triggers a protective response, leading to compensation or avoidance behaviors that change movement.

Even after inflammation fades and tissues heal, those natural protective loops of signaling don't always settle back to their normal state. The longer or more frequent the signaling loops persist, the more likely those movement behaviors become reinforced on the neural level. Just as we can train motor control patterns to learn a new skill, the brain can learn and train protective patterns to the point where they interfere with function.

We've come a long way in our understanding of the physiology and neuroscience of pain, but the effectiveness of our methods of treatment haven't made the same leaps as our knowledge. We still spend too much time chasing pain or trying to manage inflammation, which is like trying to mop up a spill without plugging the leak.

That's not to be interpreted as "Don't treat pain or inflammation." I deploy whatever techniques and tools I can to reduce inflammation or irritation, but I don't necessarily attack the pain because it's a gauge I may not want to change directly.

We don't need to fix pain using movement, but we need to understand pain with movement. Discovering the relationship between pain and dysfunction can prevent me from muffling the pain and moving someone into greater dysfunction rather than restoring function and seeing if those areas indirectly change pain. That's making someone "better" by removing risk factors and restoring function rather than simply removing pain.

If someone reports pain on intake or with the FMS, the question that should arise isn't "Can we exercise away the pain?" but "Is there a health deficit at play?" When you collect a history, patients are focused on what hurts. They want your attention there because they came in with a clear narrative of their symptoms, but are totally unaware of their signs.

We see this all the time. Someone with knee pain will look up a solution online and use a well-thought-out mobility or strengthening program. There's a misappropriation that a painful area must need more mobility or strength and that it requires more corrective exercise. Then the person is frustrated by the lack of results. Most patients and clients can't appreciate that if they have a degenerative hip or stiff ankles, there's a good chance the knee will hurt before the hip or ankle does, and all the knee exercises in the world won't solve that kind of problem.

Symptoms—Subjective evidence of disease

Signs—Objective evidence of disease

We need to think more like veterinarians: They can't treat based on symptoms because their patients can't talk. They can't do the job well unless they collect data and signs through measurement or observation of the animal.

When we treat a person who gives an extensive narrative about the painful knee, it's hard to stay on track and do a thorough head-to-toe exam. When presented with a client or patient with pain, we too often go for efficiency over effectiveness; we zero in on the painful area. Placing all our efforts on a painful spot makes our patients happy, but there's a better-than-average chance that a distant body part is impacting the map of movement and is contributing to the problem.

Then, when we don't see predictable results, we need to ask ourselves if we're using bad methods or if those methods are simply misappropriated because an over-valuation of symptoms is clouding our signs.

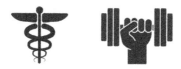

DON'T MISS PAIN ON THE SCREEN

Many professionals rush through the screens or initial examinations so they can get right into treatment or training. Some of that's in pursuit of efficiency, but some might also be fear-based—the belief that if someone is there because of pain or for a workout, they won't return if 80% of the first visit was testing. Some of that rush to train or treat can be driven by an uncertainty around the real problem and a need to provide something of value to the patient or client.

However, the most successful trainers and clinicians don't worry about that because they understand the additional time spent getting a clear picture on the frontend makes them more effective and more efficient with everything that follows.

Remember that the first goal of the FMS and the SFMA is to uncover pain in functional patterns. In your testing, the last line out of your mouth before every movement should be, "Please let me know if you have any pain while performing this movement."

In our 20 years of working with professional athletes, it's still amazing the number of high-performing people who experience unexpected pain in these simple postures and patterns. They won't always say it; people want to please us or perhaps just be tough, so always watch their faces for signs of discomfort or the body language of rubbing or touching painful areas. Without purposeful attention, even clinicians trained to be hyper-focused on pain often get lost in dissecting the nuances of the movements and fail to recognize which patterns provoke pain.

Clinicians identify patterns in the SFMA that are dysfunctional and painful (DP), functional and painful (FP), dysfunctional and non-painful (DN), and functional and non-painful (FN). This naming convention is a linguistic and visual separation of pain behavior and dysfunctional behaviors that enable improved communication and accountability. That relationship of pain and movement plays a significant role in a clinician's treatment plan.

If a patient can demonstrate a good quality of movement through a full range of motion without significant asymmetries, we label that as functional. Any departure from that standard we label as dysfunctional.

	Functional Non-painful (FN) Full, unrestricted movement without pain	Safe to Develop
	Functional Painful (FP) Full, unrestricted movement with pain	Protect
	Dysfunctional Painful (DP) Limited, restricted movement with pain	
	Dysfunctional Non-painful (DN) Limited, restricted movement with pain	Correct

For those trainers or coaches without a medical background, how you identify pain is less important than simply identifying that pain is present. No matter your role, the presence of pain with movement should always influence your first action—protection.

DON'T TRAIN A PAINFUL PATTERN

People who present with pain on a movement screen need some level of medical care. That could be a school athletic trainer, manual therapist, physical therapist, chiropractor, or doctor—but the cause and source of pain needs to be addressed. This scenario will test your trust in the second movement principle, because even as a fitness or sports professional, you should be operating under the same principles of medical professionals.

1. **First, do no harm.**
2. **Protect, before you correct.**

Pain and dysfunction are different. Often, the painful body part a patient focuses on—the symptomatic one—isn't where we find a source of dysfunction, and a movement pattern that provokes pain may or may not be dysfunctional.

If we measure full range of motion in a shoulder but pain is present, we shouldn't look at that as dysfunctional; we should see it as symptomatic or pain-provoking. If we say something is dysfunctional, we need exercises to push into that dysfunction to correct it. With a painful joint or pattern, laying corrective exercises on top is like slamming your fingers in the car door hoping your hand will feel better.

When pain is uncovered in the FMS, *protection* demands that we seek a deeper assessment in health, and in the meantime, avoid those patterns or activities that generate pain.

That doesn't mean the presence of pain requires everything to come to a full stop. While that client waits to be medically cleared, the screen provides the mechanism to recognize other patterns to address. You can train around pain, but you're not likely to stumble upon a solution for it in fitness. As a trainer or coach, letting a painful area cool off while addressing other dysfunctional areas doesn't mean you're eliminating anything—training those other patterns or areas of the body that don't provoke pain can often support the body's ability to self-correct dysfunction in the long term.

As a clinician, when a patient arrives at the clinic, we get to deliver a deeper assessment to see the four quadrants of movement and pain behavior (FN, FP, DN, DP). While we have the tools to protect and address the joints and soft tissues of those dysfunctional and painful patterns, we have the same opportunity as the trainer or coach who referred the client to correct those dysfunctional, non-painful patterns.

Sometimes people see these dysfunctional patterns and write it off as, "Oh, he's 50, or she's stiff, or he's played rugby all his life," not realizing that every crack in the foundation could be a contributing factor. There's no reason to make those assumptions when we can treat a DN pattern with much greater acceleration and safety than we can work on painful patterns. Then we can go back and see if the provocation of the problem is improved.

You can deploy your set of skills and training to address pain, soft tissue restrictions, poor motor control or joint mobility, but identifying those dysfunctional, non-painful (DN) patterns through the assessment creates the connection for the patient and the professional. Whatever correctives or strategies you prescribe to address DN patterns can be relayed and reinforced during the training session. Instead of worrying about a potential tug of war on whose instruction to follow, you and the trainer or coach are working off the same score sheet while providing a blended and proactive approach to recovery.

"DON'T LET THE MEDICAL DIAGNOSIS DRIVE THE BOAT"

That quote from Dr. Hulme captures where many clinicians struggle in delivering and communicating effective treatment plans. Patients often end up labeled by a medical diagnosis with little additional functional or behavioral context. Sometimes, through their own research or talking with friends and family, people walk into a clinic with expectations of what they need.

How often have you been asked, "What are some good exercises for my (fill in the body part) pain?"

Would you do the same treatment for every patient who walks in with the same diagnosis? Of course you wouldn't, because you recognize there can be other impairments or issues beyond the painful joint or injured muscle. We don't treat the diagnosis; we treat the person. The medical diagnosis provides perspective of the physiology or biomechanics of what may be going on from a local level, but it doesn't provide clear guidance on what to do.

Those of us practicing medicine know that, but patients don't. That's why we need to have that conversation right out of the gate. People are sold on the idea that a particular stretch, exercise, or treatment is the solution for a problem. They're searching for someone to confirm their beliefs.

The medical diagnosis doesn't tell us what to do; it tells us what *not* to do—the positions, loads, and sensations to avoid and the lifestyle behaviors that may be contributing to impaired healing or an elevated pain response.

A functional diagnosis, established through the SFMA, tells us which movements may need to be avoided, but also which movements can benefit from a corrective path. Using the variables at play can help patients appreciate that pain isn't the problem—*pain is the signal.*

PROVIDE AN AWARENESS TOOL

As you've no doubt experienced, patients and clients can be unreliable in recounting their history of injuries or surgeries, and even those who are actively in pain aren't always connected to it in such a way as to appreciate its impact. Even though it can provide valuable information on the behaviors that might be contributing to the pain, asking 10 questions about pain might not always be time well spent during your history-taking.

With our first order of business being protection, what we do to protect them matters less than what *they do to protect themselves*. Diving deeper into the aspects of the biopsychosocial model is necessary because you'll struggle to resolve pain if steps aren't taken to manage the other 23 hours of the day.

Unfortunately, it's unrealistic to believe you'll have an hour or more to spend on a patient's history, so the situation calls for a more systematic and efficient approach. Several years ago, Dr. Hulme created a "mindfulness/pain journal." The journal provides the information he'd normally gather by a probing conversation about pain, but the patient can complete this at home.

It's a better option than asking the questions in person for two reasons. First, when people are actively monitoring and recording symptoms and the activities they're performing throughout the day, it can illuminate behaviors or activities they may not have been consciously aware were hurting them. Second, having a record facilitates the conversation during follow-up visits, connecting their experiences back to the functional diagnosis.

Knowing if or when pain is modifiable by a position or activity significantly increases the odds of being able to help. You can drive home the point of where movement is helping—and which postures or positions may need to be abandoned to provide better ways to manage pain. You're able to take their experiences and connect those back to dysfunctional or painful movements and take a targeted approach in peeling away those layers.

KNOW WHEN TO WAIT

By positioning the movement scale of the FMS alongside the in-depth assessment of the SFMA, we can look at movement dysfunction and pain to reconcile disagreements between the parts and the whole. We see these as frontline tools in capturing the global vital signs of movement to better direct our care, but no matter what setting you practice in, when someone is in pain, there's no obligation to perform the movement screens during your initial examination.

When someone experiences pain with the FMS and the FCS, we'd rather you immediately refer to a healthcare practitioner and save the screens for another time. Function isn't the concern of the day; quality of life, safety, and vital signs are.

Even though the SFMA is valuable in detecting dysfunctional patterns that may be contributing to painful movement, it is also inappropriate under certain scenarios. Ask yourself if the baseline data is worth the risk of collecting or if a movement screen or assessment will provide relevant information to direct your actions.

When someone is clearly in pain or struggling with basic functional movement, what valuable information can we gather from an assessment—or really any test that's likely to provoke more pain?

We know that pain and inflammation will alter the expression of movement. Acute injuries or surgery often produce so much inflammation that not only is that person not ready for the SFMA, but it may even take multiple visits just to provide that readiness.

The first order of business isn't the SFMA—it's getting the health and vitals of rest and regeneration to a minimal level. This means ensuring that patients are breathing appropriately, getting enough sleep, hydrating and fueling their bodies for recovery, and appreciating ways to provide temporary relief through better positioning or pain management.

The Secret to Sustained Success?

Use your cycles wisely.

Use your patterns wisely.

Use your stresses and stressors wisely.

Use your production wisely.

My goals for those patients are a lot less ambitious than what I accomplish on stage at a seminar, but a lot of my cases start that way. They aren't ready for fancy stuff. I need them hydrated, sleeping, and out of the recliner chair and into bed. For people who need to move a little, I might even put them in a brace, not because I want their muscles to get weak, but because I need to provide a degree of integrity and lifestyle protection before I try to correct anything.

Use the Functional Movement Systems to make sure you don't miss the big picture as you're analyzing and connecting the dots between parts and impairments. When we encounter pain or acute health issues, the screens are there to tell us which movements to protect while our local tests and measures provide more actionable information.

Moving a patient or client through that progression of *Awareness and Protection* offers the opportunity to gain control over the situation.

Our responsibility is to foster that development as the obligation shifts to us to deliver meaningful change to their conditions. Before we can decipher what the global picture of functional movement has to say, we need to teach our patients and clients how to interpret what it's telling them.

OPPORTUNITIES FOR CHANGE

Perceptions

- How can you separate or connect painful movement and dysfunctional movement?
- When can you safely pursue other qualities of movement while working to resolve pain?
- What is your role when the person in front of you needs help outside your scope? How strong is the professional network you can access?

Actions

- Focus your attention on uncovering and guarding unprotected parts, patterns, loads, and skills. Offer a simple tool or process for someone to monitor their pain and its response to behaviors or activities.
- If possible, wait to address pain directly towards the end of a session—as long as you see the gauges of movement trending in the right direction without an increase in pain, your confidence in a positive outcome should go up.
- Build a medical referral network and use it.

Reflections

- Review awareness or pain journals with your clients to help them identify and understand trends in the data. Do you see them taking ownership of the variables impacting their pain?

- **Clinicians:** After you address a non-painful, dysfunctional pattern, retest the painful pattern and see if movement quality or pain are improved. Did improving dysfunction elsewhere impact pain?

- **Trainers and Coaches:** Track how many "healthy" clients have pain exposed with screening. Would you have caught that pain without testing for it?

CHAPTER TEN

MASTER YOUR COMMUNICATION. OWN YOUR ACCOUNTABILITY.

- ▶ What feedback do you ask from your clients and patients?
- ▶ How do you gauge if they're understanding and retaining what you tell them?
- ▶ Is it easier to change behavior through instruction or perception?

One of the truest lines I've ever heard came from Alwyn Cosgrove, the owner of Results Fitness, when he said, "A confused customer doesn't buy." He meant if you have to sit people down to educate them about your menu of offerings or explain why they need you so much, they aren't going to pay for your services—and some may not even show up in the first place. He was talking about it from a business sense, but I also see it applying to our every interaction.

A confused consumer won't buy what you're selling. A confused student won't learn what you're teaching. A confused athlete won't receive what you're coaching. And confused clients won't follow through with your treatment or training plan because they don't appreciate the value.

You don't need to teach clients the language of Functional Movement Systems, but as you practice and refine the mechanics of your screening, you'll want to refine your communication in how you speak about both the screens and movement.

If there's one topic in this book you'll see again and again, it's communication. From the beginning of my career, I recognized that the central breakdown between performance training, fitness, medicine, and rehabilitation came from a disconnect in communication and accountability. We teach the language of the Systems to professionals because we wanted to develop a simpler way to be more communication-friendly and accountable for those global movement measures across every phase of growth and adaptation.

Some people act like their education level or status absolves them from communicating well. They can't understand why someone would ever doubt their diagnosis or question their methods. But if anything, status should increase the burden because there's a double-edged sword to effective communication.

On the one hand, we as professionals need to be more thoughtful and intentional in the language we use to communicate with our clients and patients. But to foster that self-awareness in our clients to help them change movement, we also need to shut up and get out of the way.

It comes down to enhancing the economy and accessibility of the language we use and how we capitalize on the teaching moments created by our actions. Those require conscious development and, sadly, our professional educations are heavy on developing our ability to solve physical problems, but not on how to teach and connect.

Because we're all products of teaching environments where we were lectured to, we default to that same approach of largely one-sided interactions. When you're talking the equivalent of calculus and trigonometry to somebody who hasn't learned algebra, no amount of technical explanation will help the message be received.

That first time working with a client or patient might be the only opportunity you get to establish a connection. Expecting them to decipher your language means that talking may be the first barrier to putting them on the path to success.

MEET PEOPLE WHERE THEY ARE

If I have a talent in changing movement, it's not in my hands; it's that I've personally been on the treatment table and under the knife. I understand what it's like to be on the other side of the conversation. Maybe you do too.

The words and language you use when teaching or coaching are more important than you might realize. The way a client wants to be talked to might not be in the language you feel comfortable with. More often than not, you'll uncover the best language by talking less, by asking questions and listening to the answers.

In the first interaction after collecting a client's history and going through an assessment or one of the screens, you'll need to fight every professional urge not to describe what the movement screen showed you. Your inner voice will be screaming that you need to explain the score, what it all means…and your plan to justify whatever exercise or intervention comes next.

The screens may provide enough information to chart a course forward, but they also provide that first window into someone's physical self-awareness. So, instead of doing the talking once you've completed the screen, ask the question, "How do you think you did?"

Client: "I did terrible!"

You: "Really? Why do you think you did terrible?"

Client: "I couldn't do that one," or "That was so hard…"

You: "I actually think you did pretty well on that one. Which do you think you did the worst on?"

Sometimes they're spot on, but often they're way off. If they think they have great balance on their right foot and you just showed them they don't via the hurdle step or single-leg balance test, you need to either adjust their awareness or illuminate it. That shift in awareness doesn't come from being told the score was low or the movement was dysfunctional. The awareness comes from having them present their words and perception of what they experienced.

Let your client own that awareness and experience. If you don't have to translate their language into your terminology, don't. Make that translation in your head, as long as you feel confident that their words, like "stiff, tight or misaligned," match with your objective measures.

If you believe the ankle is stiff and the patient tells you it feels "locked up," that's the phrase to use. Anything you can do to change what that feels like is now perceived as value. When you perform a mobilization, the person tells you it feels less locked up and you then show a measurable improvement, you'll never again have to lecture on the biomechanics or physiology at play. In your patient's mind, you suggested something; the patient felt the response, you measured it—and you both saw it improved. Now you look like a genius.

You can't verbally coerce people or educate them to be compliant or to buy in—they have to feel it. Those elements you ask them to participate in—the self-stretch, the self-mobilization, or the exercise routine—is where they become your ally. It can save a lot of stress later if you take that time on the frontend to align their subjective evaluation with your actions and your objective measurements. If they can't understand or explain what you're doing, you'll always be explaining and justifying the value of your service.

SHOW, DON'T TELL

If we need to challenge an opinion of the root cause of client issues, listing the objective evidence can help support our case, but rarely will it convince anyone if the experience or belief doesn't match. Instead of trying to minimize someone's perception with facts, we need to engage in a conversation…not a lecture. When people believe they're mobile but they're not, we need to reveal that through an experience that allows them to discover things of which they might not have been aware. That's where we too often miss out—by not doing a good enough job mapping out a strategy with their active involvement.

Think about the typical experience of an initial visit at a medical clinic. The patients come in, fill out the paperwork, have a history taken, go through a battery of tests they don't understand, and then have all that information condensed and explained before diving into a treatment.

Even for an initial training session, most of it *hopefully* consists of testing and history-taking to establish a baseline before jumping into exercise. When the pitch comes at the end—why they need to keep coming back to work with us—we may believe that the more explaining we do, the more confident they'll feel in our skills.

In reality, the more we talk, the more likely they are to mentally check out.

TACTIC—Video Feedback

We mentioned how using video can be valuable as you learn how to screen, but it can also be useful as you work with clients. Change occurs when people gain a new perspective layered onto what they feel and are able to put in their own terms.

There are plenty of mobile phone applications that allow you to draw lines and angles on video so when you tell people you're going to measure their ability to squat or the ability to extend the neck, you can provide immediate feedback. You can draw a line where the body falls and another line where everything should be.

You can show the range of motion and say, "This is where you are now. We need to get to XX degrees."

When they can see where they need to go, do another video to show the change after you perform an intervention. You're reinforcing the functional model in their heads by connecting actions with the movement experience.

Creating that experience can gain much needed buy-in as you lay out the map of what their journey might look like—communicating a functional perspective and saving yourself time and words.

How often have you given the standard "Come three times a week for six weeks," or sold a package of training sessions and been confused when people suddenly stopped showing up?

Not everyone will give you the time you need to restore physical function if you haven't established trust and provided proof they can see or feel. Taking the client's perspective into account, did you both agree on the limiting factor, the weakest link, or the bottleneck? Prioritizing your plan without communicating your rationale or having a dialogue runs the risk of you never getting a chance to put that plan into action.

If you believe an ankle is tight, you can test the theory that restoring motion to the ankle and improving a lunging pattern may result in a successful deep squat or less back or knee pain. If you made the right decision and delivered a local or global action to elicit a positive change, you now have the opportunity to deliver the input and the feedback to foster greater awareness.

Have you ever had someone look at you, stunned, and ask, "How did you do that?!?" after something you did resulted in an immediate change in pain, movement, or strength? When people can feel a change or can visually see the "before and after," you won't need to convince them it's better—they'll tell you.

They now understand your value more deeply than if you'd spent 15 minutes explaining anatomy and biomechanics. For the medical professional, you can now confidently explain the prognosis and recommendation on the frequency and duration of treatments. If you're a trainer or coach, you can speak to what their program will initially look like and the planned progression to unrestricted training. The ability to communicate the end goal and to lay out someone's past, present, and future is a big deal. Communicating that process means the message is clear; your client feels engaged and invested in the process—and as a side effect, you look smart.

COMMUNICATION GOES BEYOND VERBAL INSTRUCTION

These strategies mostly detail the initial interactions with clients and patients, but the same rules apply as you continue your work. We automatically think being a better communicator means doing a better job of explaining, but explanation has no assurance of understanding.

Proper communication means succeeding in conveying ideas to ensure understanding by others. The master communicators are those who understand the value of their words and use them sparingly and tactically. They succeed by creating environments and situations where self-learning can occur, and providing context, guidance, and encouragement in fostering those moments of self-realization.

The language of movement isn't a spoken language, which is why trying to change it through verbal instruction or coaching is inefficient at best. That's where conscious skill training and subconscious movement correction differ. You have to explain a new movement or skill so that someone can gain a conscious level of awareness, but qualities like mobility and balance show up as responses to movement tasks and obstacles and are rarely at the level of conscious awareness. They resolve and become engrained through successful repetition of challenging activities, not from coaching someone through what to squeeze or how to accomplish it.

Mastering your communication requires delivering just enough instruction and guidance to allow for success, but it all starts with creating environments and experiences that raise self-awareness and facilitate effective self-learning. Communicating well means getting out of your own way.

OPPORTUNITIES FOR CHANGE

Perceptions

- Do your patients/clients/athletes value you for how much you know or for how much you involve them in the process?
- Do you believe your client could communicate the weak links and the plan you outlined if someone were to ask about them?
- Are you dedicating more time to explaining, or more time to fostering physical awareness and self-discovery?

Actions

- Before explaining the findings of your tests and screens, ask for their perspective.
  - What did they feel was most difficult? What do they feel they need to work on? What do they suspect the problem to be?
- Take their perceptions and beliefs and either prove or disprove them through a movement experience. More on this in the next chapter.
- At the end of your first interaction, ask your clients to restate the area or areas they need to work on and what they plan to do to address it.

Reflections

- Track how many people don't return for a second visit. Did you learn why they didn't come back?
- Track how many don't complete their course of care or training program. Did they achieve their goals sooner, or did they leave you?
- Track how many are compliant with their "homework." Do they not understand the value, or are they not experiencing a benefit?

CHAPTER ELEVEN

CREATE AN EXPERIENCE.
INSTILL AWARENESS.

- ▶ Can you change behavior more effectively by adjusting your instruction or adjusting someone's perception?
- ▶ How are you gauging someone's level of physical awareness?
- ▶ What actions are you taking to improve that physical awareness?

Before exercise and before education, people need an experience. An experience of something they're unaware of or an experience of a connection between breathing and movement may present your best chance to sample the current level of physical awareness and reestablish a connection to their body.

Perception drives behavior. If your client doesn't perceive a problem or doesn't believe in what you've identified as a problem, long-term change is unlikely to occur.

When people believe they can't perform a movement and they can't, you don't have a problem—they want a solution just as much as you want to provide one. But when people aren't good at self-regulation and can't reconcile their confidence-to-reality ratio, to change a movement behavior—or any behavior, really—you need to deliver just enough information to generate reflective questions, just enough to get them intrigued.

The ability to recapture awareness may not come easily, but it has to come from directing our actions to put someone in a place of self-discovery. If we put people through an experience that's information-rich, challenges their awareness, and illuminates basic breathing or motor control, on the other side of that experience we should be able to deliver an intervention that produces a measurable change.

If we can't, the neurological system didn't appreciate what we did or there's some other limiting area at play. If there's a measurable, positive response, something similar to that experience can now become the exercise or activity path that lays the groundwork and confidence for the adaptation we hope to see unfold.

THE THREE RS: RESET

When discussing the SFMA, I talk about the system of directing interventions through a process of Reset—Reinforce—Redevelop. When I first proposed the concept of the Three Rs, I did it in a medical context to make sure clinicians who wanted to understand our unique approach didn't think exercise was designed to reset movement. Exercise can reset movement—and we've all used it that way—but we shouldn't assign people exercises and just hope they self-correct.

This Three Rs approach creates the environment for better self-learning and self-regulation by organizing your layers of intervention into a strategy. Even though it grew out of the SFMA, the process and stages apply whether you're a clinician, trainer, or coach.

	Test	Action	Retest	Delivery
RESET Local Global	Subjective Local Objective Global Objective	"Experience"	Subjective Local Objective Global Objective	Passive Active-Assisted Active
REINFORCE Protect—Don't Correct—Do	Subjective Local Objective Global Objective	"Corrective Activity"	Subjective Local Objective Global Objective	Packaged Self-Reset with Protective Structure
REDEVELOP Modulate Stress and Recovery for Homeostasis	Pick a Primary: Heath Cycle Movement Pattern Physical Capacity Skill	"Whole Activity"	Subjective Local Objective Global Objective	Whole physical activity, with corrective supplementation for unstable vital signs

We have to rechart movement starting from a client's subjective awareness in a way supported by objective measurements from our global and local testing. The reset occurs when our course of action causes a positive change at a local, global, and subjective level.

Where a reset for a clinician might mean dry needling or manipulation, it might mean mobilization and repatterning for the fitness professional. Whether it's passive like a stretch or a manual therapy intervention, active-assisted like a motor control technique, or whether it's completely active and independent, like a breathing exercise or a mobility progression—it all can work. But it's not on the client to create that experience.

The responsibility lies with the practitioner to create an experience that points down the path of reinforcement and redevelopment. It's through that progression that the responsibility shifts from the professional to the client until ultimately, a client is independent or working with a coach to chase greater production.

THE THREE Rs IN THE 4X4

	RESET	REINFORCE		REDEVELOP
	Awareness	Protection	Correction	Development
Production	Skill or Performance Measures	-	+	=
Fitness	Functional Capacity Measures	-	+	=
Wellness	Movement Risk Factors	-	+	=
Health	Vital Signs	-	+	=

An upfront baseline screen or test tells us who they are. After delivering our brand of reset on the opportunity we find, a second screen tells us how much we helped. We need that first quick feedback loop to tell us, and the client, if this movement nutrient we're providing is what they need before we lead them down an exercise path. Beginning the journey with tight feedback loops on our actions protects us from setting off in a direction where we lose sight of what's working and what's not.

PARTS AND PATTERNS

Once you've completed a screen, do you have a clear direction on the next steps or actions to take?

People often struggle with that first step; where many people fail with the screens is in looking at the patterns as exercises. They assume that if we find dysfunction in the pattern of a squat, lunge, or push-up, we need something that looks like a squat, lunge, or push-up to fix it. There's an extensive library of exercise videos at *functionalmovement.com* and we find that people get very focused on finding the "best" exercise for a pattern without first identifying the root of the problem.

After you perform a screen in combination with local testing, take a moment to put together a movement picture. The point of the SFMA and the underlying local biomechanical exams aren't to treat every mobility and motor control problem you find. The point of the FCS isn't to create a laundry list of exercises to improve a loaded carry or standing long jump.

The point of the screens is to find the common thread linking everything together—from the areas lacking the freedom of motion or the pattern or patterns lacking control that are throttling the full expression of movement quality and capacity.

We want to remove assumptions and instead test hypotheses. If a client demonstrates asymmetry with the inline lunge and dysfunction on the overhead squat, we can start making all sorts of assumptions about the weak link: tight hips, weak stabilizers of the trunk or pelvis, ankle mobility restrictions, or poor motor control, balance, and weight-shifting.

I've seen people operate off assumptions by picking and choosing a few exercises for each of those problems to send home with a client, or simply mixing the correctives into the training program without ever dialing in a specific plan of attack. Taking this approach and trying to cover as wide an area as possible means they're just hoping to hit on the actual problem.

The opposite can be just as bad. Chasing every faulty pattern and exhaustively assessing every possible part to roll out 10 different exercises for a corrective strategy isn't a solution clients will follow.

Trying to solve 10 different issues at once makes compliance challenging and is only going to make people feel like they're broken.

> ### Don't "Practice" the Test
>
> When we want to make a change at the level of parts, we often end up with tests and exercises that look the same, particularly in healthcare. Take the example of the typical test for rotator cuff strength, where the elbow is bent by the side. When we do a muscle test in that position and determine those muscles are weak, we cut off a piece of rubber tubing and proceed to have the person practice the test as an exercise. You can easily come back and demonstrate improvements in strength, but does that mean you've restored function?
>
> If the exercises we deliver amount to practicing the test, how do we know we aren't just changing the metric without changing the output we actually want to change? That's why, whether we are talking about the movement patterns of the screens or other tests, we can't rely on practicing the test to change the behavior of movement. It works on a service level, but not deeper where we need it to work.

PATTERNS HELP MAKE DECISIONS

Looking for patterns doesn't mean we don't value getting into the details, but we only need to investigate details when the bigger picture doesn't look right. We want to efficiently eliminate possible causes by turning our assumptions into hypotheses. We can rely purely on local tests and spend 15 minutes working through measuring the motion of the ankle and hip or muscle testing the hips and core, or we can zoom out and observe the global picture of movement and filter through more information that might prove valuable.

If you see the same client with an asymmetrical lunge and a dysfunctional overhead squat demonstrate symmetrical leg raises and hurdle steps, you can eliminate or at least steer away from hip mobility and stability as a limiting factor. If the patient demonstrated adequate control on the push-up and rotary stability, you can possibly move away from weak stabilizers as the cause. You've now gone from five possibilities down to one strong possibility (the ankles) and four less-likely possibilities. Now you can use one local test—maybe the ankle clearing test or a true joint or motion assessment—to see if you're right.

Testing one hypothesis at a time and targeting the one or two areas you believe to be the weak link can be like nudging that first domino in the right direction that allows everything else to fall into place.

You'd have to deal with the ankle first, but only because the questions and testing led you there. If you find "bad parts," there's no reason not to do something for them, but you need to show the person that what you did locally not only increased the motion by a measurable amount, it also improved the quality and control of the movement, or resolved the pain. You can work on the part and see if the pattern changes, or if there are no limiting parts, work on the pattern and see if the movement fixes itself.

Differentiating between when to work on parts versus patterns shouldn't be more than a three-step process: Test—Take Action—Retest. You don't need to solve a problem in a single session, but when you make better decisions, the client will begin to appreciate how a weak link in a seemingly unrelated area can create a cascading effect on movement.

MOBILITY COMES FIRST

You may be familiar with the joint-by-joint approach I developed along with strength coach Mike Boyle, but it bears revisiting as a tool in helping you be more effective in looking at parts. We designed this as a simplified concept to allow practitioners to take a global view at the local relationships between mobility and stability of the joints. The appreciation for the anatomic structure and sequencing of the body's joints helps on the front end of an evaluation, and also later with exercise choices.

THE JOINT-BY-JOINT MODEL OF MOBILITY AND STABILITY

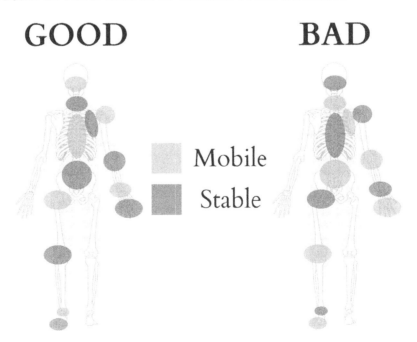

In the anatomical design of the body, we see an interwoven system of mobility and stability. All joints require a combination of mobility and stability, but there's an elegant structure to the alternating sequence where those that allow greater degrees of freedom are typically preceded by those that are structurally more stable.

That system allows for efficient transfer and absorption of forces. As the foot hits the ground when running, a stable arch allows a mobile ankle to adjust to the surface, while the stable knee absorbs and transfers force up to the mobile hip. If those adjustments can't be made effectively because of a restricted ankle or hip or an unstable arch, dysfunctional patterns can lead to compensations in movement.

When it comes time to perform in an environment or activity that exceeds the body's ability to compensate, the relationship between mobility and stability breaks down. Fail to succeed in that environment or activity often enough, and the ripple effects up and down the chain can often end in pain and injury.

TACTIC—Prioritize Mobility of the Foot and Ankle

Maintaining the mobility and stability of all the joints is critical in maintaining function, but the most common problem areas lacking freedom of movement are the thoracic spine, hips, and ankles. If we had to choose one area to prioritize for a client, patient, or ourselves, it would be the feet and ankles. Everything starts from the ground up, and one of the strongest indicators we have found of future injury is a lack of ankle dorsiflexion.

When dysfunctional movement patterns point us toward a local problem, appreciating the relationships between mobile and stable joints can help identify the areas to assess more deeply. What tools or techniques you use to assess or correct a faulty part is up to you, but you need to know whether your local intervention on a muscle or joint had a global effect.

Whatever mobility intervention you choose needs to be run back through the filter of the screens to see if it globally influenced movement. If the action didn't produce a global effect, you have to ask if you were in the right place, or if the person needs added exposure or integration time.

When someone comes in with multiple dysfunctional patterns, poor lifestyle behaviors, and a history of injury, it can take a week or two to demonstrate significant changes in functional movement. But the instant the ankle has enough motion to allow a squat or lunge, it no longer can be the excuse for the inability to squat or lunge.

Ensuring that mobility restrictions within a pattern are addressed first renders subsequent exercises for motor control, balance, or improving capacity more effective. When people lack the freedom in the ankle or hips to perform the squat pattern, they can't feel and react to input from the environment as effectively as possible. This also means they probably aren't able to apply the coaching and cueing you're trying to deliver. A targeted mobilization aimed at the hip or ankle can improve both the quality and capacity of a squat simply because it removes the barrier to both.

MOBILITY STRATEGIES

Passive	Active Assistive	Active
Manual Joint mobilizations or manipulations, acupuncture, dry needling, soft tissue interventions (ART®, Graston®, trigger point, massage) **Self-Passive** Static stretching, self-mobilization, foam rolling or self-soft tissue work (stick, etc.)	Active motion with assistance from an external source (person or machine) to reduce the bodyweight demands to the movement pattern. *Examples* Supported squats, ASLR with a resistance band	Dynamic stretching or self-mobilization Proprioceptive neuromuscular facilitation (PNF) or contract and relax techniques

The options for improving mobility come in many forms; the choice of which to use largely comes down to your skills and how engaged you need your client to be. We think of the progression of interventions moving in much the same way as we do the progression of physical learning. The entry point for introducing clients to new experiences, positions, or activities is where the professional controls the exposure to the stimulus and the client is passively engaged. As a client becomes more comfortable and awareness grows, so does the level of involvement and independence in self-regulating exercise and activity.

You don't need to begin with passive mobility work like manual therapy, foam rolling, or self-mobilization. However, beginning passively can reduce mechanical resistance, improve input to the nervous system, and create familiarity with new positions. Some type of soft tissue intervention is often required to reset movement because tissues adapt to the lifestyles we lead. Expecting three sets of 10 repetitions of exercise alone to change movement is a tall order when you're fighting against the hours of poor movement (or lack of movement) some people perform in a day.

In many cases, the patterns of tightness and weakness we see in opposing muscles are actually a manifestation of imbalances in the signaling of the involved nerves, inhibiting one group of muscles while protectively activating another. A soft tissue intervention can immediately affect muscular activity, whether through blood flow or reduced neural tone. That's why people can sometimes hop off a treatment table with massive changes in available range of motion.

But they don't immediately own that newfound freedom. They may now be exploring degrees of movement that have been untapped for years. Here's where active-assistive and active mobilizations can begin to bridge the gap between mobility and control of it.

Resetting tissues and then layering active motion on top reestablishes the natural sequencing of parts on the way to reclaiming a movement pattern. Active-assistive interventions with assistance from another person or an external source allows us to scale our work on mobility in two ways.

First, it allows us to focus on quality by facilitating better alignment, support, balance, and sequencing of a movement. Second, it allows us to focus on quantity by scaling the loads to introduce the volume of exercise needed to reinforce better patterning and motor learning. As tissues and responses improve, transitioning to active engagement sets the stage for a cleaner exercise approach and a shift toward control.

https://qrco.de/bcasLv

Let's Empower People

You can improve mobility of joints and tissues with your hands or any number of tools and exercises. Where we can all do a better job is providing people with the knowledge of how to independently monitor and manage the quality of their bodies.

Breaking down dysfunctional patterns into parts and delivering an intervention to improve mobility at the local level can have profound effects on a pattern, but only when mobility is the weak link. Don't fixate on mobility interventions if mobility is already present because the impact on your client's experience will likely be minimal. If mobility isn't the issue or you delivered the right intervention that produced an immediate improvement, it's time to move on.

CONFIRM CONTROL

Beginning with patterns can quickly uncover a faulty part when a screen is followed by an organized assessment.

But what if we can't find a problematic part? What if the intervention we deliver for mobility doesn't globally change movement?

When someone presents with dysfunctional movement but no clear injury or physical restraint to executing a pattern, many clinicians are unsure of where to go from there.

Addressing movement is like solving a math equation.

$$\text{Local Freedom} + X = \text{Movement}$$

Freedom of movement of a local part is only half the equation. If we rule out local freedom—mobility and flexibility—as the weak link, we then need to solve for X. In this movement calculation, X represents global control, which comes from awareness, breathing, and motor control. Those three elements are difficult to quantify and hard to coach into improvement, but without those three components operating at or above a minimal threshold, movement suffers.

$$\text{Local Freedom} + \text{Global Control} = \text{Movement}$$

$$\text{Local Freedom} + (\text{Awareness} + \text{Breathing} + \text{Motor Control}) = \text{Movement}$$

If we've asked the right questions, we should have some idea of a person's awareness. We can train someone how to move or control breathing, but those processes ultimately occur on a responsive, subconscious level.

The language of movement is written in feel—which is why restoring movement goes beyond just getting the parts moving better. We need to intentionally engage the perception and control of the nervous system at a developmental level if we want to reset function.

As you strive to create an experience for a client, I want you to mentally work through the examples laid out in this diagram. The postures described on the left side follow the developmental progression (and specifically the orientation of the spine) from lying supported on the ground to standing. Any activity more complex than lying flat on your back or stomach requires postural control. The fundamental stability in that prone or supine position is initially what allows infants to move and control their heads and limbs, and sets the stage for the complex movements to come.

Postures	Static Stability	Dynamic Stability
Standing	Standing, Single-Leg Stance	Locomotion Stepping, Striding, Kicking, Lunging, Squatting
Stacked	Sitting, Half-kneeling, Tall-kneeling	Transitions Up/Down from Sitting, Half-kneeling, Tall-kneeling
Suspended	Quadruped, Plank (Side + Front)	Creeping, Crawling
Supported	Reaching (Arm or Leg)	Rolling

Postures are described in relation to the orientation of the spine.

Moving up and to the right through the postures and patterns requires the ability to first hold and stabilize the body in progressively more challenging postures, and then maintain that posture while using the extremities to dynamically crawl, reach, carry, kick, and run. It's the bottom-up approach in which children develop their motor skills, and it can also be the most effective way to illuminate the gaps in an adult's current abilities.

When we encounter clients who lack control, we need to go back to the most fundamental pattern where they failed, and find the boundary where failure is no longer present. That boundary is in the posture that puts them at the edge of their ability. This is where they bump against the limitation or asymmetry of that position and use their internal processes to solve the movement problem for themselves.

> ## TACTIC—Confirm the Integrity of Rolling
>
> Rolling is ground zero for movement patterns. When we see poor control with multiple movement patterns across different postures, we often use rolling to re-establish the reflexive control of the trunk and pelvis.
>
> You'll find most people fall into two groups: those who feel that rolling is too easy, and those who find it too difficult. When we discover that someone struggles with this simple movement pattern, most often the difficulty that arises is the result of a lack of mobility.
>
> To get a valid sample of rolling and fundamental stability—and to deliver better correctives—we need to eliminate significant deficits in mobility to the hips, shoulders, and spine.[16]

Deconstructing a pattern to find the right level at which to work is where we find the Goldilocks zone—not so easy as to be under-stimulating but not so difficult that the task can't be accomplished. It needs to be just right. The better your pattern recognition becomes, the more quickly you can find the right position for your clients.

But how will you know when you've chosen the right position or intervention? You'll know you've found the ideal area in which to work when you see *breathing change*. You're operating just at the edge of that barrier of control when you find that level of effort where breaths start to shorten or become shallow.

Reduced freedom in a joint can rob the brain of feedback from the extremities—and shallow breathing or breath-holding can rob the brain of information as well.

The brain uses subconscious strategies to provide stability where none exist by holding the breath and triggering the autonomic nervous system to increase nervous system output. The bracing strategy of those muscles offers stability, but drowns out the more nuanced signals the body requires to finetune movement control.

As you create an experience, allow your client to find the most challenging position or pattern where breathing can occur normally. Remove that disruption to normal breathing and you can then manipulate motor control by adjusting feedback or assistance and allowing the brain to become acquainted with the limits of stability.

---

16 *https://youtu.be/wzS2E28fmzk*

I watched many of my peers trying to solve the equation by chasing gold standards of freedom and control. But I decided to look to the right of the equals symbol and work backward. To restate the equations: Demonstration of basic freedom + demonstration of basic control should = a demonstration of basic movement.

The burden on you is to hold yourself to the standards established for all three parts as you try to solve your clients' movement problems.

STABILITY STRATEGIES

We can address stability as we did mobility—by uncovering the level of dysfunction where we need to begin, and then scaling our interventions appropriately. We can make the demands of the position easier by providing assistance, additional support, or proprioceptive input to the system. Small perturbations, external pressure, and joint compression or distraction can all work to restore reflexive stability on the way to more dynamic interventions.

Once people can maintain a posture, adding the challenge of active motion forces the brain to sample and respond to a changing center of gravity. When they can successfully move while maintaining a posture, we can then add the external forces to challenge the body to maintain or control movement.

https://qrco.de/bcasLu

Some combination of work on mobility or control is often enough to see an appreciable change in movement, but the clients may only be borrowing the changes to movement—there's no guarantee the gains will hold. Here, our purpose isn't to correct movement as much as it is to raise awareness and help people experience that rapid change in pain or the quality that can be made in their movement.

When clients experience a change in the depth of the squat, the stability now felt with rotation, or the decreased pain in their back, they begin to feel the connections of the parts back to the whole. We're simply setting the stage for a larger corrective strategy.

Assisted	Active	Reactive Neuromuscular Training
External Support for Balance: Using hands for support, making the position less taxing (less range of motion, wider base of support) **External Load for Proprioception:** Manual pressure or approximation, weight held in the hands, distraction forces	Active motion of the extremities, head, or torso to change the center of gravity and increase demand while adjusting base from wide to narrow	Dynamic work at one point of the body to create perturbation or torque from an external load. Base should be adjusted automatically based on intensity and load

TACTIC—Deliver the Same Action in Different Ways

I used to wonder if I had one good mobility or stability exercise, should I do three sets of that or three separate exercises? I used to just do the one, but now I see that giving someone the same task but working in three different patterns or three different postures has a more profound effect on the nervous system.

If I manually work on ankle mobility on the table, then move to an active motion in kneeling and then squatting, I'm delivering the same message three ways.

When coming out of the first attempt, I know what screen or test sent me there and I go back to retest it. Adding a layer or two to the first experience can increase the odds of greater awareness and change in the movement.

DON'T PUT YOUR PERCEPTION ON SOMEONE ELSE'S EXPERIENCE

Creating an experience implies that in your testing, treatment, or coaching, you can't work only at the conscious level to help people become more self-aware. They have to feel it and see it and digest it themselves to connect with the experience and subconsciously internalize it. The screens and corrective strategies magnify dysfunction to guide people along a path to become more self-aware by running them directly into the problem.

When you do things right, both you and the client get to see if something changed. However, the reason you know it changed and the way the client felt it change may be different. That language must be reconciled.

We covered the importance of using the same language as our clients when it comes to how they describe what they're feeling—our "tight" is their "locked up." That's how you communicate in response to what they say. But how do you communicate as you're teaching or guiding them through an experiential movement or a new exercise in a training program?

Are you teaching in their language?

As an example, if we're testing multi-segmental rotation in standing, we can ask two subjects to turn their bodies as far as they can. We ask the first, "What did you feel?" He says, "I felt pressure on my ribs on the left side." We ask the second, "Is that what you felt?" She replies, "No, I felt stretching on my back on the right side."

Now imagine you're teaching people a movement; you tell them to twist until they feel tension in the ribs. That might be your experience when you twist, but not theirs.

It seems like a trivial thing, but your words matter. If you rely primarily on teaching through intrinsic or internal cues, you run the risk of laying your perception onto your client's experience. If they're experiencing something different than what you describe, it's a missed opportunity for connection.

The other option is teaching through extrinsic or external cues like, "As you turn your body, lead with your eyes and go as far as you can." Externally placing focus takes your perception out of the equation, but it might not foster as much self-awareness for the person performing the exercise.

Let's be thoughtful about the words and language we use because this also comes down to operating in a Goldilocks zone—just enough external cues to provide direction and just enough internal cues to stimulate awareness. That means asking people to focus on what they're feeling or experiencing with a movement or exercise and communicating it in their own words.

With that reference point, you can begin to direct their attention internally on their breathing, alignment, or sensations to foster awareness, and then bring their attention externally to the task.

Your instruction can be as simple as, "Lead with your eyes, turn as far as you can, and breathe in that position. If you feel unsteady or uncomfortable, breathe and find a position you can maintain."

You're not asking them to feel anything specific; you're asking them to move and use their internal processor to self-correct. A simple breath cycle is often overlooked as the quickest way to reduce unnecessary tension and allow exploration at the edges of their movement.

When we do the toe touch "magic trick" at our seminars that gets people touching their toes after they haven't touched beyond their kneecaps in years, we don't tell them what to feel or where to feel it. We instruct them to pinch a foam roll between their legs, reach and extend up toward the ceiling, and then go down to touch their toes, breathing and listening to their bodies along the way.

Other than "Slow down and breathe," the most important internal cue you can offer is to suggest what *not to feel*. We need to protect against injury and the exacerbation of pain, but we often don't explain anything other than, "Don't go into pain, and when it gets hard, stop and breathe." Beyond that, whatever happens, happens, and whatever they feel is their experience. When people touch their toes for the first time since childhood, they care less why they can now do it…and a lot more about the experience that got them there.

GET BUY-IN

Getting buy-in from patients, clients, and athletes is always a topic of discussion. I've heard hundreds of people lay out methods to get clients personally invested in working with them, but I've always been inclined to look for professions who don't worry about getting buy-in… like eye doctors.

After we go through the battery of tests and measurements at an optometrist's office, they spin us through the wheel of prescription lenses and don't tell us which lens is better—we tell them. Eye doctors perform a self-evident, practical, realistic test that supports the reinforcement we need for visual ability. If you have a significant enough visual deficit, it becomes immediately clear what you need before you walk out the door.

When you can demonstrate change in the way movement behaves during a single session, you have a similar opportunity. Getting buy-in from clients, athletes, and patients isn't accomplished by convincing them of what's wrong and what they should do about it. Buy-in comes after delivering a positive movement experience against a baseline you set. If you can clearly demonstrate that you took away a limitation and replaced it with better physical production and can show the steps that produced it, you'll make a new fan every time.

It's no different with athletes or active, competitive clients or patients. They can sometimes be challenging because they need proof that you're better than previous coaches or trainers with whom they've worked. Particularly if they've experienced success in the past, suggesting something that will challenge their confidence-to-reality ratio always runs the risk of being poorly received.

We've found that most honest people with information presented in a straightforward and tangible way are ready for change. That information is received most easily when it's delivered through an elevated awareness of their movement.

For many athletes, the a-ha moment is when you can tie your testing to an area in which they were struggling. Say this is a baseball pitcher with a poor active straight leg raise:

You: "Does your coach keep telling you to get over your front leg?"

Client: "Yeah, how did you know?"

You: "Well, that test we did, where you had to lift one leg up in the air…that's basically the same thing you're doing when trying to throw the ball. But if you can't do it slowly and easily on your back, how do you expect to do it when standing on one leg throwing a pitch?"

Or a runner with back pain at a chiropractic office:

You: "We found you don't have adequate control when you stand on one leg, which means every time your foot hits the ground, your body's working overtime to hold you up straight. Do you find your back feels different depending on the running surface?"

Client: "When I run on the track at the high school, I don't feel too bad, but as soon as I try to run on the sidewalk, my back starts to hurt within a few minutes."

Working on the leg raise or balance for a session, and then retesting the movements that matter the most to them can tell us if the issue we addressed is contributing, is unrelated, or is the root cause of the problem. We might not have the complete solution yet, but continuing to align their experience alongside our data allows a two-way conversation in the process of change.

The challenge is that clients aren't there for a single positive response—they want a long-term solution, which requires positive adaptation.

SET CLEAR EXPECTATIONS

A long time ago, a physical therapy assistant who worked for me said it best when he told a patient, "You're going to move better two or three days before you feel better. I wish it were the other way around, but it's not. And if you're moving better but not feeling better outside of a four-day window, we'll look at this again."

He didn't need to have a pain science discussion or lecture on the intricacies of what was going on. Most people care less about why the problem occurred and more about what they need to do and how long it will be before they can get back to the activities they enjoy.

For some, that might only require adjusting their awareness, breathing, and control, while others may need supplemental work or a targeted intervention. Ultimately, you can try to convince someone of the best course of action by providing more information and more explanation, or you can do the work upfront to link the changing physical awareness back to your actions. Then you can communicate what the journey will look and feel like.

There are few solutions in the health and fitness world that are simple, but risk factor reduction often provides greater return on the investment of time and effort than a fitness strategy. The fitness gains we seek come much more readily when the foundation is ready to support them.

Strength or fitness gains may not change the quality of life, activity, or support the work you're doing as much as removing areas of risk in movement or lifestyle. Removing dysfunctional movement patterns or delivering something that changes behaviors can offer far more value in protecting against a greater functional debt than immediately chasing a greater return. Stacking up positive changes can produce a compound effect on the quality and quantity of the work someone can perform—all because you're lowering the barriers to success.

Getting buy-in doesn't come from "talking" someone better—it comes from providing opportunities for people to feel and see change and letting them tell you it's working.

PUT YOUR REPUTATION ON THE LINE

The most uncomfortable piece for many professionals taking this approach comes from making yourself vulnerable. When it comes time to deliver on your plan of action, you need to capitalize on a teaching moment with an action that's transferable back to the area of concern for your client. The vulnerability comes from working on something you believe is the root cause but that might not be clearly connected to what your client believes is important.

The patient has neck pain and you work on a dysfunctional thoracic pattern. The client wants to improve running performance and you choose to first work on breathing. We must get that agreement—that awareness—by changing someone's subconscious dysfunction into conscious dysfunction.

That's where the subjective and objective come together and that's the experience we're trying to generate.

You must be comfortable in your metrics, feedback loops, and the measurements you take because your clients will only provide you with so many chances to demonstrate that you have the answer to the problem.

Show your work and explain what you believe is the weak link and why it's important to address. There's an inherent risk if you make an incorrect decision without having the systems and processes to back you up. The good news is that "I'm looking to gain better information" is a magic line because there are three possible results that can occur when you take any action, good or bad:

1. *Pain, movement, or production gets worse—better information of what to avoid*

2. *Pain, movement, or production doesn't change—better information that this isn't the main cause*

3. *Pain, movement, or production improves—better information on what you need to do*

Any of the three outcomes provide a teaching opportunity, but to really work out the kind of logic that will prevent a lot of questions, *provide one experience and make the call.*

It's an empowering moment when you can create a positive change with a single action aimed at the weakest link. There's an elegant way to play it, and all we're talking about is an extra five minutes. If you're taking a single action on something you and your client agree on, you're simply interested in the outcome. If a retest shows a positive outcome subjectively, locally, and globally, you're both now aware of the limitation, and you're also both aware of what's changing. It's in those moments when your clients' and patients' eyes get big.

You don't need to say anything—there's no debate and there's no discussion. They're onboard.

The sum total of your collected subjective, local, and global movement data should point to at least one area where you can take action. If you're systematic in your collection of that data and in the selection and delivery of your first action, 85% of the time you should have a measurable change to build upon.

All you want to see is a positive change so you can move to training or something to reinforce the new position or added control or mobility you uncovered. When you become consistently effective in delivering on the initial experience for your clients, your path forward will be clearer and you'll find yourself doing a lot less selling of your value to clients and patients.

OPPORTUNITIES FOR CHANGE

Perceptions

- What does your testing point to as the most likely root cause of dysfunction?
- Do you suspect limited local freedom or impaired global control as the primary weak link?
- When reset, what part or movement pattern do you believe may untangle dysfunction from more complex movement?

Actions

- Based on what your testing shows, choose one path of either mobility or stability, deliver your intervention, and retest to see if change occurred.
- Communicate your hypothesis and strategy once you're clear of the direction you want to go. When you can accurately map out their experience and how you expect them to respond, you'll gain more buy-in to all of your subsequent actions.
- Don't immediately opt for passive or overly conservative postures to address mobility and control. Choose the option(s) with the most active participation from your client that produces a positive change in mobility or movement.

Reflections

- Commit to taking action on one layer of dysfunction. Are you able to produce a measurable change in the quality of movement? Are your results telling you to continue on that path, or that you need to pivot?
- Reinforce no more than three correctives for your patient/client/athlete to perform between sessions with you. Are they able to sustain or improve the positive change the next time they see you?
- Try coaching an exercise solely by guiding the breath cycle. Did it change the exercise's effect on the quality of movement? On client awareness?

CHAPTER TWELVE

PROTECT THE QUALITY YOU FIND

- ▶ Do people learn more effectively from more information or from a more conducive environment for learning?
- ▶ Can our clients out-train a bad diet? Can they learn effectively when sleep-deprived?
- ▶ What can you remove from someone's lifestyle to help with success? How can you "detoxify" a lifestyle?

After you identify and confirm a client's weak link, the next step is to reinforce the change you created. When most people hear the word "reinforce," they think about strengthening or supporting something through addition—by adding exercises or healthy behaviors. But in the Systems, we think of "reinforce" in the context of our ethical movement principle of *Protect–Correct–Develop*. Before trying to *correct* by adding new behaviors, exercises, or activities, we need to *protect* by removing barriers to success. Those barriers aren't just the mobility or stability problems we measure; they're the negative factors driving the deficits we see.

Rather than looking at what successful, durable performers all do the same, it's more important to look at what they similarly avoid. This speaks to the idea of managing the minimums to promote non-failure. Ego tells us it's more impressive to teach or provide people with something new to do or use. The truth is, we're almost always more effective by focusing on stripping away those things that may be counterproductive.

It doesn't matter how effective the methods or techniques you have at your disposal; your success will be limited when people are only sleeping five hours a night, are living off Red Bull and processed food, and trying to train five days a week while managing the stress of school, work, or family. You aren't obligated to change these weak links when you find them, but they're getting ready to sabotage you at every turn if you don't ensure the basic standards of essentials like sleep, hydration, or nutrition are being met.

You may already be providing the right treatments, but the body won't hold changes made in the clinic or gym when the other 23 hours a day are spent in a toxic environment or lifestyle. A lot of professionals don't realize how many negatives they probably need to remove before they can vet the quality of a treatment or training program. Depending on the number of lifestyle or environmental changes that could be made, you might do nothing more than help clients change the way they're breathing, eating, sleeping and being active for a week and have a better chance of seeing changes in movement than giving them five of your "best" corrective exercises.

	Test	Action	Retest	Delivery
RESET Local Global	Subjective Local Objective Global Objective	"Experience"	Subjective Local Objective Global Objective	Passive Active-Assisted Active
REINFORCE Protect—Don't Correct—Do	Subjective Local Objective Global Objective	"Corrective Activity"	Subjective Local Objective Global Objective	Packaged Self-Reset with Protective Structure
REDEVELOP Modulate Stress and Recovery for Homeostasis	Pick a Primary: Heath Cycle Movement Pattern Physical Capacity Skill	"Whole Activity"	Subjective Local Objective Global Objective	Whole physical activity, with corrective supplementation for unstable vital signs

Even if you're able to make positive changes in function or production, without ensuring the minimal standards for those variables, you're unlikely to solve movement dysfunction in the long term because clients will never own those gains.

	RESET	REINFORCE		REDEVELOP
	Awareness	Protection	Correction	Development
Production	?	Remove Stressful Activity	+	=
Fitness	?	Remove Harmful Exercise	+	=
Wellness	?	Remove Movement Risk Factors	+	=
Health	?	Remove Health Risk Factors	+	=

REMOVING NEGATIVES TO MANAGE RISK

Our movement screens provide one measure of risk, but if you aren't addressing all the modifiable risk factors at play, it might not matter how good the FMS score is or how well you design a training program. Most clinicians don't know how many risk factors their patients have. Many of those patients are out of a painful episode, but are ultimately discharged from rehabilitation with the same level of risk factors at play. Removing pain while ignoring the other risk factors doesn't significantly reduce the likelihood of symptoms returning later.

When I speak about the role of the screens in injury prevention, there's inevitably a surge of critics who question the validity of our tools. That conversation always leads to a dead-end because their interpretation of our message is that achieving a certain score on the FMS or FCS implies someone is less likely to get injured. That's not what we're saying.

Plenty of people with a perfect 21 on the screens still get injured. At an NFL Combine presentation, I pointed out every professional football player has a 100% likelihood of getting injured regardless of the FMS score. The goal of the screens is to identify those at a greater risk of future injury because people don't meet a required minimum for the environment they're entering—we're screening for the likelihood of failure. Lower screens are associated with slower recovery because the risk factors complicate recovery.[17]

---

17 Butler RJ, Contreras M, Burton LC, Plisky PJ, Goode A, Kiesel K. Modifiable risk factors predict injuries in firefighters during training academies. Work. 2013 Jan 1;46(1):11-7.

Former NFL Strength Coach Jon Torine oversaw an Indianapolis Colts team that was first in the league for fewest games missed due to injury. He reminds us that running a 40-yard dash in 4.3 seconds doesn't imply that someone will be a successful wide receiver in the NFL, and there are plenty of examples of guys who ran it in 4.5 or 4.6 seconds and became Hall of Famers. But if a wide receiver runs a 4.7-second 40-yard dash, we can confidently say the odds are against having a successful NFL career because he doesn't meet the minimal standard.

A high FMS score doesn't mean people will excel at their chosen activity or will be more resilient because it's just one variable. We'll stake our reputation that when 1s, 0s, or asymmetries show up on a screen or the lifestyle is counter-productive to sustaining function, your clients are significantly more likely to encounter trouble when it comes time to perform—on the field or in life.

Identified Movement Risk Factors[18]

Non-Modifiable

- Age greater than 26 years
- Prior history of injury plus time lost to that injury

Modifiable

Health	Wellness (Global Function)	Fitness
• Pain with movement • Perceived recovery • High BMI • Grip strength asymmetry or below age standards • Reduced physical activity	• YBT asymmetries • YBT composite score below the cutoff • Ankle dorsiflexion asymmetry • Multiple 1s on the FMS • Multiple FMS asymmetries	• Muscle strength asymmetry • Low cardiovascular fitness

---

[18] See Appendix pages 357–359 for the research and rationale behind these risks.

Understanding these objective data points alongside undesirable behaviors found on the intake survey can help target areas of greatest risk before creating a treatment or training plan. Rather than a conversation about risk reduction or lifestyle choices when progress stalls or frustration sets in, we can bring early recognition to the qualities, activities, and behaviors provoking the symptoms or hindering production. Some of these we can take action on as part of our treatment or training programs, while we empower patients and clients to take ownership of others by offering the tools for them to measure change. That's the beauty of so many people currently using activity trackers or apps on their phones and watches—the ability to monitor and track physiologic responses when we alter our activity, sleep, and diet should help reinforce our work.

Deploying a larger plan built on removing negatives to manage risk ensures that the good work in the clinic and gym isn't immediately undone as soon as they leave. There's no foolproof method or strategy to ensure that your patients/clients/athletes sustain the effort required to keep those risks from returning, but managing people through their behaviors is the best way to get them bought into everything that comes afterward.

DON'T SACRIFICE FUNCTION FOR FITNESS

When it comes to removing negatives, one of the hardest conversations you'll have is when telling people they should stop training or exercising. Exercise and training have become a big part of people's identities today. Telling people they need to temporarily put things on hold or implying that the bootcamp class or running club they've been participating in may have actually been eroding their production can be a touchy subject. If you don't believe me, try telling an injured runner to stop running.

We often find people who have the illusion of fitness. They find or modify environments so they can move in isolated ways or participate in group training or endorphin-producing activities that may cloud their perception of dysfunction. They're chasing more plates for an exercise or a faster time in a workout, but in their pursuit of fitness, they're sacrificing function. Function and fitness should grow together—but giving up function to get fitness won't let you keep fitness for very long.

For example, after ACL reconstruction, we've seen high school athletes trying to return to running who demonstrate single-leg balance measures four standard deviations below those of a 70-year-old adult. They're good compensators and may be able to accomplish the act of running, but if we looked at them as 70-year-olds, we'd consider them unsafe to even take a walk for risk of falling.

Plenty of people can perform with a medical or functional problem by gritting through it or compensating around it, but suffering through activity shouldn't be our standard operating system. That medical or functional problem might not improve and may actually get worse, creating even more problems.

The connection between exercise and health is so drilled into our brains that we continue to pursue fitness activities, believing they'll improve health or function…even to our own detriment.

No matter if your clients are with you to improve their health, fitness, or productivity in a given activity or sport, your responsibility is to protect the integrity of all of them. When someone scores below the acceptable thresholds on the movement screens, if the conversation doesn't address pushing pause on exercises or activities that jeopardize that integrity, then you're part of the problem, not part of the solution.

TACTIC—Confirm Your Corrective Stuck

Want a quick example to see if an exercise or activity is working against function? Correct a dysfunctional pattern, have the client run a mile on the treadmill or perform whatever activity you believe is counterproductive to their movement, and then retest the pattern.

When you recheck that pattern, did your correction stick?

If dysfunction returns, you have another teaching moment to elevate someone's movement awareness, and another chance to refine your corrective strategy.

Of course, telling adults they aren't allowed to do something works about as well as it does for teenagers. If you're continuously telling them "You can't do this. You can't do that" and don't allow them to work out or participate as they envision, they're going to go find someone who will tell them what they want to hear rather than what they need to hear. You need to communicate that having a movement pattern or body part that's painful, dysfunctional, or asymmetrical doesn't mean they need to scrap their fitness plans—just the fitness that's counterproductive.

I often ask patients and clients, "Can you commit to temporarily not working on your fitness while we work on other things that may have a bigger influence? Can we put your fitness goals aside for a bit, hit a corrective strategy for a week or two, and then come back and reassess?"

If you've done the work on the frontend to gain buy-in of the process, asking those questions and vetting the potentially counterproductive exercise or activity choices will be less painful. Guiding clients and patients through that experience can produce massive change with no added stress because better perception drives better behavior in both the short and long terms.

Education is best invested once better awareness is in place, because once awareness is set, protective behaviors should be clear, simple, and actionable. The conversation moves from one of "You shouldn't" to "Why would you?"

RED, YELLOW, AND GREEN LIGHTS

We can't allow people to proceed down an exercise path unless we've established what activities or behaviors need to be restricted, where we know they'll likely do more damage than good. Convincing people of the need to stop doing the thing they probably care most about is an effort in futility if you can't clearly communicate that message.

If we've performed a full screen, we should have two buckets of patterns: one set of patterns where they demonstrate competency that can potentially be loaded and trained, and one set of dysfunctional or painful patterns that need to be modified or handled through a corrective strategy. We can maintain and maybe improve the clean patterns while we bring up the messier ones, but always first with respect to protection.

It doesn't have to be all or nothing—and in practice, that may even be a counterproductive approach.

Your exercise and activity decisions and those of your patients and clients can be intelligently guided by filtering the results of the screens through a system—one that's similar to a traffic light system. Taking this approach can make the transition to training and exercise selection straightforward.

- **Red Light**—Exercises that need to be avoided because they directly challenge a painful or dysfunctional pattern

- **Yellow Light**—Exercises to use with caution because even though they don't directly challenge a painful or dysfunctional pattern, they may not produce a positive effect

    - Rescreening after programming yellow light exercises will give you an idea if they're positively or negatively impacting the pattern.

- **Green Light**—Exercises that can be safely used because they either don't impact a dysfunctional pattern or may positively impact the pattern

First, identify red light exercises for the patterns that were scored as 0s or 1s or were asymmetrical. These should be avoided whenever possible until the patterns have reached a minimal standard. Do nothing more than this and you've already helped that client because you won't often get immediate feedback when doing something contraindicated. A shoulder may not hurt while doing an overhead press, but lacking adequate shoulder mobility or control, by the time that cumulative stress eventually makes itself known, the damage may already be done.

Examples of Red (Protection), Yellow (Correction), and Green (Development) Light Exercise. For a more complete list, see page 361.

	Red Light (0s, 1s, asymmetries 1 / 2*)	**Yellow Light** (2s, asymmetries 2 / 3*)	**Green Light** (3s)
Active Straight Leg Raise	Running, Sprinting Deadlifts Cleans, Kettlebell Swings	Squats Step-ups	Half-Kneeling Chop or Lift Upper Body Training Core Work
Shoulder Mobility	Overhead Pressing Pull-ups Handstands Snatches	Rowing Horizontal Pressing	Deadlifts Cleans, Swings Lower Body Training
Hurdle Step	Running, Sprinting Single-Leg Exercises	Symmetrically Loaded Squats Deadlifts	Half-Kneeling Chop or Lift Suitcase Deadlift Upper Body Training
Deep Squat	Loaded Squats Clean Snatch	Single-Leg Exercises Split Squat, Lunge	Deadlift Turkish Get-ups Half-Kneeling, Tall-Kneeling Chop or Lift

*½ and ⅔ are scores representing asymmetrical movement on the tests performed on both sides of the body (leg raise, shoulder mobility, rotary stability, lunging, and stepping)

Second, identify the yellow light exercises for those dysfunctional patterns and make a judgment on the relative risk to reward of challenging their production. When we see a poor push-up, we need to question whether it's worth the risk to have clients training on their feet. If they've demonstrated they can't connect and stabilize their top and bottom halves in a horizontal position, is the reward worth the risk to stand them up and load them, hoping they can organize and stabilize the spine and trunk stability in a more demanding vertical position?

Following the traffic light approach respects the natural development of movement in exercise selection. It protects your clients from themselves and from the wrong course of action.

Sometimes circumstances in competition or training don't allow for completely avoiding certain patterns, but that demands an even more watchful eye and being flexible in your exercise selection. Training and loading a mistake and then having to over-coach the solution is frustrating for everyone, and also more likely to result in greater dysfunction and potential for injury.

> ### Don't Compromise Integrity
>
> Bad form shouldn't be repeated, and absolutely shouldn't be repeated for a conditioning effect.
>
> In competition or on a testing day in the weightroom, form is expected to deteriorate during a maximal effort.
>
> In training, we need to always strive for maintaining the integrity of movement. Adding repetition of exercise, skill training, or behaviors on top of dysfunction means you're likely to lock in a pattern you'll never get rid of. That's one reason it's a good idea to leave a little in the tank and strive for quality first.
>
> Prioritizing training time, volume, and intensity over integrity eventually results in less integrity over time.

Because promoting fitness and activity are vital parts of physical development, we need to protect the movement our clients have before we try to correct and develop the movement they need. Promoting an active and robust lifestyle should never come at the expense of the quality of fundamental movement. Leaving negative movement or lifestyle factors unmanaged will constantly derail your best efforts in changing movement.

When we elevate our clients' awareness and protect them from the negative physical and behavioral influences on their movement and production, it allows us to see more clearly and work further along the path of adaptation with as close to a blank canvas as we can get.

OPPORTUNITIES FOR CHANGE

Perceptions

- What behaviors or environmental factors can you remove to protect your patient's/client's/athlete's health, wellness, fitness, and production?

- What can you offer to provide a deeper appreciation of how they can protect health, wellness, fitness, and production for themselves?

- How are you choosing exercises to be avoided, approached cautiously, or leveraged to reinforce your work?

Actions

- Always look for variables you can remove (permanently or temporarily) to reduce risk and create a better environment for positive change to occur.

- Don't train 1s or painful patterns. Resolve the quality of movement before adding quantity (volume, load, speed).

- Don't train people into worse movement—quickly rescreen dysfunctional patterns after training to catch negative changes. Better yet, teach people how to screen themselves.

Reflections

- Using the same awareness tools, check if your patients/clients/athletes report any impacts from lifestyle or behavioral changes. Can they see or feel a positive or negative change?

- After a week or two of intervention, formally screen if lifestyle changes are creating a measurable change in movement. Are the signs of health, function, fitness, or production improved?

- Compile a library of different exercise or training variations to account for dysfunctional movement that still addresses the goal of treatment or training. Do you have at least three variations of an exercise to allow someone to perform the movement successfully?

CHAPTER THIRTEEN

CORRECT THE QUALITY THAT DOESN'T MEET THE STANDARD

- ▶ Is what you're observing a problem with a part, a pattern, a capacity, or a skill?
- ▶ Do you have the tools and tests for each to give you a definitive answer?
- ▶ What actions can you take to correct the issue?

Corrective exercise has gotten a bad rap. Many exercises labeled as "corrective" aren't even really correcting anything, and that's left a bad connotation for many trainers and coaches. Most target a single part of the body or tissue physiology, with little challenge to the sensory system or the movement of the body as a whole. That type of corrective ends up as rehearsed movements that are awkward or given arbitrary training volumes and loads, hoping they'll somehow create strength, integrity, and competency.

The role of corrective exercise is to address the intention, purpose, and behavior of movement—not the muscles of movement. It may seem counterintuitive, but the more verbal correcting and coaching someone needs to activate a particular muscle through exercise, the less likely it is to be corrective. Correcting poor movement patterns occurs at the edges of ability, performing an activity scaled to allow adaptation to occur naturally.

As a medical, fitness, or sports professional, the same process and techniques we employed in the reset of movement apply when it comes time to correct movement. We need to scale the delivery of the interventions and correctives targeting the weak links to make those changes stick. If we did an effective job of uncovering the interventions that produced a positive change in movement or pain, we should already have a clear direction forward.

However, the weak link is more than just faulty parts and patterns. Our movement screens and assessments look at the patterns for growth and development at a fundamental level because once children achieve those patterns, they naturally begin to crawl and climb, lift and carry, and run and jump with increasing frequency, volume, and consistency.

As we confront unique obstacles, habits, and injuries over a lifetime, our natural capacity to perform these human movements often diminishes alongside the quality of movement. Lacking the capacity to perform or sustain an activity can default into compensation and knock a pattern out of balance just as easily as poor mobility or stability of a single joint.

Correctives aren't just mobilizing an ankle, rolling on the ground, or doing exercises with an elastic band. Correctives are any exercise or activity delivered with the intent of reestablishing and maintaining a fundamental awareness of mobility, stability and movement, as well as an appropriate baseline of the quality and capacity of movement.

	Test	Action	Retest	Delivery
RESET Local Global	Subjective Local Objective Global Objective	"Experience"	Subjective Local Objective Global Objective	Passive Active-Assisted Active
REINFORCE Protect—Don't Correct—Do	Subjective Local Objective Global Objective	"Corrective Activity"	Subjective Local Objective Global Objective	Packaged Self-Reset with Protective Structure
REDEVELOP Modulate Stress and Recovery for Homeostasis	Pick a Primary: Heath Cycle Movement Pattern Physical Capacity Skill	"Whole Activity"	Subjective Local Objective Global Objective	Whole physical activity, with corrective supplementation for unstable vital signs

> **Dysfunctional**—lacking the minimal standard to respond and adapt to environmental stimuli
>
> **Deficient**—lacking the minimal environmental standards of other successful performers who are where your client wants to be
>
> Once screens are established in a population, we can look for the minimum screen scores associated with acceptable risk and production across the population. Here the screen is no longer general—it's helping define failure.

Movement is considered dysfunctional if the human organism lacks the minimal standards to adapt and respond appropriately to basic environmental stimuli. Movement is considered deficient if the individual cannot meet the standards of the particular environmental demands of other successful performers in that same environment.

Any debate on acceptable levels of physical capacity or skill are always in relation to others in the same role or activity, as well as the goals of the individual. Does your client need to be strong enough to succeed as a linebacker in the NFL or strong enough to succeed as a firefighter?

Do clients need enough endurance to work on a construction site or enough endurance to compete in an Ironman triathlon? Our movement screens tell us if people are functional enough to respond and adapt, and our capacity and skill tests should tell us if they meet at least the average standards for each population or environment.

- **Competency**—measured against the baseline of a movement screen (demonstrated base function)
- **Capacity**—measured against normative data for a particular population or category of activity (sustained function against a particular environmental stress)
- **Skill**—measured by coaches and experts who grade through observation, special tests, skill drills, and previous statistics when available (specialized function against a particular environmental situation)

	RESET	REINFORCE		REDEVELOP
	Awareness	Protection	Correction	Development
Production	?	-	The Expressed Totality of Health, Wellness, + Fitness	=
Fitness	?	-	General Physical Capacity	=
Wellness	?	-	General Physical Competency	=
Health	?	-	General Physical Vitals	=

STANDARD OPERATING PROCEDURES FOR CORRECTING MOVEMENT

Before maximizing your layer of movement—health, wellness, fitness, or production—the preceding layer needs a minimum to be present. Pain, poor health, questionable function, or negative lifestyle behaviors will never support optimal fitness or productivity for long. Correcting movement demands that we respect this hierarchy in the larger strategy. Identifying an underlying health or movement concern doesn't mean we can't train—just that we need to change the expectations and approach. How we address each dimension depends on our particular set of skills and expertise, the standards to be met, and what our tests and observations tell us are the areas of opportunity.

Our professional success lies in how quickly and effectively we can scale our corrective strategies and tactics. Understanding the systematic way to allow our clients' internal systems to reorganize to a balanced state puts us on the straightest path for additional training or environmental inputs to mold them from there.

SFMA—CORRECTING PHYSICAL VITALS OF DYSFUNCTION AND PAIN

If you have the skills or training, the first order of business for any corrective strategy is getting a patient out of pain. If local and global assessments uncover painful or inflamed joints or muscles, the SFMA provides the opportunity to look for the dysfunctional, non-painful patterns where you can focus your attention. That doesn't imply that you're delaying action on painful or inflamed parts, but if you deem this patient appropriate to take down the path of exploring the dysfunction, you need to identify the highest-value DN patterns to address.

The breakouts for each top-tier pattern of the SFMA point toward either a loss of freedom in soft tissues or joints, or the loss of integrity, stability, or motor control. It's a rare occurrence when a patient presents with a single dysfunctional pattern or a problem that's purely tissue-related or only a motor control deficit. Knowing that you're likely to overturn more than one area to address, it's up to you to decide how deeply you want to engage with dysfunctional patterns in a single session.

If someone presents with more than three DN patterns in the assessment, it's more valuable to limit yourself to focusing on just the one or two most fundamental patterns. This usually offers a better approach because the likelihood of a related painful area becoming irritated increases the more testing you perform. Luckily, if you select the right pattern to focus on, improvements can often manifest in the other DN patterns as well. Narrowing your choices to the most critical patterns comes from understanding how to scale the demands of movement shifting from simpler to more complex patterns.

Cervical Spine → Shoulder → Multi-segmental Flexion or Extension

→ Multi-segmental Rotation → Single-Leg Stance → Squat

Forward bending—multi-segmental flexion or extension—is often the most obvious and common DN pattern we see in our testing. The thinking often goes that aggressively breaking down and correcting that pattern is more efficient because it involves body segments linked to the other patterns. That logic isn't wrong, but initially attempting to correct a more complex pattern can present another instance where looking for efficiency first limits our effectiveness. Because that larger pattern consists of simpler patterns of the neck and shoulder, dysfunction of those patterns may actually be driving poor movement of more complex patterns.

For that same patient with dysfunctional forward-bending who also demonstrates a DN in cervical mobility, spending three minutes addressing the cervical spine could:

- Take DN multi-segmental flexion or extension to FN—confirming the neck was the weak link
- Produce some improvement in the quality of movement—suggesting the neck was part of the problem
- Produce no change at all—telling us that dysfunction at the neck was unrelated to the multi-segmental pattern

The starting point of correction is to break down dysfunctional patterns into parts and to progressively integrate the parts back into the patterns of movement. The effectiveness of a single intervention can spread across multiple patterns, making the person more efficient as a by-product. At worst, it just provides valuable data to continue to drive the treatment.

RESOLVE FREEDOM OF MOVEMENT

We covered why mobility precedes motor control in the developmental progression and why we should hold to that same progression as we move to restore functional movement. While we first need to recapture adequate mobility, we can't fixate on mobility interventions as the only options. Mobility restrictions we observe don't always represent changes in the quality of joints or tissues. Rather, it's the natural protective response of the nervous system to stiffen and contract soft tissue around joints where strength and control can't provide sufficient stability.

The freedom of motion of local structures and the sequencing of the surrounding muscles play a role in mobility, which is why "mobility" and "stability" interventions can both produce improvements in motion. When we see a larger difference between the passive and active range of motion of a movement, that's usually the best indicator of when focusing on stability and control may yield more rapid and sustained benefits than a more mobility-focused intervention.

Regardless of the root cause of mobility deficits, regaining it without layering motor control onto that new motion means you're neglecting to hit "save" on the metaphorical document. The patient needs to own the pattern in a slightly new way that comes from reinforcing mobility gains with stability interventions—adding mobility without adding the strength or control to manage it increases the risk of injury rather than reducing it.

As always, test, apply your intervention, and retest to confirm if a change was made. Seeing dysfunctional, non-painful patterns improve from your intervention is valuable for prognosis and planning, but for the patients, reexamining those other painful patterns has far greater value in driving connection and compliance.

If they see and feel immediate improvement in motion, control, stability, or pain in movements that weren't directly addressed, they can easily appreciate the value of your strategy and skills. That's important because one of the primary goals during a first visit is to establish the first layer of correctives to send home that day. That initial homework, when completed, is another tool to help determine how quickly you'll be able to make rapid changes in the quality of movement.

How Much Homework is Enough?

There's no magic number of correctives to give as a home exercise program—it will always be patient- and problem-specific. Think of it in terms of the minimal effective dose. If you made a positive movement change with three correctives, do you need to send them home with six? Is more always better?

Initially, your goal is to maintain the changes made in the clinic or gym. Keep the burden low and put it on them. Asking how much time and effort they're willing to commit can dissolve excuses that often accompany poor compliance.

When pain is part of the calculation, we can't be as certain of the response as we would be if the patient was just demonstrating poor motor control or mobility. When we send someone home with one or two correctives, the initial focus is always on the simplest dysfunctional non-painful patterns because we need to be confident the person won't return 48 hours later, worse than before.

If we send people home with two correctives and they return looking like we didn't give them anything, that's a different person than if we sent them home with a couple of correctives and the corrected pattern improved. If the change persisted, we have permission to proceed full speed ahead. If it didn't, it'll probably take a little longer; we might have chosen the wrong correctives or we need to re-examine the patterns.

If you captured the change before, you can capture it again—it's just a matter of revisiting those factors and activities to protect against and the corrective actions and behaviors that will move things forward.

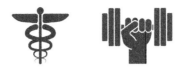

FMS—RESTORING COMPETENCY TO SUPPORT CAPACITY

The SFMA treatment hierarchy progressively moves from simple to more complex movement patterns in the same manner as correcting movement using the FMS. Addressing fundamental patterns where we can easily identify and correct mobility bottlenecks unlocks the functional postures and patterns. That's why the active straight leg raise and shoulder mobility patterns take top billing along with ankle mobility—they provide a first filter of mobility and control that drives the other patterns.

ASLR → Shoulder Mobility → Ankle Mobility[19] → Rotary Stability → Push-up → Lunge → Hurdle Step → Squat

When mobility is measurably improved or taken out of the equation, we need to recognize when there's significant inefficiency in the system. If someone can't control that mobility or maintain a posture without altering the breath or bracing the muscles to hold a stationary position, improvements in that efficiency come more readily from challenging the brain, not the body. Long before we worry about getting muscles or movements stronger, the neuromuscular platform of awareness, breathing, mobility, timing, coordination, and control needs to refine itself. We achieve this by providing a rich sensory experience that stimulates the sensory-motor memory with a challenging experience that's not mistake-free, but free of compensation.

Don't fight movement. Sometimes position is the only disadvantage you need, and by compressing the environment you allow movement to grow out of that hole. Developmental positions like kneeling or being on hands and knees aren't just to reacquire balance; there are systematic disadvantages to those patterns. Without providing an answer or telling them what to activate, guiding people through challenging positions they can overcome allows them to climb out of the box and reinstall their internal software.

There are people who have enough strength to muscle their way through sloppy movements, and there are plenty of professionals trying to coach lifts with clients who can't achieve or control the required movement or shape.

---

19 Ankle mobility is a clearing test within the Motor Control Screen, but is presented here in the context of the FMS because of its importance to movement quality in the higher-level patterns.

Before worrying about progressing into more dynamic movements, ask if we see mastery of those postures. Can they maintain a posture when simply holding the position of a plank or a squat? Can they take slow, controlled breaths while balancing in a kneeling position?

Taking a high-performing or active person and asking for less rather than more can feel like a regressive approach. We're all searching for the shortest, fastest path to see change, but we forget that creating change in many of these instances doesn't take long because so much of it is tied to the nervous system.

The first four weeks of weight training often produce the biggest strength gains, but it isn't due to significant changes in muscle tissue and structure. Those gains don't come from physical changes in the muscle, but from the improved efficiency of the nervous system in the new exercise or activity.

If harnessing the nervous system creates the sudden, drastic changes we see in fitness and production, we're missing an opportunity to maximize that change if we don't dedicate the initial effort to tuning that natural movement system.

CONTROL BEGINS WITH THE BREATH

Eastern traditions of meditation, yoga, and the martial arts recognize the role breath plays in engaging the nervous system. The breath produces the control and balance seen in yoga, the power and speed of a karate kick, and the relaxation and recovery of meditation.

We know the influence breathing has on the body's biochemistry, the balance of our emotional and stress response, and the biomechanical function and tone of the spine and muscles, but we rarely dedicate adequate attention to it in a health or fitness setting other than shouting "Breathe!" as a client's face turns red.

There are plenty of good clinicians and trainers who recognize that breathing is an indicator of stress to the CNS and work to reduce that stress response through dry needling, spinal manipulation, or deep breathing exercises. Then they send their clients to the gym to do an exercise where they struggle and hold their breath, jacking the system right back up. If you don't dedicate just as much attention to early exercise interventions as you do your last manual technique or needle placement, what was it for?

As clients explore movement at the edges of their ability, the first sign of dysfunction and struggle is likely to be a change in breathing. Breath-holding or fast and shallow breaths are unconscious strategies to excite the nervous system for more output and control, particularly in cases of pain or dysfunction. Unfortunately, those strategies are compensations. While holding our breath is valuable for stabilization when lifting or squatting a big weight, it shouldn't come into play when simply standing on one foot or moving submaximal loads.

Diligently monitoring your clients' breath and bringing their awareness and conscious control to the depth and speed of breathing will maximize the effort you put into improving freedom and control. It's the most effective tool to dump unnecessary tension from the system.

Coaching 360-degree breathing—expanding the rib cage in all directions—as you move someone from fundamental to functional postures charts the same path to function as other corrective strategies. If you can teach someone how to breathe for softness in a three-to-one ratio of exhale to inhale, you can incrementally transition to a one-to-one ratio as the complexity and demands of movement increase.

Breathing to perform a kettlebell swing is different than breathing for yoga, but learning how to breathe in the most effective way for each makes both activities fundamentally and functionally better.

The most valuable coaching cue in your arsenal might simply be "Slow down and breathe" because the minute people can't breathe normally, they're losing the compensation battle and their competitive advantage.

TACTIC—Invest Time in Breathing

In the Systems, we've been using breathing techniques to get people reacquainted with their breath and have seen a positive change to movement roughly 70% of the time in response to the most basic breathing drills.

https://qrco.de/bcasLt

REINTEGRATE THE PATTERNS

Stability doesn't mean lack of movement. Stability isn't stiffness. Stability is the reflexive or reactive timing needed to create integrity around a joint. The less effort required from the nervous system, the better.

Training stability and motor control is distinctly different from training strength. Most of the stability that aligns the joints, creates dynamic posture, and produces the axis of rotation for the prime movers to fire occurs at about 20% of the maximal voluntary contraction of the muscles.

In athletes, what we often mistake for stability in movement patterns is abdominal bracing or high-threshold strategies. When people get into the mindset that they need to strengthen something to correct dysfunction, they train sequences that over-activate the prime movers and under-activate the stabilizers. Rather than training strong, responsive stability of the trunk and pelvis, they're reinforcing a hard, braced core that limits the simultaneous balance of breathing and movement.

When it comes time to move and perform, teaching rigid bracing strategies trains the body to throw on the parking brake rather than tapping the brakes to regain control. The parking brake may stop you on a dime, but if you aren't able to take it off as you continue to drive, you do so at the expense of the brake pads and fuel economy.

Reestablishing stability starts with the reflexive control of the nervous system. When interference is withdrawn from the system by removing pain, addressing breathing, and improving mobility, we lower the barriers to recapturing motor control because the signals are now clearer.

People typically think of the output of the nervous system as the demonstration of strength, power, or speed, but the relative strength of a person doesn't always reflect how well that reflexive system is working.

We regularly work with athletes with above-average muscle strength who fall over trying to perform a simple chop or lift in a kneeling position. We no longer assume people possess enough stability just because they demonstrate superior production or capacity in a particular activity. When an athlete lacks stability, that incredible bench press, sprinting speed, or vertical jump might not even be close to their true capability.

Here again is where the movements of the SFMA and FMS are intended to help confirm the quality of stability within the postures of the developmental sequence… literally from the ground up. Can people demonstrate the most fundamental stability qualities of control when lying on their back or stomach? Can they hold a posture with good integrity of breathing and control? Can they control that posture when adding motion or added complexity?

Postures	Patterns	
	SFMA	FMS
Standing	Squatting Single-Leg Balance Multi-Segmental Flexion/ Extension Multi-Segmental Rotation	Squatting Lunging Stepping
Stacked	Movement Breakouts *(Long Sitting, Seated Trunk Rotation, Half-kneeling Narrow Base)*	—
Suspended	Movement Breakouts *(Prone Rocking, Lumbar Locked Rotation)*	Push-up Rotary Stability
Supported	Rolling *Shoulder Mobility *Head and Neck Motion	ASLR *Shoulder Mobility

While we screen these motions in standing, they develop in fundamental positions. Assessing and correcting them in supported positions often reveals a more complete picture of dysfunction.

We should be able to see the movement patterns of the FMS and SFMA within that framework as checkpoints to progression. If someone can demonstrate the mobility and pain-free static and dynamic stability in a measured movement, we can call that "functional" and have greater confidence in the integrity of the foundation we're trying to build upon. We can begin the work of redeveloping greater health, wellness, fitness, or production only when we can positively answer "Yes" to those questions for each movement pattern.

BUILD STABILITY FROM THE GROUND UP

Understanding how to systematically confirm stability in these positions is simple. Delivering and scaling the interventions to improve stability across those postures is where the systematic approach often breaks down.

One of the common requests we hear from clinicians and coaches is for specific exercises for correcting a particular pattern—a magic bullet that clears dysfunction in one move. They're asking how to ace the test, rather than asking how to interpret their findings.

We've shared many of the exercises we find most beneficial for improving particular problems or patterns on our FMS website, but as with any good system, you should be able to take your preferred exercises or something you learned from a course or seminar and be able to identify where it can be plugged into the system to yield the greatest effect. A larger resource of tools can be valuable, but not as valuable as understanding how to apply the tools you already have to find the best solution in the near term, and how to solve more challenging questions in the future.

The Corrective 4x4 Matrix is a tool we present in our SFMA courses as a more refined decision-making tool for choosing the postures and positions to work on based on a client's ability. The best exercise is the one that produces the most profound change in the quality of movement. That's not a satisfying answer for those professionals looking for a handful of solutions, but exercise is a multisensory experience and should be taught using as many forms of input as possible.

THE CORRECTIVE 4X4 MATRIX

Posture	Assisted Movement	Independent Movement	Reactive Patterning	Independent, Resisted Movement
Standing				
Stacked				
Suspended				
Supported				

This corrective 4x4 matrix came from my work with Dr. Greg Rose, a chiropractic physician, as we tried to create a framework respecting how we dealt with movement from both a neurological and an orthopedic standpoint when reinforcing mobility or static and dynamic stability. Each box provides a marker for delivering interventions at the appropriate level to help reeducate the sequencing and internalization of the patterns. Someone may require passive assistance to successfully perform a pattern. Adding some level of resistance can actually help activate stabilizing muscles. Your job is to consider where on the grid the exercises or activities you can deliver fit.

Are we covering this matrix with all our clients? Absolutely.

Are we hitting every box? Not necessarily.

It's because the movement should tell you where to start and where to go next. Adding resistance and active motion is always the goal to reinforce the integrity of movement, but if you find yourself needing to deliver constant instruction and cueing for someone to train with load or intensity, it should be clear that you need to regress the demands of the task.

On the other hand, if you observe rapid change in a pattern, you may be able to skip a level of assistance, move into a more challenging posture, or add a layer of resistance. Progression or regression comes from making those small adjustments to position or assistance to place a client in the posture and position where the movement can only be performed correctly. Where we observe successful self-correction tells us when we can advance a stage.

TACTIC—Prioritize Symmetry

Here's a scenario that confuses a lot of new practitioners.

On the bilateral screens like a straight leg raise or a lunge, a client presents with an asymmetrical 2 / 3 score. A week after working on correcting the movement, you rescreen and see a symmetrical 2 / 2. Did you make this person worse than before?

The answer would be no. Restoring stability to one side may temporarily remove some range of motion, but now the opportunity is there to build that person back up with integrity.

Improvement isn't always just taking a movement pattern from a 1 or 2 to a 3. Symmetry should be more important than a 3 because that 3 might be on an unstable or hypermobile side.

We always want to progress toward reinforcing those postures and patterns through increased demands and resistance because the increased feedback and neural demands from those interventions help a person own a position or pattern. All our corrective strategies build toward adding load to the patterns, because loading the pattern is like hitting save on the newly written movement.

When we load a movement, the added stimulus and repetition hard codes that movement pattern into the brain, which is why prematurely loading patterns or postures and training with poor form before achieving a functional threshold is so counterproductive. There's no need to demand technical perfection of a skilled movement before adding load or speed, but we need to verify efficiency with the underlying movement patterns the client has available.

Facilitation Techniques	
Reactive Neuromuscular Training	Performing the movement independently with added demands to challenge stability and provide greater feedback
Active	Performing the movement independently with focus on improving the quality of breathing, control, and timing
Assistive	Performing the movement with additional support, feedback, or environment to reduce the demands

We need to be thoughtful in delivering corrective interventions at the level they can be most readily received. That may initially mean assisting to give an advantage in stabilizing a position or pattern, or offering cueing and coaching to bring greater control through awareness as someone works through a stability problem.

When entire body segments don't maintain alignment or contribute to dysfunctional patterns, magnification of the dysfunction by introducing light resistance or perturbations can drive a corrective compensation by "feeding the mistake." Providing an external load such as a band around the knees or hips or applying manual pressure to push people further into dysfunction when they can't maintain the alignment of their knees or base of support when squatting or lunging are examples of this reactive neuromuscular training (RNT). Rather than trying to activate specific muscles, we're trying to elicit the body's reactive response to reorganize and connect the system of moving parts.

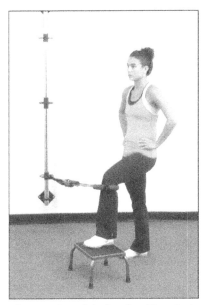 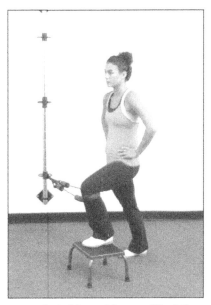

The stimulus of the band pulling the knee into an undesirable position can "feed the mistake"—helping the nervous system consciously and subconsciously respond to resolve a dysfunctional part and restore global control of the lower body and trunk.

THE CORRECTIVE 4X4 MATRIX

As control improves and the client moves into more upright positions, we continue to recycle the process of facilitating static and dynamic control until we retest the patterns of the FMS and find them to be functional. If progress plateaus, we may need to look for another weak link or revisit mobility or those behavioral risk factors to see if we've hit a new barrier to progress.

Checking the boxes of the 4x4 can show you where you may need to dedicate more time and attention, but a need for correction doesn't stop when someone "passes" the FMS—it just provides a bridge to pass through health and wellness to explore greater fitness and production.

Possessing an acceptable level of movement competency only tells us someone should be able to reasonably respond and adapt to the environment. But if we hope to build a resilient, consistent performer within that environment, we need to deliver the same corrective strategies to reinforce stability within a larger program of training fitness and skill.

Example of interventions to correct the multi-segmental flexion pattern

Posture	Assisted Movement	Independent Movement	Reactive Patterning	Independent, Resisted Movement
	Passive or Active-assistive	*Active*	*RNT*	*Static and Dynamic Loading*
Standing	Toe-touch Progression with Heels Elevated	Reverse Toe Touch	Resisted Standing Trunk Curl with Pattern Assist	Full Turkish Get-up
Stacked	Half-kneeling Chop with Band Assist	Half-kneeling Trunk Curl	Resisted Half-kneeling Trunk Curls with Pattern Assist	Full Turkish Get-up
Suspended	Quadruped Trunk Rotation with Band Assist	Quadruped Trunk Rotation	Resisted Quadruped Trunk Rotation with Pattern Assist	Partial Turkish Get-up
Supported	Supine Curl Up with Band Assist	Supine Curl Up	Resisted Curl Up with Pattern Assist	Partial Turkish Get-up

* *In these examples, "Band Assist" denotes a resistance band used to complete the pattern more easily. "Pattern Assist" denotes a resistance band used to provide additional activation of stabilizing muscles.*

> **Correcting Behaviors**
>
> The examples outlined are specific to correcting movement, but don't forget that the principles remain the same when working to correct other client behaviors. Trying to correct a client's diet, or sleep, or hydration can be addressed in the same manner—provide assistance to make the change easier, empower independence, and then add complexity or challenges to make those new habits more durable.

FCS—REINFORCING CAPACITY TO POWER SKILL

At this point, you're probably thinking you should always be working to maintain movement competency. That's the message we are trying to communicate, but fixating on scrubbing out every speck of dysfunction is counterproductive when the real barrier to success may be a deficiency in capacity or skill.

When we load a pattern, the goal is just as much to see at what point that pattern falls apart as it is to reinforce it. We can run someone through the best corrective strategy, but just loading or training a pattern may not be enough to expose a weak link when the time comes to perform in a more demanding environment than the clinic or gym.

The FMS can tell us when we have enough function to move well, but doesn't provide as much guidance on how to move often. If a movement falls below our standard as a vital sign, that's dysfunction. When it falls below the demands of an environmental standard, that's a deficiency.

Most sports and work or activity requirements have accepted standards of fitness capacity to gauge people's ability to perform in their specific environments. Tests like a two-mile run or a one-rep max on a lift need to meet the standard for an athlete's sport, and the same for the ability to lift and carry a specific amount of weight or stand for a particular amount of time for many work or activity requirements.

These minimal quantitative movement standards are much easier to determine than our qualitative movement standards, but the two are inextricably linked. Someone who cannot meet the minimum capacity measurements is treated like someone with a fitness problem, but the deficiency they exhibit may actually be functional.

We introduced the Fundamental Capacity Screen as a tool to measure those movement minimums for capacity in the same way the Functional Movement Screen did for movement competency. Through the FCS, we can measure whether the fitness problem we find is due to a lack of strength, endurance, or power, or whether the individual lacks the ability to fully express those qualities.

Without screening functional capacity, it's easy to assume that deficits in production will naturally resolve if we apply the stresses of fitness or performance training. That's why it's often challenging for trainers and coaches to see the need to implement correctives. The fitness and performance metrics they're tracking tell them all's well, and that getting a client or athlete to jump higher or run faster just requires training those qualities of power and speed.

It's easy to migrate toward tests that look like the things we want to improve. Testing a vertical jump or speed or how much someone can lift in isolation tells us what the output looks like, but it doesn't tell us if that output is a representation of a person's true ability.

Good athletes and high performers can often mask deficiencies because they compensate well when moving at faster speeds. However, adding an additional filter like the Fundamental Capacity Screen exposes weak links by testing a higher degree of movement control.

QUANTIFYING THE CAPACITY FOR MOVEMENT

Reinforcing capacity picks up alongside loading movement patterns—we may know competency exists in the patterns, but we want to challenge those patterns and energy systems. Screening and conditioning capacity within the developmental model respects the concept that crawling and climbing precede walking and carrying, which then grow into jumping and running.

Movement control, postural control, explosive control, and impact control are the developmental tests in the FCS for determining the general capacity to perform these foundational activities in a measurable way. All of the specific fitness and performance tests we deploy are precisely that—measurements specific to a particular environment or activity.

The data we collect provides the opportunity to understand where deficiencies exist in these global patterns so we can dedicate our attention appropriately during the initial design of a training program. Leaving those deficiencies unexamined increases the risk of those first weeks of a training program resulting in less than expected results.

Movement Control → Postural Control → Explosive Control → Impact Control
(Motor Control Screen)   (Carry Screen)   (Broad Jump)   (Triple Jump)

Can your athletes demonstrate balance and control in multiple planes? Can they maintain a posture and alignment under load and fatigue? Can they produce force efficiently through the body? Can they absorb and redirect force efficiently?

If we want to bolster our confidence in those answers and in the durability and resilience of our clients, we should care less about how good people are in these qualities, and care more about how bad they are. The FCS constraints progressively expose the weak links that can limit both global fitness and production by giving us a better measuring stick to quantify the threshold qualities and compare them across groups regardless of the task or environment.

THE QUALITIES OF CAPACITY

Movement control is captured through the Motor Control Screen (which consists of components of the Y Balance Test; see page 354) as the initial link between the FMS and FCS because it examines control at the limits of stability where dysfunction becomes magnified.

Our research tells us that testing movement control through the Motor Control Screen and the Y Balance Test may provide better insight than jumping, bounding, or skill-specific tests looking for who will have problems returning to activity because the screen restricts the opportunity to sneak by through compensation.[20]

If the screens expose dysfunction, deficiency, or a significant asymmetry when controlling the extremities in two or three planes of motion, the question of how far people can hop or how fast they can do a shuttle run is irrelevant.

Postural control asks whether an athlete can maintain integrity under load—the importance of which becomes apparent most often with weightlifters and athletes with impressive numbers in the weightroom who display inconsistency or experience chronic injury in competition.

Historically, most team-based strength testing has consisted of a one-rep max on the squat, deadlift, or press, a comparison of whether they're above or below average compared to their peers, and then more sport-specific measurements to design a training program.

---

20 Teyhen, D. S. et al. What Risk Factors Are Associated With Musculoskeletal Injury in US Army Rangers? A Prospective Prognostic Study. Clin. Orthop. Relat. Res. 473, 2948–2958 (2015).

Teyhen, D. S. et al. Identification of Risk Factors Prospectively Associated With Musculoskeletal Injury in a Warrior Athlete Population. Sports Health 1941738120902991 (2020).

Often when we test the postural control of those same athletes using a loaded carry, we find relatively unimpressive results compared to their weightroom numbers. We're only asking them to carry 75% of body weight, which is a fraction of the weight some of them are lifting in training or competition. When we see these kind of loaded carry results, we can't help but question whether their impressive single-rep results in the gym are representative of their true maximum.

Findings like these indicate the athletes are probably producing in spite of their control by relying on their prime movers to control the posture because their stabilizers aren't up to the task. It's not the load; it's the integrity under load that creates the evidence of strength. For this reason, we always emphasize that our clients learn to carry before they learn to lift.

When we see people with a below-average carry and an above-average lift, we know they're close to a plateau in their production because carries are a great barometer for the organization of the system. With this additional layer of information, we can see if dedicating time to improving postural control will produce bigger lifts or improved capacity purely as a result of improved efficiency of the system.

Moving up the movement hierarchy, *explosive control* looks at power generating capability, while *impact control* takes it a step further, looking at the ability to absorb and redirect that power.

If we observe dysfunction or measure a deficit in either ability, trying to "train to the test" by implementing a power or plyometric exercise that looks like the tested movements is rarely the best option. Exercises like barbell cleans or kettlebell swings are great for training the body to generate and absorb force, but those are learned skills.

Even plyometric hops are skilled to a certain degree and, even with a scaled approach, we don't need to add complexity when basic control is already compromised. What that person needs is the physical experience in an exercise that provides immediate visual and proprioceptive feedback with a significantly lower learning curve.

That's why battling ropes can be such a simple corrective to develop explosive control. I doubt anyone who's used battling ropes would say it feels like a corrective exercise, but when delivered with intention, it can have a corrective effect. As we scale it, moving from kneeling to standing or increasing the thickness of the rope, we allow the body the opportunity to find and internalize its newfound control in more functional positions.

If it's necessary for a client's goals to transition to exercises like kettlebell swings or barbell cleans for power development, the established minimal capacity can support the skill required for those exercises.

> ## TACTIC—Random Practice
>
> When correcting motor patterns, we're not trying to target muscle physiology. We're trying to target a feel and improve the carryover effect of that movement, so we shouldn't just repeat the same exercise. We need to facilitate more random practice if we want to dust off and reinstall those patterns.
>
> Coming up with three or four exercises that accomplish the desired goal of patterning a particular movement, and then having the person randomly practice those exercises with four or five repetitions is more effective than just focusing on a single option. Switching the stimulus trains the brain to respond and access that motor pattern to meet the changing demands.
>
> It's kind of like learning how to shoot a basketball. Shooting from the same spot on the floor will help you learn more quickly, but if you want it to carry over to performing in an actual game, you'll need to vary how far you are from the hoop, how high you jump, and how quickly you release the ball.

Strengthening a movement like a squat or press can elevate the threshold of where those patterns may ultimately break down, but to translate that into production, it's necessary to go deeper than just strengthening patterns to make them more durable. Exercises like walking a balance beam, bear crawls, six-position loaded carries, rope waves, or swinging Indian clubs don't look like a particular sport or activity, but they all allow us to work on correcting and integrating control of the whole system while simultaneously enhancing capacity.

When we recognize that the neurologic systems are more sensitive and faster than the tissues to adapt, we see where a quick, tangible benefit can be gained from a corrective endeavor. It allows us to build on a body operating as a cohesive unit. Integrating those functional components within a sport- or activity-specific training program can sustain that functional capacity on the way to even greater physical development.

DO YOU NEED THE FCS?

The FCS is a more recent addition to the Movement Systems, which leads many professionals to question whether it's a necessary tool to add to their repertoire. Depending on the dimension of movement where your services and skills fit, the required components of the evaluation process depend on the presentation of the client and the goals. It comes down to whether you can identify the physical barriers that are standing in the way of greater production, and how to best measure and value that information.

The FMS (and modified versions of the FMS) are human tests appropriate for everyone from a grandmother in a PT clinic to a professional athlete. The SFMA is a necessary tool for those working in healthcare dealing with patients in pain or those who may need a deeper assessment when struggling with function.

https://qrco.de/bcasLs

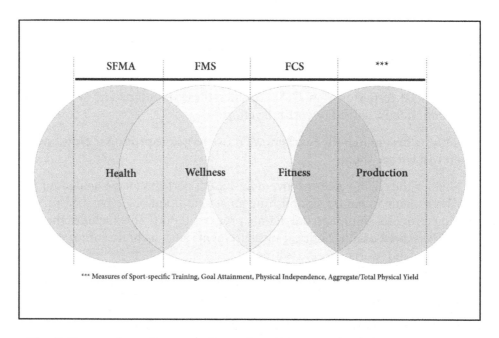

*** Measures of Sport-specific Training, Goal Attainment, Physical Independence, Aggregate/Total Physical Yield

The FCS is goal- and activity-dependent because it bridges the gap between movement competency and movement capacity and skill. A 60-year-old woman coming in for personal training may not need to complete an FCS—but she might if she's also a runner or pursues other competitive or performance-related activities. When there's a question about the ability to perform well in a particular environment, we need to ensure that capacity is adequate before engaging in higher-intensity training to prepare for those demands.

The biggest questions to ask yourself as the basis for your decision-making on the necessity of the FCS are:

- Does this apply to the goal?
- Is it safe to do the test?
- Will the information I collect make a difference in the program I design?

At a minimum, everyone should do the FMS. If you find that a client has pain in the FMS, significant risk factors in their medical history, or has been given restrictive parameters by a medical professional, an FCS is probably inappropriate. If you observe 1s in any patterns that make you concerned about safety in performing the tests, it's also best to forego the FCS.

If dysfunctional or painful movement is present, the data you collect from the FCS will likely be flawed, so the value of the screen may initially be minimal. In those instances, there are more pressing needs to address just to restore a functional baseline. If the client is a person looking for general fitness without the specific demands needed of a particular sport, activity, or occupation, the screen may also not be necessary if the results wouldn't dictate the programming.

The capacity screen is a way to gain more information. Whether or not you feel the need to perform an FCS, consider these questions and whether the information to be gained is worth the effort:

What tests best match the markers we'll use to gauge progress? How and when will we use them?

Whether the client's goal is movement-based, performance-oriented, or primarily aesthetic in nature, establishing an agreed-upon objective measure as a baseline provides an unbiased dynamic progress report. This includes the FMS and FCS, as well as other critical measurements such as body comp, strength, endurance, and sports-specific testing.

What environment do I need to prepare this client for and what energy system or systems do we need to develop?

Should a wrestler be able to run four miles? Does a swimmer need to perform Olympic lifts? Does this person have to perform under certain climate challenges—weather, terrain, and other elements? If there's a performance-based goal, at what level of competition, and when will your client need to be ready?

Understanding the environment under which a goal must be met is key to appreciating how to program effectively to reach your clients' goals. Lifestyle, activity, or sport demands all dictate the need for more specific development of aerobic or anaerobic systems. Each requires a specific application of training, so the program should be aligned with the functional capacities and energy systems required to compete. If those training or environmental demands are going to tax the qualities captured within the FCS, would that baseline data dictate the programming choices you make?

What are the demands of the activity? How much force will the person need to produce and absorb—how often, how quickly, and in what planes and positions?

In the same way we need to consider the energy systems, the physical challenge of training is based on creating a stress that will create the desired physiological adaptations. If you don't have a profile of your client's sport or activity demands, it will be impossible to know when you've achieved optimal levels of strength, power, or endurance to meet the demands of the daily or competitive environment.

There are plenty of resources available with normative performance data for different populations and activities, but people get lost chasing maximal strength, power, or speed, when in most cases they don't need to be maximal—they just need enough strength or speed so it's no longer the limiting quality.

Will improving the level of fitness progress them toward a performance goal? Probably—but we can't know if people are producing as well as they could be. Until we define the markers that say competency and capacity are present and sufficient to support the full expression of movement, we may be leaving some of both fitness and production untapped.

TACTIC—Capture Function with Capacity

Once you've established a baseline, performing both the FMS and FCS on the same day can be incredibly valuable. If you see dysfunction in the FMS or the Motor Control Screen and then apply a corrective that creates a positive change, quickly rescreening the FCS can sometimes demonstrate a significant gain in capacity.

How does changing an FMS by a couple points or improving arm or leg reach by a few centimeters add strength and capacity? Think about it as jumping or running in tight jeans or with a taped ankle. A lack of mobility or misfiring of stabilizer muscles can rob the body of the ability to fully express the capacity at its disposal.

THE PROCESS OF CORRECTION

Behind every successful physical culture there's a systematic process at play. There was a systematic way to build a Spartan warrior. There's a systematic way to develop a Navy SEAL. And there's a systematic way to correct and develop movement.

Seeing growth and adaptation from the perspective of the Movement Systems is to see that we approach screening and correcting movement patterns on a continuum to chart the straightest line to greater production. Do we address each area in this order each and every time? No. But we do confirm that the quality of each progressive aspect of movement is intact and functional before we focus efforts on driving further adaptation.

The systematic process of restoring function through the patterns of movement leads us to the doorstep of developing stronger, faster, and more powerful bodies. When each of these patterns can receive a mark of approval, we should be confident we've set the stage for growth and adaptation of physical ability to occur as we expand the range of activities and exercise.

The following encapsulation of all the global patterns within the movement screens and assessments, provides the perspective of how we've tried to capture that developmental path. This progression is the connective tissue of the processes of the Movement Systems.

Foundational Mobility and Control
Cervical Mobility and Control
Thoracic Mobility and Control
Global Flexion and Extension
Ankle Mobility and Control
Breathing Screen

Fundamental Movement Patterns
ASLR
Shoulder Mobility
Trunk Stability Push-up
Rotary Stability

Functional Movement Patterns
Inline Lunge
Hurdle Step (FMS) and Single-Leg Balance (SFMA)
Deep Squat

Movement Control (Single-Limb Stressed Balance and Motor Control)
Lower Body Motor Control Screen
Upper Body Motor Control Screen
Y Balance Test

Postural Control (Motor Control—Stress Against Posture)
Carry Screen

Explosive Control (Power Dissection and Demonstrated Jump)
Broad Jump
Broad Jump Hands on Hips
Single-Leg Jump

Impact Control (Energy Storing Dissection and Demonstrated Bound)
Triple Broad Jump
2-1-2 Bound

The standard operating procedure for working with movement entails being able to move through the checklist of tests and confirm each pattern is intact with an acceptable level of quality. In my attempts to concentrate our work down to its simplest form, I often think of the process for working with movement as simply as:

Painful Movement → Treat the problem

Dysfunctional Movement Quality → Tune the system

Deficient Movement Capacity → Train the weaknesses

Impaired Production → Trim the barriers to success

DEDICATE TIME TO THE PROCESS

You as a professional may not have the individual knowledge or comfort to personally address each of those patterns or the problems that you encounter. However, you share the responsibility of protecting the integrity of all of them.

How you address the functional limitations you encounter is up to you. There are countless tools, techniques, and tactics, but honoring a process built around movement demands that you always have a clear intention and goal for the actions you take. Whenever you encounter pain, dysfunction, deficiency, or impaired production, this strategy offers a decision-making model to look back and correct gaps in mobility and stability rather than fighting those higher-level postures and patterns that can hide dysfunction.

If you're diligent in holding to the process, I promise you'll find that spending the time on the basic developmental patterns often allows movement to refine itself, streamlining and speeding up your process to greater production.

But guess when movement won't refine itself? When you don't spend the time.

Instead of rushing to instruct movement and asking people to memorize it, make sure they know what they're doing…and then keep things light.

Every corrective exercise used appropriately will create some anxiety and frustration; so let your clients get a little frustrated. Let them be wobbly. Don't rush through an exercise like a Turkish get-up. Don't rush through the chop and lift. Don't rush through the frustration everyone encounters with a single-leg deadlift. If people don't learn what a mistake feels like, they can't feel it when something is right.

What's your role here? Tell jokes. Smile a lot. Keep the environment and your input constructive. Remind the person to breathe.

Breaking down movement patterns and applying your skills to correct them from the ground up can profoundly alter the trajectory of your clients' daily life, but the change is often temporary.

When someone leaves your clinic or gym in a better state than they arrived, it doesn't mean they'll return the same. Prescribing corrective exercises to maintain those improvements isn't a solution—it's just a tool to keep that movement alive so it won't be necessary to start over the next time you see them.

Elevating production and sustaining success and ownership of movement goes beyond reinforcement and correction. The only way to leave behind the physical barriers to the activities we want to pursue is through development of this newfound physical territory.

OPPORTUNITIES FOR CHANGE

Perceptions

- How are you choosing what physical qualities to work on? What takes priority and why?
- How are you determining when someone is ready or safe to perform in their chosen environment? What are your standards?
- What's your criteria for:
  - Discharging someone from medical care?
  - Determining if someone is ready (safe) to train?
  - Clearing someone to return to sport?
  - Deeming someone ready to pursue their goals without your guidance?

Actions

- Define the minimum standards for each layer of movement that, when achieved, confirm someone can safely pursue higher levels of movement.
- Place a screen (at least the FMS) in every reassessment—every four weeks or ten visits.
- Have a referral network—MDs and clinicians who get it, or fitness and training pros who get it.

Reflections

- When you perform those reassessments, perform a full screen to look for changes in all of the patterns. Is your programming promoting or hindering movement?
- Think about correctives not as stand-alone exercises, but as components of warm-ups, recovery days, or fillers between conditioning exercises. Can you maintain the quality of movement through better program design?
- Test—Intervention—Retest. Whether it's for a single intervention, a single treatment/training session, or a treatment/training cycle, you need to catch at least a snapshot of movement to stay on the right course. Where can you start today?

CHAPTER FOURTEEN

DEVELOP THE QUALITY TO SUPPORT ADAPTATION

Patients and clients don't come to us because they're producing at their best. They come to us because they want to get out of pain, lift more weight, run farther and faster, or jump higher—in short, they want to do more activity and do it better. Because their goals of greater production rarely include getting better at rolling on the ground or improving the quality of movement, asking them to put their personal goals aside for a week or two to address their movement risk factors can feel like an overly conservative path. That's probably one of the biggest reasons so many professionals are reluctant to adopt this approach in their businesses.

Redeveloping movement is the stage many of us rush to because this is where we get to flex our professional muscles and creativity. Unfortunately, we often get there without those boring but valuable protective and corrective actions or the challenging step of elevating someone's self-awareness. Trying to demonstrate how good we are by optimizing something we only assume to be normal may impress patients, clients, and athletes in the short-term, but it's adding unnecessary risk and uncertainty to the larger process.

Regardless of the initial point of entry to working with someone, you have to continuously look back upstream to identify those weaknesses or risks that may compromise your success in developing greater resilience.

Today, we have more functional problems than healthcare or fitness alone can fix—and we see so many people showing up unprepared for the training we have in store for them. For that reason, the middle ground of wellness, between the layers of health and fitness, is one of your best opportunities to build a competitive advantage; bridging the gap between rehab, fitness, and production is wide open territory. A big reason for that is the disconnect so many professionals have in their delivery of movement correction and movement development strategies.

For health professionals, the corrective exercise piece gets magnified to such a degree, they struggle to transition into a more sustainable training program. Somewhere in the process, patients either end up in rehab purgatory, doomed to perform low-intensity exercises in perpetuity, or they receive a training program consisting of more corrective exercises than movements intended to improve fitness.

	Test	Action	Retest	Delivery
RESET Local Global	Subjective Local Objective Global Objective	"Experience"	Subjective Local Objective Global Objective	Passive Active-Assisted Active
REINFORCE Protect— Don't Correct—Do	Subjective Local Objective Global Objective	"Corrective Activity"	Subjective Local Objective Global Objective	Packaged Self-Reset with Protective Structure
REDEVELOP Modulate Stress and Recovery for Homeostasis	**Pick a Primary:** Heath Cycle Movement Pattern Physical Capacity Skill	"Whole Activity"	Subjective Local Objective Global Objective	Whole physical activity, with corrective supplementation for unstable vital signs

On the other side, many personal trainers and sports coaches try to distinguish themselves by dreaming up elaborate exercises or drills intended to simultaneously address multiple qualities, but without an appreciation for how to match those to meet a client's needs. Believing that challenging the body in as many ways as possible can correct imbalances while simultaneously developing fitness qualities, they devise new ways to make ordinary exercises more awkward or unstable.

And their clients are getting exposed to even greater degrees of risk.

Redeveloping the health, wellness, fitness, and production people have lost along the way has to respect the delicate balance that exists between each layer of movement. There are exercises to simultaneously correct and condition movement, but those can't be effectively delivered until you've first identified, protected, and corrected those dysfunctional or deficit patterns standing in the way.

Those same screens and assessments that put us on the correct path from the start now must become better tools to monitor progress and make small adjustments so those under our care don't just achieve their goals; they do so in the safest and most effective way.

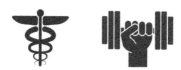

THE CONTINUUM: COMPETENCY, CAPACITY, SKILL

It's an imperfect analogy, but building a more robust and resilient body isn't so different from building a house. If you wanted to construct a new home, you wouldn't build it on a cracked foundation. You'd want to make sure the concrete slab was solid enough and level to support whatever you built on top of it. Similarly, all the protective and corrective work up to this point served to level the base of movement. When you've established the quality of the building blocks of competency, capacity, and skill, you should have confidence in the person to respond and adapt to the stress you plan to introduce.

Any time we deliver stress to drive adaptation to support greater levels of skill and production, we run the risk of upsetting the layers below. We can't live without stress, but we can't respond to stress without recovery. Those boxes of development are never fully closed because the work to maintain the balance and integrity of each layer never really ends.

	Awareness	Protection	Correction	Development
Production	?	-	+	Re-skill
Fitness	?	-	+	Re-stress
Wellness	?	-	+	Re-pattern
Health	?	-	+	Re-cycle

Maintaining homeostasis while trying to improve production requires that we continue building on the quality of each lower layer to maintain balance. For health, we need to develop more robust cyclical systems like respiration, cardiovascular and digestive function, and sleep to promote growth and recovery. For wellness, we need to repattern behaviors and movements that may begin to erode and expose risk as the stress of fitness increases. For fitness, we need to restress the physiologic systems that create a buffer of physical capacity to safely explore activities that allow us to elevate skill and production. Any addition to the top has to be met with an addition to the bottom or we risk a breakdown in the cycles of stress and recovery.

Developing those qualities is more than just transitioning from correcting to training movement. When done well, that transition looks a lot more like intelligent conditioning and programming than a wholesale shift away from corrective exercise.

The idea that anyone with movement dysfunction or deficiencies needs to stop everything and strictly follow a corrective program is misguided. You'll encounter few people who check all the boxes in covering those minimums, and even for those who can, the daily stress of life can easily upset the balance of function.

As we develop more physically robust and resilient clients, we need to develop each layer without sacrificing the foundation we've built, but we also shouldn't sacrifice the higher layers—particularly fitness or production—if it's not necessary. There's nothing worse for a patient or client with a few dysfunctional patterns than to shut them down completely and regress all of their activity and exercise. Some professionals get so wrapped up in finding and correcting one or two bad patterns, they forget they have five or six good ones to train. Focus on fixing the impaired elements, but you can still work on the good stuff.

We should be doing everything we can to keep people active and training, but we need to accomplish it safely. Avoid training or loading dysfunctional patterns; however, the last thing your client wants or needs is a program of only corrective exercises. If the client was deadlifting 250 pounds and the problem isn't linked to the deadlift, programming a deadlift with a light kettlebell or stopping altogether may only make the person weaker.

We want to see if we can sustain a pattern like a leg raise locally with toe touches or a loaded hip hinge, and globally by going on a long walk or doing loaded carries or another exercise that allows the corrections to integrate and translate into skilled activity. It's not either correcting or developing the layers of movement, but packaging our work to bolster the weak links and grow greater movement together.

Here's where revisiting the concept of the red–yellow–green light exercises can be useful. We earlier presented the concept in the context of protection and the tactics to take to avoid stress to a dysfunctional or painful pattern. Using the lights as a larger strategy applied to drive adaptation allows us to deliver a program built around both correction and conditioning.

By scaling the stress and demands of the interventions we choose, and checking the integrity of the system, we can strengthen each layer and measure responses to our choices—ensuring that we're removing the weakest link without hurting anything else. If every time we train a client we need to push reset to restore the functional baseline, something's either wrong with that body or with the stress we're delivering to it.

A LIGHT SYSTEM STRATEGY

Red Light	Score of a 0, 1, or 1 / 2 asymmetry	Address Health for 0s Protect + Correct 1s, and Asymmetrical Patterns
Yellow Light	Score of a 2 or 2 / 3 asymmetry	Correct + Develop with Caution
Green Light	Score of a 3	Develop

Take this hypothetical client's FMS breakdown:

- Deep Squat—2
- Hurdle Step—3 / 3
- Inline Lunge—2 / 2
- Shoulder Mobility—1 / 2
- ASLR—2 / 2
- Trunk Stability Push-up—1
- Rotary Stability—2 / 2

How would you work with this client? Do you need to correct each of these movements with 1s and 2s and only train the one pattern with a 3? Where do you start making those decisions?

Rather than being paralyzed by analysis of each score, see these scores as indicators of risk. Movements that are asymmetrical or have a score of a 0 or 1 on the screen present a higher risk to load and train than a movement that scores a 2 or a 3.

We should be more cautious with the exercises or activities that involve those riskier patterns. Looking over the scores, this client presents with mostly 2s and one 3, but the asymmetrical shoulder mobility and dysfunctional push-up indicate patterns to respect and exercises to avoid—these are red lights. Dysfunction in both of those patterns means the risk outweighs the benefit of performing overhead work or pressing.

Pattern	Red Light (Avoid)	Yellow Light (Use with Caution)	Green Light (Safe to Train)
Shoulder Mobility	Overhead Work Overhead Pressing	Rowing Horizontal Pressing Partial Get-Ups	Deadlift Kettlebell Swings Lower Body Work Core Work
Push-Up	Pressing Symmetrically Loaded Closed Chain Exercises	Deadlift Kettlebell Swings Core Work	Push-Up Progressions Single-Leg Deadlift Partial Get-Ups

A 1 on the push-up also means this person may demonstrate a poor connection between the upper and lower body, suggesting caution in standing exercises with bilateral loads. If you can deliver a correction that produces a measurable improvement to at least a 2, you can potentially expand the approach and address those patterns with yellow light exercises that may continue to improve quality and capacity through intelligent training.

This client could do some banded shoulder mobilizations, the downward dog, rolling patterns, and bear crawls as part of a general warm-up. Even though it may not change the rest of the program that day, retesting the shoulder and push-up after the warm-up can also show if a positive response occurred. If there's little or no change, the smart move is to avoid adding training stress to those patterns this session. If those patterns improve to at least 2s, you could attempt to introduce load to try to lock in the new function.

You could add lower body work, such as a single-leg deadlift, some sort of lunge or split squat, and a single-arm kettlebell farmer's carry. If correctives built into the warm-up resulted in 2s for the shoulder and push-up, you'd have even more exercise options such as rows or horizontal presses, but even playing it safe, you have a foundation of at least three solid exercises to develop capacity.

This blended approach allows corrective work to be built into the warm-up or rest periods between sets or exercises while you focus on the work of loading and strengthening everything else. Sneaking in correctives as fillers between sets fills time that would otherwise be passive rest for restoring movement.

Performing lower-intensity correctives like a kettlebell arm bar or a tall-kneeling kettlebell halo between sets will feel more like core exercises than correctives for most clients…and that's partly the point. A session of those combined exercises doesn't look or feel like a corrective exercise program. Yet, that's exactly what it is.

TACTIC—Don't Label a Person's Movement

Clients with fitness or performance goals who have less-than-optimal movement don't need to feel broken. As a matter of fact, they don't need to hear about an asymmetry, a dysfunction, or any movement shortcomings. In some cases, all they need to hear is, "This is your program."

Rather than labelling people (or the problems) and restricting their engagement with activity, we need to do everything we can to allow them to safely pursue positive movement behaviors.

The best corrective path is often just smart programming designed to protect and correct areas of concern, and safely reload corrected patterns to recondition the body.

A movement development program should look less like a corrective exercise program because it should ultimately grow and sustain movement competency as a byproduct of improving movement capacity. Viewing the program through the filter of the screens and stoplights asks, "Do I need to protect or correct, or am I safe to develop? What exercises and activities can best support me in both correcting and developing?"

Building that capacity through exercise and activity leads to better production and greater resilience against environmental and physical stress. It all begins by using the screens to guide the training and loading of the appropriate patterns.

Mastering that process and shifting a focus toward fitness and production metrics still requires that we continue to keep one eye on the functional metrics to know we're maintaining that delicate equilibrium between competency, capacity, and skill. Without returning to a common movement metric, it's too easy to fixate on chasing greater capacity or skill at the expense of competency. You can maintain mobility and get strong and powerful at the same time, but you can't hack it.

RAISE THE FLOOR

The goal of reconditioning capacity through training is to create a buffer zone—a physical reserve—between an individual's ability and the demands of the activity or environment. There's a common phrase in sports of someone's "ceiling" of development that aims to predict the potential maximum ability. Most successful performers exhibit greater maximums in a particular physical capacity or skill than their peers or competitors.

But ask a successful strength and conditioning coach whether the best performer in the weightroom is also the best performer on the field. You'll usually find those are two different athletes.

Make no mistake about it—pushing development and adaptation to the highest levels is critical to separating you from your competition. However, the people who consistently perform at a high level the longest are rarely the strongest or the fastest. The highest performers who elevate and sustain their level of production are those who realize that raising the floor of their weakest areas is what makes them harder to beat.

Unlike protecting or correcting movement, developing movement means amassing resources and deciding where those resources are most needed. Failure will inevitably arise when stress overwhelms the weakest link in the chain. Stockpiling resources in an area of strength rather than shoring up a weakness increases the risk of failure when a challenge arises. Because most people don't have access to limitless resources, we need to be intelligent about where we invest them. The thinner that margin between the demands of the environment and the weakest layer of movement, the fewer opportunities those people will have to utilize their full ability.

> We can use our resourcefulness to develop skill once we've built up the movement resources to a minimally acceptable level of quality.
>
> When we allow resources to fall below a vital limit, most of the resourcefulness ends up being used to compensate.
>
> The end result? Inefficiency, unnecessary stress, compromised learning, and increased potential risk of injury.

Competition, attempting to set a new personal record, or withstanding increased environmental stress will expose gaps in functional capacity by demanding physical reserves that may not exist. If training focuses on maximizing one physical capacity, such as endurance, without ensuring an adequate level of other capacities like strength or postural control, the athletes will never make full use of the resources they invest. They'll only be able to perform to the limit of their weakest quality.

The same goes for health and wellness. If people are sacrificing hours of sleep for their work without a willingness to compromise on the frequency or intensity of their training, their health and wellness will either be their breakpoint or the anchor dragging down their fitness and production.

Consider a common example of an amateur runner who shows up for performance training with the goal of improving her marathon time. She's been following a structured running program of different distances and intensities while independently performing strengthening and stretching exercises with only marginal improvements in race times. What tests would you perform to identify the weak link or links holding back her production? How would that information dictate your approach to improving her race time?

If we get swept up in overemphasizing tests of fitness and production and putting most of the focus on training to see improvements in only those measures, we're placing people's wants before their needs. Athletic skill or output are representations of how well people can utilize the resources they have, but it doesn't accurately capture the resources they have available to them.

When we aren't identifying and managing the minimums of the physical resources, we may find that following a performance-driven training program doesn't ultimately produce the changes we expect to see. Choosing exercises or interventions to add horsepower to the engine may not be what produces the greatest effect when driving on three flat tires.

To develop and sustain function and fitness in pursuit of enhanced productivity, a conditioning program should build from the bottom up just as a corrective program does. This ensures the most fundamental capacities are adequate before adding complexity and volume to drive adaptation.

Movement Control → Postural Control → Explosive Control → Impact Control
(Motor Control Screen) (Carry Screen) (Broad Jump) (Triple Jump)

These should make intuitive sense. The better you're able to control your posture and movement within your limits of stability…the better you can maintain that posture and control under load…the better you can translate that to ballistic movement…the better you can respond and adapt to the changing dynamics of an activity.

It's like saying someone should begin with simple bodyweight exercises before adding resistance and speed to more complex lifts. Developing the capacity of those movement patterns with respect to how each supports the next protects us from skipping right to training for production, and assuming the fundamentals are covered just because an athlete has been training or performing at a high level.

Improving the baseline competency and fundamental capacities of patterns before more specific training for high performance isn't always the fastest route to better production. If success was measured by how quickly you can make change, that would be a problem, but how quickly you can create change has almost no bearing on the sustained success of a program and the durability of the results. Success should be measured by how few actions and adjustments you need to take in the long term to foster steady growth and development.

You can take immediate action to develop multiple qualities at once and be forced to constantly react and revise your plan. Or you can first fortify the foundation and remove the barriers to success.

When you apply your initial efforts to manage the minimums and raise the floor beyond the threshold of failure, you'll find your path is far less constrained, with far more opportunities to explore and extend the boundaries of physical development.

INTEGRATE SELF-LIMITING EXERCISES

As you reload and retrain patterns, self-limiting exercises are a valuable subset of exercises to integrate into your plan. Self-limiting exercises demand greater engagement and produce greater physical awareness because they don't provide the painless mastery found in a fitness machine or a simple exercise. These should form the cornerstone of a corrective or developmental program. A self-limiting exercise like rolling, walking on a balance beam, jumping rope, or a Turkish get-up impose mindfulness of alignment, balance, and control by providing constant feedback and a physical barrier when those qualities aren't respected.

A self-limiting exercise requires instruction to be performed correctly and safely, but because it presents natural boundaries, it can both improve and sustain quality movement. When appropriately scaled and coached, a self-limiting exercise will show when an athlete has had enough because they're generally more taxing to the nervous system than they are to muscle physiology.

When delivered with the right level of intensity, they improve at the same pace that conscious and reflexive control improves to meet the demands, and gains are largely tied to how effectively a person can bring breathing, awareness, and control into harmony.

EXAMPLES OF SELF-LIMITING EXERCISES
Excerpted from Movement

Pain or Discomfort to Learn Body Management	
Balance Beam Walking	Climbing Activities
Barefoot Running and Training—Pose, Chi or Evolution Running	Farmer's Carry

Breathing		
Crocodile Breathing (yoga)	Rolling Patterns	Classic Yoga Instruction
Classic Martial Arts Instruction	Pressurized Breathing for Power	SeeSaw Breathing (Feldenkrais)

Grip / Shoulder / Core / Control		
Goblet Squat, to Overhead Lift	Bottom-Up Clean, Bottom-Up Press	Bottom-Up C&P, Tall-Kneeling
Bottom-Up Press, Tall-Kneeling	Climbing Activities	Heavy Rope Work (Brookfield)

Balance and Small Base Control		
Trail Running	Bottom-Up Press, Half-Kneeling	Single-Leg Deadlifting
Single-Leg Med Ball Catch	Half-Kneeling Kettlebell Halos	Tall-Kneeling Kettlebell Halos
Goblet Squat to Halos	Medicine Ball Throws, Half-Kneeling, Tall-Kneeling	Single or Alternate Leg Jump Rope

Posture and Coordination		
Jump Rope	Indian Club Swinging	Turkish Get-Up
Kettlebell Overhead Walking	Farmer's Carry	Surfing & Stand-Up Paddleboarding

Combinations		
Cross Country Skiing	Trail Running	Single-Leg Squat
Single-Arm Pushup	Chop and Lift, Half-and Tall-Kneeling	Press—Bottom-Up, Half-Kneeling
Double Press, Tall-Kneeling	Single Bottom-Up, Clean/Squat/Press	Double Bottom-Up, Clean/Squat/Press
Yoga	Pilates Mat Work	Martial Arts Movements
Climbing Activities	Surfing & Stand-Up Paddleboarding	Obstacle Courses
Sparring	Running Uphill	Running Downhill
Compressed Athletic Activities—meaning smaller areas, quicker play, increased one-on-one contract and disadvantaged activities		

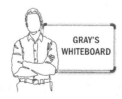

https://qrco.de/bcasLr

A Turkish get-up can be challenging to introduce to someone lacking basic movement competency, but once competency is achieved, it works incredibly well to maintain the quality of the overall movement system. Kettlebell training helps maintain full-body strength and power because it exposes weak links in strength or stability and demands the exercise be scaled to the appropriate level for success. Activities like stand-up paddleboarding or trail running are self-limiting because they demand physical awareness and higher levels of control to the changing stimulus and immediate feedback they provide.

People won't make a career out of an activity if they can't maintain the quality of movement in their training; with self-limiting exercise, mindful clients can generally trust the exercise will prevent overtraining as long as they refuse to compromise on technique. If we take the long view and think about not just developing, but also sustaining the quality of movement, function, and fitness over a lifetime, it's often these types of exercises and activities that provide natural support beyond the confines of a formal training program.

> **TACTIC—Efficiently Maintain Function**
>
> We've found that the easiest way to maintain function in programming is to always look for an excuse to include a variation of a hip hinge for the lower body and a Turkish get-up for the upper body.

WORKING WITH GROUPS

Effectively screening groups demands collecting the best quality data you can and identifying the athletes who need the most attention with the available resources. Effectively correcting and training movement in groups requires additional planning on the frontend, but the application of your efforts remains the same as when working with individuals. Work on minimums first and allow maximums to take care of themselves through intelligent programming.

It doesn't matter if it's a group of 10 or 500, if your role entails working with groups, the goal is to leave no one behind. This is true whether you're working with firefighters, CrossFit® athletes, or groups of school children.

It's more beneficial to each individual and to the group as a whole to identify minimum levels of ability across a wide array of attributes and to ensure the entire group achieves at least that minimal accepted level of proficiency. Screening always produces a distribution of functional or dysfunctional and sufficient or deficient movement across the movement patterns. Identifying those who need more support is essential, but being able to organize and scale your training program is the only way to help the entire group thrive.

What do you do when members of a group can't or shouldn't perform a particular exercise? Focusing your coaching attention on them to find the right exercise modification can be difficult to sustain at scale. Do you just stick to the plan, lighten the weight, and keep hammering that square peg into the round hole, waiting for them to gain the mobility, control, capacity, or skill to succeed?

You can either take the wait-and-see approach or you can acknowledge that using a one-size-fits-all training or corrective program for every member of a group is inefficient and potentially detrimental.

We could go to high-level fitness competitions and I could show you shining examples of some of the best FMS scores, loaded carries, vertical leaps, triple-hops—all the tests we hold dear. But many people in a class setting will try to accomplish what those athletes can accomplish without having the requisite movement capabilities.

Those competitors don't just have strength, power, and endurance—they have almost gymnastic-level mobility and control compared to most of the people they beat. Average people pursuing high-intensity training aren't just lacking capacity—they also lack the ability to adapt on the fly because they have to overcome their movement issues.

WRITE YOUR PLAN IN PENCIL, NOT PEN

Delivering a movement-focused training program to a group requires you to provide options. For example, if the training program for the day calls for back squats, how could you structure that to benefit everyone? Those who scored a 3 on the FMS can do back squats focused on finding the right load. Those who scored a 2 might be more successful with a front squat or a kettlebell squat, and those who scored a 1 would be better served doing some kind of corrective, like a toe-touch squat.

The untrained eye sees a group of people doing three different things and will probably ask why everyone isn't back squatting if that's the prescribed exercise for the day. But we aren't programming off which exercise we think is most important—we're programming off the patterns we want to train and what each person needs. Training squats means training the squat pattern—in the safest and most effective way possible.

But won't people progress differently? Won't there be muscle imbalances or a different training effect if one person is doing back squats and another is doing a corrective version of squats?

Maybe. Debates about superior exercises can only be of value once everyone achieves the same functional cutoff and demonstrates the same minimal standard of quality movement as their peers. In the short-term, it may require a more complex structure to the training plan, but if we can bring everyone up to the same standard and then sustain it in the medium and long term, your planning will get easier. It doesn't mean everyone needs correctives—just those who demonstrate a need.

We can more easily train and work in a team or group setting if we can figure out where everyone needs to be. Once we have a baseline, we can deliver our program and retest to see if we're making the impact we expect.

Don't get married to anything other than the baseline, how you use the information collected, and what intervention you choose. If someone offers you a different opinion or presents a new method to achieve your goals, you can measure it against the standard and decide if it's better than your current tools.

TACTIC—Be Flexible When Training Groups

The art of training groups is being good at progressions, regressions, and substitutions.

Have two or three alternatives for each primary lift—Deadlifts are on the program, but those who scored a 1 on the leg raise have banded leg-lift correctives, split squats, or single-leg deadlifts. Those who scored a 2 may do better with a kettlebell instead of a barbell.

Mix pattern correctives into the warm-up—Everyone whose leg raise is a 1 performs three specific correctives; everyone whose shoulder mobility is a 1 performs three others; everyone who has a 2 or a 3 has a general movement pattern warm-up.

Add filler correctives—Intersperse those same correctives into rest breaks between sets or exercises.

Retest—See how quickly you can get the person back into a full pattern.

RETRAIN SKILL AND PERFORMANCE TO ELEVATE PRODUCTION

Learning a new movement skill is difficult. Anyone who's worked with athletes or skilled professionals knows that reprogramming old or negative movement skills is even more challenging. The pain or poor production we measure in our clients and patients is often the result of the repetitive patterns of their skill, sport, or occupation practiced in poor technical or tactical ways. This is typically why they come to us looking for answers.

An already challenging task is made harder because historically, skill and performance training leaned more on the "art" of coaching rather than the science. Biomechanical measurement and analysis have broken skilled movements into more granular data, but many skill and performance coaches rely on a trained eye or intuition to coach specific drills and exercises. The same emphasis on parts or specific muscles addressed through specialized drills, gadgets, or exhaustive coaching and cueing may produce positive gains in developing a new or refined skill, but is it really the most efficient path to take?

If your role primarily exists to improve an athlete's production in competition, it can be difficult to see the value of the movement screens. The movements don't look like throwing a football or clearing a hurdle. Taking a squat from a 2 to a 3 on the screen doesn't mean you'll magically see a significant gain in the vertical jump.

But if you can find the person who screens with a 1 or a 0, or who shows a drastic asymmetry in the capacity screens, that's important information. That's the person you need to identify because with so many movement options already taken away, a breakdown is a more likely result than greater production. You need to meet people where they physically are and make sure you're covering those minimums of movement if you want the output to match the effort it took to produce it.

Think of it from the perspective of a professional strength coach. The dilemma for strength coaches is that they have a compressed time window to improve physical output, but the professional athlete in front of them probably didn't reach that level of competition in a pristine body. With four weeks to improve a vertical jump or a 40-yard dash before a scouting combine, it feels like the solution is to get right into training hard and fast.

But the best performers are often those who are also the best at compensating, and that athlete might be walking around with stiff ankles, barely able to squat to parallel. Instead of aggressive training, the option could be spending a week getting the ankles moving and the squats as deep as possible. Then adding single- and double-leg strength work along with skipping, jumping rope, and plyometrics. Time and again we've seen this kind of approach producing better results in movement…as well as in athletic production.

That's why the information from the FMS, FCS, and the YBT is so valuable alongside sport-specific or performance-based testing: The movement tests give us direction. If we observe and measure limitations in production but don't have the testing and interventions to confirm that competency and capacity are at acceptable levels, we can't be certain if the person simply lacks skill, or lacks the physical ability to achieve and sustain the required postures and patterns to express it.

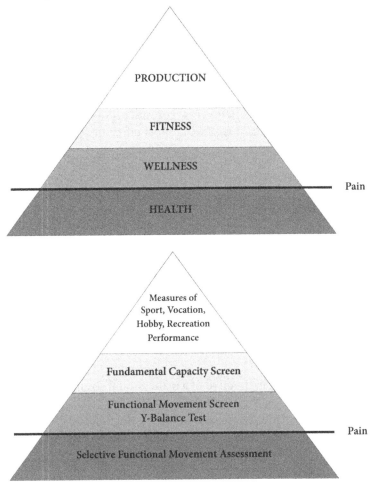

We need to establish the integrity and availability of physical resources before trying to train a person to be more resourceful.

- ▶ If we measure pain or significant dysfunction on the FMS or YBT, restoring pain-free, functional movement and reloading those patterns comes first.

- ▶ If we measure deficiencies or dysfunction in the FCS, rebuilding capacity and adequate movement resources becomes the focus.

- ▶ If we know that movement competency (function) and movement resources (capacity) are available and adequate, but specific testing shows production is deficient, we should put time and effort into retraining skill.

It's not that we can't simultaneously measure and cultivate these qualities, but without committing to the development of the most fundamental area of weakness, production will always suffer. Achieving a minimal level of competency or capacity can sometimes allow skill to reset itself, unlocking greater production as a byproduct. But applying a solution without confirming coverages of the basics of health, wellness, or fitness only adds uncertainty to the outcome.

A Movement System Case Study

I provided an example at the World Golf Fitness Summit of this progressive approach in a case study of a young golfer dealing with pain. I showed how the SFMA easily targeted the problem and brought us to the doorstep of the FMS.

The FMS went deeper into the problematic patterns, which then brought us to the threshold of the FCS, where that gave us quite a few loads and stresses to create an exercise program.

In addition to relieving the pain, his on-course productivity increased without ever specifically working on the skill of golf...because skill resets itself.[21]

SKILL FLOWS FROM SUBCONSCIOUS FUNCTION

In professional sports, the likelihood of making a positive, noticeable benefit to production in the face of practice, travel, physical strain, and competition is lower than the likelihood of negatively impacting it day to day. The coaches who understand the risk-to-reward ratio act appropriately and identify which athletes are at least average or above average in function, capacity, and skill, and which fall below. Those average and above average athletes can move forward through a thoughtful and structured training program, and those below will need more time and resources to bring them physically into safer territory.

---

21 https://www.functionalmovement.com/Articles/877/tpi_-_case_study

I love physical training, but I'm most passionate about resetting and rebuilding those movement patterns that run on autopilot because they provide a clean surface on which to build. When I talk about restoring the movements captured in the functional screens, unless people have altered anatomy, they shouldn't need retraining at the conscious level to achieve the subconscious movements they learned as a child.

That's why performing one or two corrective exercises can suddenly allow people to touch their toes. They didn't magically change the length of the fascia or the range of motion in the joints—modifying the environment and task dusted off the correct, stored motor pattern sitting on a shelf in their brains and allowed it to be accessed. Moving through a functional movement progression means moving from:

**Subconscious Dysfunction → Conscious Dysfunction →
Conscious Function → Subconscious Function**

Bringing awareness to dysfunction and reinstalling subconscious movements through correction and development makes all the difference when training new complex skills like swinging a golf club or throwing a curveball that involve more conscious control and directed practice. That's why we believe so strongly in the process of the 4x4 grid. If we get it right from the start, all the actions that follow point us toward a natural process of growth and adaptation.

Greater production sits at the top corner of the grid, and it can only grow to the extent that the qualities beneath it are developed enough to support it. Before you expend extra energy, programming and coaching to squeeze out a bit more production, spend a little extra time looking back to fitness, wellness, and maybe even health to be certain there are no cracks in the foundation compromising your efforts and the results.

	Awareness (?)	Protect (-)	Correct (+)	Develop (=)
Production				
Fitness				
Wellness				
Health				

OPPORTUNITIES FOR CHANGE

Perceptions

- Where are the potential bottlenecks in your process? Are you in control of them?

- Is pursuing greater production in some activity or sport enhancing or eroding health, wellness, or fitness?

- How are you balancing stress and recovery to maintain homeostasis in the system?

Actions

- Look for the bottlenecks upstream that could affect your outcome. Take action, where you can, to remove unnecessary stress to the system.

- Perform the FMS on the exit from rehab or the entry into fitness. Perform the FCS at the transition from fitness to sports or high-intensity training.

- Construct your treatment or training plans to emphasize conditioning and developing movement, always respecting those areas that need protection and correction.

Reflections

- As you work to push the boundaries of fitness and production, always look back for signs that the integrity of those lower layers of movement may be breaking down.

    If you see those signs of trouble arise, can you identify if your actions are the cause?

- **Clinicians:**

    Dedicate some portion of your time with a patient to identifying self-limiting activities or exercises that they can safely pursue on their recovery journey.

    Can you observe greater engagement and improved outcomes with their plan of care?

- **Coaches/Trainers:**

    Track the incidence and duration of recurrent or preventable injuries.

    Can you detect improvements in the resilience or rate of recovery after implementing consistent screening before and throughout a training plan?

CHAPTER FIFTEEN

ELEVATE PERFORMANCE OR EMPOWER INDEPENDENCE

- ▶ Are your clients looking for more performance…or for more independence?
- ▶ Are you providing the tools and education to put them on the right path?
- ▶ If you were suddenly removed from the equation, would they be able to continue toward their goals on their own?

What are your patients/clients/athletes looking for in their lives: more performance or more independence?

Those of us living primarily in the rehab world would probably say most of our patients come looking for independence. They don't want to be in the clinic any longer than they absolutely need to, and they want to understand what to do to manage their worn-out knees or cranky low backs to return to their active lives. If you've experienced moving around on crutches or recovering from surgery, you know independence is worth more than performance.

If you're a personal trainer or a coach, many of your clients come to you for guidance in achieving a leaner, more muscular body or competing and performing at a higher level. But you may also have clients who come seeking your expertise to learn strategies and tactics for managing their lifestyles, fitness, or activities. If the goal is to continue to push the boundaries of that portion of their lives, there's only so far they can make it on their own before a new goal moves the endpoint and requires new knowledge and guidance to get there.

Performance or independence is rarely an either/or proposition. The average person can't or won't rehab an injury, drop 50 pounds of body fat, or learn to master a skill through willpower alone. A therapist, coach, or trainer is necessary even though the goal may be independence. A competitive athlete wants to achieve the highest possible level of performance, but that typically requires a team of professionals to manage the facets of lifestyle and training to reach that level.

Even the most dedicated and driven athletes are rarely totally independent—pushing the envelope of performance will always require more resources, whether that's more money, more time, or more support.

Many people don't want just independence or just performance—they want both at the same time. They're looking for the shortest route that requires the least amount of resources...and ultimately, the ability to do it themselves. Tim Ferriss, who wrote *The Four-Hour Body,* rose to popularity by providing ways for average people to hack their abilities and make it look like they made the whole journey on their own, in half the time. But in almost every case, he wasn't independent getting there himself. He spent his time, effort, and money to tap into resources most people don't have access to, in order to accelerate his learning curve and get there quickly.

We can find shortcuts to better health or production, but sustaining those benefits can be hard without first spending the time to learn and appreciate the process it took to remove the steps in between. We can empower independence and teach people to follow the path to self-correction and self-management or we can maximize performance by designing and controlling the variables for them, but we can't effectively do both at the same time. Aiming too hard for one means losing sight of the other.

We need to understand what our clients really need and be able to have both conversations. Most of us already have a script for speaking to performance, but we should also have a script about teaching independence and accountability, with the metrics to let people know how they're doing with both. We should be comfortable asking, "Would you rather not have to be here? Would you rather be able to do this on your own? Or are you looking to significantly upgrade your ability?"

We should be comfortable asking those questions because both paths can end at better production. It's just that the fast track removes independence and requires a more involved guide.

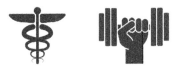

ARE YOU OFFERING INDEPENDENCE OR PERFORMANCE?

When people are on an independent health or fitness journey, they want a consultant, not a coach. They want to learn lifestyle and fitness tools they can apply on their own, and then check in when they need more guidance.

In a sense, the better you are at empowering independence in your clients, the quicker you make yourself irrelevant.

From a business perspective, there would seem to be little incentive to take that approach. However, if you know upfront that a client or patient wants independence, you have permission to be the best teacher ever. If you provide people with the knowledge to succeed, and also the tools to know when they are approaching their limits, then every time they need more performance, they know where to come to get it.

When people want independence, you should have no fear of moving them toward self-management of their own bodies; there will always be other people who either want or need your long-term involvement. When someone in their social circle is looking for a similar experience, they know where to send them.

Some people will need maintenance physical therapy or chiropractic care for the rest of their lives. There are people who, whether from a lack of motivation or self-sabotage, will be unable to maintain fitness without a personal trainer.

And it's nearly impossible to achieve a high level of skill or production without guidance and mentoring along the way. But to a potential client, if most of your success stories entail constant maintenance, you aren't going to sound like a very good investment of their time or money.

We've been taught that a successful business is built on creating lifelong customers, but restoring the health, wellness, and fitness on which our culture should be built means we can only allow a portion of those fitness enthusiasts and people looking to improve their health to be completely dependent on our systems.

It's not sustainable for patients and clients to be caught in an unending performance-driven model that withholds the tools and education required to empower self-dependence, because they'll continue to struggle to take responsibility for their physical well-being.

Is what you're providing today sustainable for your clients? Can their health and fitness survive in lean times?

We all believe we're equipping people with tools to sustain their independence, but I'm willing to bet the majority of patients and clients who stop working with you don't leave because you both agree they're ready. They leave because their insurance coverage runs out or they see a diminishing return on their time and financial investment. If their time, money, or resources are suddenly taken away, they'll cancel the gym membership or stop coming to work with you long before they give up their creature comforts.

> ## TACTIC—Promote Self-Selected Fitness (Jason Hulme)
>
> By the end of their time with us, we want people to achieve their goals and understand what they have to do to stay away from our clinics. We don't want people stuck in a model of always needing care unless they truly *need* on-going care. What drives the shift and the way we've seen the best outcomes is when they self-select fitness on the backend. It's not us influencing them to get to the gym, but their realization of and choosing of that path.
>
> We make it a point to bring that fitness element in at the tail-end of our treatment, because I want patients to gain that awareness of, "I realized that if I just do rows with a kettlebell, my shoulder pain is gone," or "When I keep up with deadlifts or make a habit of walking 30 minutes every day, I feel better than I've ever felt."
>
> Instead of providing a three-page maintenance exercise routine, help people feel and appreciate the benefit of a minimal effective dose of fitness in their lives. It's a lot easier to help them make that a part of their lifestyles.

We didn't build our business on bulk; we built it on expertise at the highest level. Following the strategies and processes of the Movement Systems ensures every action we take moves people to their desired levels of health, wellness, fitness, and production along the straightest possible route. But our long-term business interests are tied to making the majority of those clients independent.

Our waiting rooms have never been empty after making people better and more independent in the shortest time possible. The people we've empowered to be independent in developing their health and fitness tell anyone who will listen about the turning point in their lives that started in our clinics and gyms. That isn't necessarily the moment they were out of pain or suddenly moving or performing beyond their expectations. That turning point comes when we hand over the tools and the instruction manual to craft a movement-focused lifestyle of their own.

PLAY WITH A CHALLENGE—PRACTICE A SKILL—TRAIN FOR CONSISTENCY

That instruction manual on how to lead a robust, movement-rich life is hard to come by today. The inverted American approach to improving the quality of health or fitness is to first look to exercise and training. Being prescriptive with training metrics like how long to run or how much to lift often requires so many modifications and compromises that people give up from the complexity of the solution or worse, participate in activities without the ability that qualifies them to participate.

Rather than assessing a lifestyle and the risks that can be managed or removed, people try to supplement exercise into their days and, with the best of intentions, end up exercising the wrong thing, at the wrong capacity, at the wrong time, with the wrong loads, and using the wrong ideas. That approach has clearly failed us as a society, but we can move beyond viewing formal exercise as the solution to every problem by putting together a lifestyle plan to elegantly address movement quality, capacity, and skill.

The best strategy for helping people understand how to construct an independent lifestyle that supports long-term function and fitness starts by finding the form of activity that will both serve their goals and be sustainable. Notice I said the form of *activity*, not the form of exercise. It's easy to let exercise rules govern our lives, when instead we should be letting the principles of movement govern our exercise.

There are world cultures without formal exercise as part of the lifestyle that are healthier and more fit than most Western cultures. This tells us that not everyone you meet needs a long-term periodized training plan. The path to optimal health, fitness, and production doesn't need to be dependent on exercise if we can find the physical activity each person needs and wants.

Are we talking about someone looking to make running, lifting, or competitive sports a part of life, or someone who just wants to be physically independent and able to play with their kids? Will this person benefit from an approach based on self-discovery with scalable, exploratory activities like those espoused by Erwan Le Corre at MovNat®? Perhaps this person would be better off with a more authoritarian, structured approach like the Russian kettlebell environment of Pavel Tsatsouline. Or do your clients just need guidance on how to protect their long-term success from their own self-sabotage?

Psychology, goals, and motivation all play a part in finding the right direction. The simplest strategy we use is to focus less on finding the right type of exercise and focus more on whether the person needs more play, more practice, or more training. These three levels of engagement with activity mirror the process by which we learn, and can help you and your clients navigate a path forward together.

PLAY

When we find safety, we start playing and exploring. Play means doing an activity for its own end, just for the fun of it. Play is running on new trails or hills just for the enjoyment and experience of running, or participating in physical activities like paddleboarding, hiking, or recreational sports for enjoyment more than a training effect.

Creativity and problem-solving occur when the environment isn't unduly restrained, and room to explore and experience new postures, patterns, or skills offers intrinsic and extrinsic feedback. We aren't interested in technique or metrics as much as we purely want to promote a sensory experience. We're engaging and exploring limits. Learning occurs most easily in a positive emotional state, where we can turn the activities someone enjoys into motor learning and movement-sustaining interventions.

PRACTICE

When we more deeply and deliberately pursue the thing we like doing, we engage in practice. Where play is less goal-oriented, practice represents using feedback to work toward greater mastery of an activity or skill. It's work, but it pays. Practice might be trying to run as quietly as possible, or working to refine technique in tennis or skiing to improve the quality of the effort.

When my daughter saw her big sister do a cartwheel, she spent the next six weeks trying to cartwheel herself through every room in our house. She played with a lot of moves and latched on to one she wanted to master. With better quality as the goal, practice introduces a risk of failure, and practice under the eye of a mentor or teacher can chart a safer and straighter course.

TRAIN

Training comes when we're "good enough" with a movement or activity and our focus shifts toward elevating physical capacities through consistency and volume. Training is entirely goal-oriented because it requires a baseline, measurement for consistency, and the manipulation of physical volumes and intensities to facilitate and measure progress. In training, we take that running activity and manipulate it with the intent of elevating the capacity to run longer or faster. Training requires more work than practice, and there's no guarantee of recouping the investment.

Ask most people in the gym why or what they're training, and the answer rarely fits the criteria. What most people are doing at the gym probably shouldn't be categorized as "training."

We need to recognize that the problem might have less to do with people not understanding how to exercise, and more to do with the fact they're being told to do something they'd rather not be doing. The motivations of each individual play a tremendous role in the different levels of engagement with activity. Understanding what people actually want and need can help align a better physical lifestyle.

FIND OPPORTUNITIES FOR PLAY

Play is emotionally driven and random and yet there's full engagement—more engagement than often seen in a gym workout. When we find activities enjoyable, things we love so much that we want to practice them, we may need a little assistance to stay engaged, but with deliberate practice and outside guidance, we get the right feedback and attention to detail to improve. Once we've practiced something enough, we may want to elevate our status and have organized training for it. As long as that activity has been practiced to a degree where movement quality is consistent enough to minimize opportunities for failure, the organization and monitoring of a training program can be a valuable solution.

It's a problem when people see something like a kettlebell for the first time on a Monday and are "training" with it by Thursday. They completely skip the steps of safely playing with it long enough to learn what they can and can't do, and then practicing it with precision until a coach or trainer gives the thumbs up to proceed.

We miss the mark when we start worrying about volumes and intensities of training without the stages of play and practice to connect with movement.

People used to go to a gym to practice a skill, and the workout was a side effect. That's what we see when kids enjoy playing an activity—the conditioning is a by-product, whereas in training, conditioning is the focus. Training is absolutely a priority for people looking to compete, but for everyone else, let's reexamine its role. Rather than first thinking about the training program we can design for a client, maybe the first step should be identifying those areas of play and practice we can leverage to develop and sustain both function and fitness.

For people looking for independence, the goal isn't to get them to train—the goal is to use training to support the activities they want to engage with more deeply. Training should fill the gaps and raise the baselines wherever we measure a deficit or dysfunction, while promoting play and practice of activities sustains function and fitness.

When we create a program that looks more like once or twice a week of focused training, and two or three days of focused practice or playful enjoyment of an activity, it looks a lot more like holistic fitness than a corrective exercise program. But you need to be able to define "play," "practice," and "train" with respect and integrity for both the people you train and for yourself.

Maybe we should ask our clients to "play" running first (exploring trails, hills, new environments), "practice" running second (not making noise while running), and "train" running if that's what their goals require. If running is something they want as part of their lives with no intention of competing or elevating the output, a three-day-a-week training program will have them focused on details rather than their enjoyment.

Maybe we could use a play day as a recovery day. Stand-up paddleboarding is something I love. It's constantly challenging and totally engaging, but it's play. It's a workout and it might even look like practicing skills, but I do it purely for enjoyment.

Let's consider giving up one of our training days to have a practice day for those activities where we're not as proficient or wish we could do better. What if we engineered a workout one day a week where we only practiced a single lift or a Turkish get-up? This workout wouldn't be about how much or how many we do; instead, we'd be working toward perfection. We aren't just doing the activity, but *practicing it*. Maybe it's working with an instructor or with a partner and videoing each other, reviewing the video, and focusing on the precision and the technical aspect. There will be a workout and conditioning as a side effect, but the point is to get better at a movement.

SUSTAINABLE ACTIVITY PROGRAM > CORRECTIVE EXERCISE PROGRAM

We can better impact health and movement not through constant correctives and training, but by better conditioning through playing and practicing activities with just enough supplemental exercise or training to shore up the weak links. Those one or two weekly training days can fortify movement patterns, the proficiency of a lift, or developing physical capacities. The rest of the week can be filled with enjoyable activities that fortify engagement and connection with the body.

Some people may have such a permanent alteration in their structure that they need to refresh the system with correctives every day. For almost everyone else, a well-designed lifestyle should only require corrective efforts to counteract the environment or behaviors when we stray too far into stress or inactivity.

Without a doubt, we all benefit from training toward a goal or competing against ourselves or others, but that doesn't diminish the importance of designing a movement-focused program that extends beyond the boundaries of the gym. If we want our clients to embrace a lifestyle that promotes and sustains movement, we need to engage them through the dimensions of play, practice, and training.

Moving people toward independence in long-term function and fitness is no different than moving them toward independence in their nutrition. Movement is a nutrient; we need to replace it with whole foods before we try supplementing. The expectation of a nutritionist is to guide and educate people toward autonomy; as movement professionals, we should operate with the same expectations.

TACTIC—Use Play to Develop Awareness

People building a youth development program around movement often encounter vocal opposition from parents because a lot of the activities they see look like play. Most of that resistance comes from parents going into the experience with different goals.

If the goal is to develop physical self-awareness, movement competency, and grace and poise in active daily life, we probably have that covered. If the goal is to train an Olympic gold medalist, we'll probably be behind in that regard—but realistically, we'd already know if we had a gold medalist on our hands.

Parents often don't see the value if something doesn't look like a high-performance training program. When I work with kids, I explain to the parents that they're spending their money on a way to let the kids become physically involved and aware in the way they would if they lived on a farm or played outside on an obstacle course. It's those experiences that help children naturally develop their physical qualities.

That doesn't mean just letting kids play without turning it into a physical lesson—but there's a way to make sure a child plays and receives a level of instruction and precision without it being overdone. Fusing that instruction in an environment of play yields a training effect that doesn't require looking at a Fitbit.

It should be something that feels seamless. Structured, purposeful activities that feel like play should provide the chance to teach in a nonverbal way. I've done half-foam-roll balance flows with kindergartners, with professionals in Beijing regardless of the language barrier, and at conferences with three or four hundred people.

When someone thinks, "Wow, I'm more flexible, but that didn't feel like stretching" or "I'm more balanced, but that didn't feel like engaging my glutes," you're reinforcing the physical awareness that flows naturally from exploring and playing with movement.

The trainers and clinicians of the future won't be counting reps or reminding people to book their weekly appointments. They'll be managing hundreds of people in designing a lifestyle plan to sustain health, fitness, and production—some with only three visits a year; some with three visits a month, and some with three visits a week.

That can only happen by breaking the cycle of dependence for those who don't need it, and that doesn't come from more effective treatment or training alone. It comes from understanding that sustained health and resilience rely on developing both a lifestyle and an exercise plan that empower the pursuit of movement-rich activities across a lifetime.

OPPORTUNITIES FOR CHANGE

Perceptions

- How do you know if your clients *want* independence or performance?
- How are you communicating whether they *need* performance or independence?
- Where are your opportunities to deliver more play, better practice, and broader training to sustain or progress adaptation?

Actions

- Ask to what degree people want to engage with exercise, activity, or sports. Do they want to pursue the efforts for enjoyment, mastery, or competition?
- Look for imbalances between the time and effort dedicated to play, practice, and training relative to the ultimate goal.
  - Realize that in almost every case there's a longer-term benefit to be found by encouraging more play, empowering better practice, and delivering less but more thoughtful training.
- Deliver value in line with what people want.

  Either teach them the tools and knowledge to find their own way or take ownership of the planning and management of their journey.

Reflections

- Empower those who want independence with ways to self-manage their physical state.

  When an independent person returns to you, is it to pursue a new goal or to work on the same issue as before?

- Over-deliver for those who come to you to elevate their performance, but make sure that the integrity of the system is wholly dependent on you.

  Do they know how to take complete ownership of their behaviors and self-care, or are they completely dependent on you?

- Replace some degree of training and structured exercise with purposeful play or mindful practice.

  Can you measure an improvement in compliance and engagement with exercise or activity?

CHAPTER SIXTEEN

KNOW WHERE YOU'RE GOING

If you've made it this far, no doubt you've detected repetition in how we approach promoting physical growth and adaptation. That's intentional. Everyone enters their movement journey at a different point, so describing exactly what to do isn't ideal because there's no precise combination of exercises or interventions that guarantee a good outcome. Instead of stating what will work, we ascribe to the humble approach of asking ourselves, "How do I know I'm right?"

Demanding radical transparency in our decisions sends us back to the 4x4 grid to lay out our perceptions and behaviors for inspection.

The system is built on asking what movement tells us and it always honors our principles:

- Move well before you move often.
- Protect before you correct.
- Correct before you develop.

If we identify the tools to help us establish minimal thresholds, we can move our decisions closer to a binary yes or no:

Does this person demonstrate, in the present, the qualities of health that support the safe pursuit of physical development?

Does this person demonstrate the behaviors and function of wellness that reduces the risk of future failure to respond and adapt?

Does this person possess the physical capacities of fitness to withstand the demands of the environment and activity?

Does this person exhibit the performance and skills to succeed in their chosen role, occupation, sport, or physical activity?

| Awareness | Protect | Correct | Develop |
| ? | - | + | = |

Production
(Movement performance + skill or activity-specific measures of success)

Fitness
(Movement capacity + specific strength, endurance, power, speed)

Wellness
(Movement patterns + physical and behavioral risk factors)

Health
(Life cycles + vital signs)

Movement represents a single measure within each level of physical growth, but it can also serve as a flashing red light on the dashboard indicating something may be amiss. The movement screens tell us if a client is obligated to compensate, and provide tools to let us know if a change will quickly occur after a protective or corrective strategy.

My expectation is that working to eliminate or mitigate barriers to better health sets the stage for greater growth. Removing physical and behavioral risk factors will improve the likelihood of a more physically complete future. And building physical capacity can unlock the development of new skills and elevate future production. People who present with movement dysfunction have the potential to become more physically effective, efficient, resilient, and robust—but only if we first remove that dysfunction.

Early on, you'll have to keep telling yourself to follow the system. When your goal is to accelerate the growth of your business, getting people better, faster, is the logical fuel for that growth. Holding your actions up to the standard of the Systems can look like the long route, but getting clients who come seeking greater fitness or production off their feet, down in developmental positions, or in front of a healthcare professional will often help them adapt quicker and more completely.

Instead of growing frustrated and over-coaching, we'll know when to step away from complexity to reestablish a solid foundation of patterns or capacities to build upon. This model points us to the area of weakness in physical development, allows each of us to look across the full expression of human movement and over the fence at our fellow professionals to understand where their expertise and actions can support our own.

COME BACK TO AWARENESS

Look at the 4x4 grid and the layer(s) where you believe your greatest value lies and ask simple questions like:

- ▶ What's my standard for saying someone "passes" each layer of health, wellness, fitness, and production?
- ▶ If someone "fails" a layer, can I fill that need, or will this person benefit from the assistance of another professional?
- ▶ What information do I need to choose the best strategy to protect, correct, and develop each layer?
- ▶ In which column of adaptation can my knowledge, tools, or skills be improved? In which layer or layers of growth can I provide additional value?

	Awareness (?)	Protect (-)	Correct (+)	Develop (=)
Production				
Fitness				
Wellness				
Health				

If we apply that organization, the progression directs us toward the greatest need—for both our clients and ourselves.

Is this person healthy enough to focus on wellness?

Is this person well enough and safe enough to pursue fitness?

Is this person fit enough to chase greater production?

Wherever our investigation doesn't provide a clear "Yes" is the layer that should be the primary focus. We need awareness of the most fundamental weakness because that is the area that needs our fullest attention. Without a dedication to rebuilding each layer to support the rest, you're trading sustainability for short-term results.

We can't correct or protect or develop what we can't measure and we can't be confident in anything that flows from that layer.

Your Tactical Filters

The 4x4:
Where are the weak links in health, wellness, fitness, production?

Screening:
Do my measurements indicate an acceptable level
of each layer of movement?

Stop Lights:
Do I need to: stop and protect, cautiously correct,
or am I safe to develop?

The Corrective 4x4:
What's the highest posture or pattern that allows me to create change
and allow adaptation for my client?

PUTTING YOUR PRACTICE INTO PRACTICE

The FMS, SFMA, and FCS weren't built for anyone else—they were built for my colleagues and me to be more effective at our jobs. The process of building the Movement Systems forced us to critically evaluate every decision we made and learn from our mistakes and misconceptions. Only recently have we come to realize that moving clients through the system provides a natural learning process for them to gain awareness of the upstream complications to their movement goals and take control of their bodies and lifestyles.

Taking the time to move ourselves through the 4x4 creates that same opportunity to gain greater awareness and control over our own skills of evaluating, correcting, and developing movement. It takes more than just dropping new tests or tricks into what you're already doing—it requires that you open yourself up to asking, "How do I know I'm right?" and receiving the feedback and realizations the Systems produce.

Some of our greatest lessons from the movement screens and our work in developing these systems have come from the incredible opportunity to work with military service members. To become a SEAL, Army Ranger, or paratrooper, you can't fail and you can't quit. If you fail, it means you got injured or your body couldn't physically meet the demands. If you quit, it means your mind "checked out."

Looking at our database, the lowest movement group were those who consistently didn't make it, but only 50% of that group didn't make it due to injury. The other 50% quit before their bodies broke down—I think that's because for many of them, their minds wrote a check that their bodies couldn't cash. Some people quit before an injury occurs and some push right through all the red flags and signals the body sends before they blow up and fail.

When we work with professionals in the health and fitness space, we see many who follow a similar path. Through sheer will and effort, they push and grow their businesses, always looking to add more without doing a self-assessment of their weaknesses or processes until they start to get buried under the strain. When people try to implement the Movement Systems into a practice, it creates such a drastic shift from the paradigm that got them where they are, challenges and conflicts arise so quickly that they're likely to stop before hitting the point where the picture starts to come together.

If our ego is tied too tightly to our methods and we find the reality of our effectiveness doesn't match our confidence, it can be incredibly challenging to remain open-minded and diligent in the pursuit of new knowledge.

Confusion, doubt, and struggle are all natural phases we must move through as we try something new, but it shouldn't require throwing away what got us to our current position. Instead, it requires stepping back and looking at the processes of the business and actions through an objective lens that can reveal where our strengths and weaknesses lie.

BETTER DATA BEATS MORE DATA

For those who choose to follow the path of a systematic approach, the next questions inevitably become, "How long will it take to be proficient? How long before I get to the point where I don't need to do the entire SFMA or FCS, or it doesn't take an extra 15 minutes I don't have?"

Although it's always an unsatisfying reply, the answer will always be, "It depends." The individual and the dedication to applying the process plays a huge part in how quickly people can develop ability, but it ultimately comes down to how well you can learn to read and recognize those patterns of information.

The 4x4 seems like information overload, but for some context, I like to give an example of a study done on horse racing. The study looked at the effectiveness of horse prospectors—the professional gamblers who predict which horse will win a race—and their process for decision-making. The successful prospectors used a huge database of historical information to make their decisions—everything from the jockey, to the horse's lineage and racing history, to weather conditions, to the type of racing surface, and beyond.

Researchers systematically stripped away that mountain of data to the point where the prospectors could only make their predictions based on the five pieces of data they always looked at first. They ultimately found that although the prospectors' confidence levels in their predictions plummeted, their effectiveness didn't significantly change.

In my mind, this study tells two stories. First, time and experience collecting and analyzing all that data allowed them to identify the five most important variables driving their decision-making. Second, the barrier to efficiency was less about the amount of data they needed…and was more about their confidence. Prospectors had a blanket of comfort from a data surplus, but their effectiveness wasn't affected by their reduced confidence.

There are parallels in the health and fitness space. Some clinicians and trainers try to collect more data points to boost their confidence in their decisions, but end up lost without a hierarchy to process and prioritize it all.

Others on the opposite end of the continuum pride themselves on the efficiency of their processes, but haven't done the work to identify if the pieces of data they collect are the most important in driving better outcomes. Putting in the time to make this system of logic a consistent part of your practice is the only way to become both effective and efficient.

Through our journey constructing the Systems, we learned to recognize our mistakes—and to recognize them quickly. We had to train ourselves to be emotionally detached from the plan for that day if the feedback was pointing us in a different direction. All that mattered was using each session to narrow the gap between where our clients were and where they needed to be.

All of the steps and actions outlined to this point were intended to help you build a more effective model. As you progress to routinely performing the screens and checking the boxes of the 4x4, you'll recognize that the immediate feedback chips away at that larger aggregate of data you may have been previously collecting.

If it initially takes 15 minutes of your examination time, there's likely at least 15 minutes worth of things you could remove from your process that won't impact your effectiveness one bit. Dedicate a few months to sacrificing some efficiency to become a lot more effective, and your perspective will only sharpen to the extraneous things that can be stripped away.

Do we still follow all the steps outlined in the past 250 pages with every patient and client we see? Absolutely not. The better we became, the more fluid our approach became. We now know what we can skip and what our next move is based on the outcome we see.

But we've earned that opportunity because we built the screens and assessments and put them through the paces over the span of almost three decades. We can now use a fraction of the full process at any given time because, like those horse prospectors, we've learned what metrics provide us the greatest clarity and confidence in our decisions.

That's how standard operating procedures end up making things more efficient in the long run. By first making the process more effective, they provide time savings in the ability to remove unnecessary steps.

For those who follow the process as we've laid it out, efficiency comes at about six months. In the first month, proficiency with greater effectiveness comes quickly, and in the next four months you'll get smoother and tighter without losing your effectiveness. By six months, you're doing things as fast as ever…at a higher level.

Isn't that what happens to athletes when they go from amateur to pro? They're effective at a higher level of efficiency and they can reproduce it consistently. Even if you aren't where you want to be at the end of six months, take a look at your books and you'll see that greater effectiveness at the same level of efficiency will still have an effect on your outcomes and your business.

BE FIRM IN YOUR STRATEGIES, FLEXIBLE IN YOUR TACTICS

The strategies outlined thus far will make you systematic in how you view and approach your work. We've laid out a framework to guide you, but we aren't asking you to be a slave to the system or to change who you are. We want you to take what you're doing, plug it into the 4x4 matrix, and measure your results on the same scoreboard.

https://qrco.de/bcasLq

	Awareness	Protect	Correct	Develop
Production	Skill or Performance Measures	Remove Stressful Activity	Special Environment or Special Task	Re-skill
Fitness	Functional Capacity Measures	Remove Harmful Exercise	General Physical Capacity	Re-stress
Wellness	Movement Risk Factors	Remove Movement Risk Factors	General Physical Competency	Re-pattern
Health	Vital Signs	Remove Health Risk Factors	General Physical Vitals	Re-cycle

Take your current tools and techniques and drop them into the system. Look for those boxes on the grid where your knowledge or confidence is weak and seek new tools and tactics to make you more effective in that dimension. You can gain the confidence to experiment and grow, knowing that by reinforcing each layer from the bottom up, you're delivering holistic care.

New doesn't always equal better, not until it can measurably demonstrate itself as superior to what you're currently doing. Don't just take our word for it—put the 4x4 into practice in an objective and open way, and measure the results for yourself.

PART THREE: EXAMPLES

TURNING PRO

- Where are your opportunities?
- Do you have a strategy backed up by proven tactics?
- What does your business need—more resources… or more resourcefulness?
- How effective and efficient are you with the resources you have?

For a book titled *The Business of Movement*, it might seem like there hasn't been a tremendous amount of ink dedicated to "business." That's misleading. Specific business strategies are worthless (or at least unsustainable) if what you're trying to sell doesn't stack up to your competition.

Word of mouth is how we built most of the success we've achieved with Functional Movement Systems. That's purely a product of a lot of dedicated clinicians, trainers, and coaches who used the Systems to elevate their technical skills and refine their business practices before they went out to spread the word.

Becoming a better practitioner is the most important thing you can do for your business because 80% of your business success lies in being more effective than your competition at improving the lives of clients.

Just as with practical skills, we often ignore our areas of weakness and dedicate our efforts to learning business tactics to plug into what we're already doing, rather than focusing on strategies and ways to measure which tactics are the most valuable. If your practical skills are the weak link, any benefit gained from business or marketing strategies or tactics will be fleeting.

Implementing a new system such as the Functional Movement Systems into an established business can be painful. No success happens on a beautiful linear graph, and the thought of the time required to implement the systems thoroughly and completely may seem daunting.

If you haven't seen or experienced the System beyond just fixing a leg raise or changing a toe touch, you may not value it enough to take the next step in integrating it into a larger operating model for your business.

LEARN TO BE RESOURCEFUL

When there are challenges implementing the FMS—or really any new system—we often hear the excuse that there isn't enough time, enough money, enough space, or enough staff to succeed. Possessing more of those resources certainly provides more opportunities, but history is littered with the stories of failed teams, businesses, and individuals who had access to greater assets or capital and squandered it away.

A real or perceived lack of resources is a common explanation for most of the struggles people encounter, but we should be questioning whether we're being limited by a lack of resources or a lack of resourcefulness with what we already have. Rather than asking ourselves, "What more do I need?," we should be asking, "Am I working on the right things?"

If you found the perfect business strategy and added 40 new clients tomorrow, would you be able to maintain the same quality of care, exceed expectations, and continue growing? Or would it overload you and your team?

The growth and longevity of your business require more than a dollar analysis—you need a minutes analysis and a free will analysis to understand where misappropriated time and effort are preventing you from growing professionally and robbing you of your freedom. Sometimes you do need more resources. But what I've found is there's often something right under your nose that, if done differently, could change your world without a single extra piece of equipment or additional team member.

> Coach Jon Torine always likes to reference Tony Dungy, his former head coach with the Indianapolis Colts, who said, "When you think something is important, you'll make time for it."

It comes back to crafting your personal standard operating procedures.

In the early days of the aviation industry, despite the advancement of technology, plane crashes were a common occurrence. Rather than looking at it as purely an engineering problem, the proposed solution was to institute a pre-flight checklist as part of a standard operating procedure. They didn't change pilot instruction and they didn't overhaul the equipment. They simply added a few steps that seemed mindless and remedial. Within a year, fatalities from plane crashes were drastically lower without making a change in resources.

No matter how naturally talented you are, you need standard procedures because you'll forget things. It won't be the big things—it'll be the little things that only become important when the 1,000 other moving parts need to work together. Being consistently successful comes from automating the checks on those little things and initiating action rather than constantly reacting or overhauling your approach when human error or complexity suddenly creates a barrier to advancement.

Even though we all hold different positions, providing different services in different roles, we can all benefit from adopting a similar standard operating procedure. Despite everyone's professional journey being unique, we all proceed along close to the same line. Our common threads: Know your group, identify what won't work, establish awareness, deliver positive change that's always responsibly measured and is appreciable to your group.

YOUR PLAN WILL BE TESTED

Dr. Hulme's perspective on the splits in building a business described on page 105 illustrates those inflection points we all encounter. Our initial focus is tied to how we believe the world will perceive us and the false expectation that people will come to us because we possess the latest techniques or the most impressive gym or clinic.

For everyone, there comes a day when the excitement and expectation of how they expected things to go meets the more complex reality of the marketplace. Every medical provider isn't begging to refer their patients to you based on your credentials. Clients may come in because you have an impressive training space and a good marketing campaign, but they won't stick around if the experience and outcomes don't match the environment.

If you overcome those early obstacles and grow your business, at a critical point you'll need to build a team to meet rising demand. To expand the scope and scale of an operation, you'll need to make the difficult transition from being a practitioner to being a manager, and from a manager to a leader. Those who come into the health and fitness world expecting that path to naturally materialize without guidance or mentorship end up with a rude awakening.

Everyone building a business will encounter the same obstacles, albeit at different times. You can make it pretty far professionally without a systematic process to help navigate these transitional periods in your career, but each will challenge the resilience of your principles, values, and non-negotiables.

If the structure and processes you have in place can't withstand those challenging times to keep you on the right track, reactive decision-making will inevitably set off a chain reaction of compromises and potentially negative consequences.

In Part Two, we offered strategies for building a standard operating procedure to drive physical growth and adaptation for your clients. Part Three offers the same, but in the context of those who've applied those strategies to their businesses.

We benefit from others because we all drink from wells of knowledge we didn't dig; this portion of the book draws heavily from professionals who charted their courses by being more resourceful with the same resources everyone has. In each of these examples, the storyteller is looking upstream at problems and solutions. They aren't just measuring to be measuring. They're proactively managing risk before it's part of a professional standard operating procedure.

Sometimes it takes hardships in your practice to bring out your best—successful memories are fleeting, but painful memories stick around. Look back at your list of non-negotiables and know that each will be tested more than once in your career. Each time you'll have two options: compromise your core values or find a way to challenge your perceptions and your resourcefulness to guide you forward.

Following the path others have successfully traveled won't guarantee a journey without struggle, but it provides a better map to avoid getting lost along the way.

CHAPTER SEVENTEEN

MEASURE WHAT MATTERS

- ▶ What's the amount and quality of data you're collecting?
- ▶ What objective tools are you holding up against your actions to determine if you're overestimating or underestimating your effectiveness?
- ▶ How will you know when it's time to change your tactics or reevaluate your strategies?

Most business owners view the financial bottom line as the primary indicator of both the health of their enterprise and the effectiveness of their processes. It's hard to argue that making enough money to both sustain and grow a business isn't the most important metric. Revenue is an important data point, but rarely does it tell the whole story on the health of a business because it's also susceptible to influences outside of your control.

If you made a record profit in your business last year, was it because you're getting superior outcomes?

Was it because your patients and clients love working with you?

Was it because of the relationships you've developed in the community?

Those same questions could be posed if last year was a particularly bad year for your business; the theme is the same. Without data that measure the different qualities and dimensions of your enterprise, you can construct the "why" behind the trends you observe based on assumptions rather than evidence. The amount of money a clinic brings in can be an indicator of success, but it doesn't provide actionable information about which processes are having the greatest impact on that number.

Building a successful business is largely the result of viewing it as an engineer would—with a focus on identifying and addressing the weak links in systems and processes. Sound familiar?

It's easy for students in our courses to be intimidated by the volume of information presented and it's just as easy for business owners to be overwhelmed by the volume of data they're trying to process. We don't all have the ability or resources to process mountains of data, but we can all protect ourselves from overvaluing one data point at the expense of other important information. Are you allowing your personal biases or theories to convince you to act on potentially false assumptions? Or, based on limited data, are you convincing yourself you don't need to take action at all?

Striving to collect more data won't slow down a business. Done well, it will simply reallocate your attention and effort to where you need to work. If you reapply the same level of effort from one area to another, it costs no more time or money, and you can gather the feedback to know if you made the right choice.

Dedicating 15 minutes to talking with a patient and understanding the lifestyle behaviors around sleep or hydration may provide more actionable information than 15 minutes of testing range of motion and strength. In the worst-case scenario, you learn the person is positively supporting the recovery and you get to reinforce the importance of those behaviors. It's a rare occasion when you won't uncover other valuable information.

Spending even a little extra time implementing a smarter data collection strategy provides the best return on investment. The more thoughtful and pristine you are with the data you collect, the better you can manage each client and the whole of your practice from start to finish; the actions you can take are more informed as a product of tighter feedback loops. When you start collecting different metrics, it may take some time to hit a critical mass where you can appreciate what's valuable and what isn't, but the more reliable and the more robust your objective measures, the greater your awareness of where to dedicate your efforts for maximum effect.

TACTIC—Find and Fix the Foundation First

When people look at the movement screens, the testing we do, and our exercise library, they often don't realize that at any given time, we're only looking for the weakest link and the most effective exercise to change it.

Once someone flunks the leg raise, we don't worry about anything else. Once we see cervical pain on forward bending, we work to fix the neck before we fixate on another area.

All of our testing may produce data showing us that an individual is also weak, poorly conditioned, and lacking skill, but that's all data that might not matter today. The most fundamental risk is the greatest risk. It takes precedence…always.

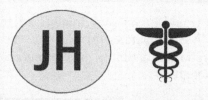

CLINICAL OUTCOMES—JASON HULME

Clinicians often hate that they have to collect and report a host of measures to show an insurance company why a patient needs their services. It's frustrating to feel like your value is tied solely to numbers on a page, and I'm sure there are therapists and chiropractors who'd choose not to collect any of those figures if they weren't required to do so. The insurance-driven health model has conditioned us to look negatively at a lot of data, but gathering and recording that information provides insights into how we're performing, and it also helps create awareness and context for a patient to gauge recovery.

I don't love that insurance companies mostly care about those numbers, but I'm always trying to do a better job of measuring and communicating progress to a patient. Once they get beyond showing someone the range of motion is better or strength is improved, too many clinicians rely on outcome surveys or subjective reporting from the patient to tell them they're doing a good job. I don't know a single clinician who hasn't been frustrated by patients focusing solely on the pain level or a single measurement as the indicator of how well they're doing. But that's because most patients only have the context for what they can physically feel or see—and often a short memory on where they began the process.

I was seeing success by helping patients understand their problems within the context of the movement screens from my first interaction with them, and I wanted to apply that same context to the larger picture of their physical status to merge the two. My primary use of the SFMA is always to help direct the path of treatment and the selection of interventions. By putting the assessment in a slightly different context and treating it like one more data point in a profile, it made it easier for patients to understand what "better" looked like from my perspective. By being transparent with patients about what we were clinically monitoring and valuing, we expanded our patients' awareness of the improvements they might not immediately see or feel.

We present a composite score from various movement tests alongside other metrics, like reported pain and the scores from a functional outcome form. That collection of objective data to measure change was summed like you would if you were totaling a letter grade in school. Someone with an A demonstrates pristine movement on their screens, no pain, and no reported disability, while someone with an F is bedbound and incapacitated.

Those findings dictate how we deliver care, but for the patients, it works as a quick snapshot of where they are relative to where they want to be. If we're doing it right, every time we do a reexamination, we're getting better data and a clearer image of progress to communicate, "Today you scored a C, but when you first came in, you had a D. Here are the areas that are better and the areas that still need work."

We had a college thrower in the clinic who'd been doing his rehab with us and was making great progress. His initial intake score on our sheet had him as a C+, and when we retested him at five weeks, he was a C-. His SFMA had now improved to nearly perfect. His FMS was better. He was beginning to work with significant exercise loads in the clinic. But his reported pain and his outcome assessment scores had gone down.

At first, his frustration was clear, but as we talked, it became apparent the scores reflected his self-assessment of activities in which he was noticing soreness or discomfort with activities he couldn't even perform before. It didn't take much to review all he'd been doing in the clinic, the improvements in his movement, and the gains he'd made in exercise intensity and volume. His self-reported metrics were throwing the picture askew, but that was the only metric he personally had to go on.

That scenario isn't unique to our practice, but shows how if you only focus on a patient's subjective reporting and don't have objective measures tracked and presented in an understandable way, you have to work hard to convince them of progress. You need to have these tools at your disposal because patients quickly lose track of where they were relative to where they are, and they fall victim to whatever story they're telling themselves. When they can see that snapshot, understand it, and realign their perception with the markers of progress, you can engage in better conversations and take more purposeful action.

That's where applying this process within the functional model shines—when you're trying to communicate and make difficult things familiar. Developing a system of your own for tracking patients' progress in a comprehensive but easily communicated and transparent way will help quantify your effectiveness and value.

Instead of spending your time trying to convince patients they're better or at least on the right track, you can separate the subjective and objective data to tell the full story of where each person is in the journey.

TACTIC—Everything in the Clinic is an Educational Opportunity

It's frustrating for therapists when doctors don't read their evaluations or progress notes to approve rehab visits. I realized early on that doctors wouldn't read a written narrative because they don't have time, but they're trained and often love to read graphs and charts.

I decided instead of a narrative, I'd send something visual that involved those areas I wanted to highlight, like range of motion, strength, or return-to-sport testing. At first, I just used an Excel spreadsheet and a color printer to show range of motion on a circular gauge like a chronometer, or a chart with red, yellow, and green to show where the patient was relative to normal ranges. Instead of being afraid they'd miss something important in the note or trying to impress them with fancy-looking graphics, I just wanted to educate them.

Providing something visual and easily digestible made it easier for me to justify whatever I needed to communicate. Whether it was slow progress or maybe that I was going to discharge early, I presented the data on one page, along with something simple like "X test confirms your diagnosis. Rehab is going very well. I estimate we're probably 50% through the recovery and will need about six more visits. If it's okay with you, I'd like to space those out and close the gaps shown above."

It was practically 100% foolproof. I developed deeper relationships with the doctors I worked with and developed new relationships as soon as I started providing those notes. I'm sure it wasn't because my outcomes were better than the other clinics in town. I just shared information in a practical way that educated them on what I was doing, and made them feel like an important part of the process.

See Appendix page 265 for an example.

INSTITUTIONAL OUTCOMES—MIKE CONTRERAS

When I was initially exposed to the FMS, I was running the wellness program at my fire station. I was also involved in running the fire academy and making sure new recruits were physically able to complete the training on the way to becoming full-time firefighters. By the end of my first FMS seminar, it became clear there was value on an individual level to optimize movement in the hope of keeping our firefighters healthy and resilient to meet the demands of their work. It was especially important to me because in both my station and the academy, we'd seen injury rates steadily going up and nobody knew what to do.

In the academy, we believed a lack of physical conditioning was the biggest predictor of failure, but all of our innovation in the physical training program didn't make a dent. We brought in a physical therapist to get our injured firefighters back in action faster, but that also didn't significantly change the trends in our injury statistics.

After the workshop, I made the decision to implement the screens, but in truth, it still took almost two years of using it before I could appreciate its full value. Part of that was tied to the fact that firefighters weren't required to participate in the wellness program and I had to do a lot of selling to get them to opt in to the screening and the overall program.

But I also personally had a hard time letting go of the view that better training would protect people from injury, despite the fact that our fitness and injury metrics were telling different stories. That was a bigger barrier to success.

Looking back, our scoring was bad, our setups were inconsistent, and there were a lot of missed opportunities in how we delivered the screens.

Luckily, we realized we were still collecting a different type of data that was producing valuable information as we saw people moving and feeling better. Because I was limited to working only with those who voluntarily participated, I didn't have clear or powerful enough information to demonstrate that value for everyone to adopt this approach at an organizational level. To make that larger change, I had to carry the banner myself and take advantage of the opportunities I could control.

Fortunately, because rank has its privileges, I had control over the 16 weeks of fire academy—each new batch of 30 recruits had to do what I told them to do. I implemented the FMS at the beginning and end of the four months…and tracked the changes. To keep it simple, I wanted to identify three groups: those who had 0s and were in pain; those who had 1s on the screen or a total score of 14 or below; and those who had a total score above 14. That approach allowed us to provide group correctives because, at scale, I could show three variations of one corrective exercise, but I couldn't effectively or efficiently show 30 individual correctives.

We realized the best use of our time and effort was to focus on those people in pain or with a low movement score so we could monitor them more closely and more effectively adapt their training. For everyone else, we could sprinkle correctives into the movement prep or provide targeted areas of focus as part of the warm-up to maintain the quality of movement, and then focus our efforts on promoting better movement through the physical training aspect of the program. We fine-tuned how we delivered the correctives and our training to fit each individual while allowing for the success of the group.

Fire Service Testing

***16 Weeks Prior to Fire Academy*:**
FMS screen, 1.5 mile run, physical agility test
Corrective/training program assigned

Eight Weeks Prior:
Retest, adjust program if necessary

Start of Academy:
Retest, academy fitness training to match the functional level

End of Academy:
Retest, work to establish a longer-term movement-focused program

FOCUSING ON A BETTER PROCESS PRODUCED A BETTER OUTCOME

We continued to collect and track the data, and then one day our risk manager informed us our academy injuries had gone down significantly. I didn't notice it at the time because my primary focus for almost two years had been to develop a robust training program—my primary metric was how many recruits successfully passed the academy. I knew our success rates were up, but when we reviewed the data collected across several academies and followed those who graduated and went into the field, we saw undeniable gains.

We looked at the original screen scores and the workers' compensation utilization from the time they got hired to roughly three years from when we implemented the Movement Systems. We distributed questionnaires that asked about behaviors and compliance with training and corrective interventions. Guess what we found? Those who scored a 14 or below on the FMS and didn't keep up the corrective and development behaviors to maintain the quality of their movement had injury rates and costs to the organization three times that of those who moved well.

The biggest takeaway was not that those with poor screens were more likely to get injured because just like football, the physical toll of being a firefighter means the likelihood of getting injured is about 100%. The important piece was that it showed that the 20% of those with poor movement screens and behaviors required a significantly greater amount of

resources than the 80% with acceptable movement screens and behaviors. That was valuable operationally, but we were also able to put dollar signs on the impact of the program. It then became easier to convince the people in charge of the larger significance. It totally changed how we looked at the Systems, how we implemented them, and where we could continue to compound our successes.

We saw these benefits from implementing the screens during the academy, but we asked, "What if we could intervene even earlier to get people on the correct path?" For the time and money dedicated to taking recruits through the academy, we needed to show a good return on investment by maximizing the number of people graduating.

Waiting until people got to the academy meant we might not be able to fully address issues we could have corrected ahead of time. I can design the academy's greatest training program, but if someone showed up physically unable to lift a ladder or if someone was super strong but couldn't move and efficiently apply that strength, not only were people more likely to get hurt, they were also more likely to wash out of the program.

So, 16 weeks prior to the start of each academy, we instituted a Fitness Fair where we'd meet with the next class of recruits to help them prepare for the rigors of the academy. We met with all the recruits, screened them, and identified those who needed a lot of work, those we needed to do a little work with, and those who could continue to do what they were doing.

Based on their problematic patterns, we gave people a training and corrective program with instructions of, "Do these seven things before you work out," and then screened them eight weeks before the academy. When they came back at eight weeks, their production went up: their power, their physical agility, their 1.5-mile run time. Then we gave them a little more to work on and tested them at the beginning of the academy and then again at the end of the academy. The positive results we saw across the board meant we had just written our new standard operating procedures.

THE DATA TELLS THE STORY

Institutional change rarely occurs without a clear financial driver, and although organizations talk about risk reduction, most don't take action until something goes seriously wrong. The additional data we collected demonstrated clear changes in functional and performance measures from 16 weeks before starting the academy, which provided two valuable things.

First, it justified the value of our pre-academy program by increasing the graduation success rate. Second, once it was part of the academy, it justified our physical training program because we were able to see a reduction in injuries both in the short and long terms.

Ultimately, the power of the model translated into less money lost to attrition from the academy, less money spent managing injuries and lost work time, and more money budgeted to expand and strengthen the program across the fire service.

Personally, that success translated into the creation of a separate business, helping organizations build risk-reduction programming through screening, data collection, developing an actionable plan, and then implementing it at scale. That work has produced data from close to 70,000 screens with around 400,000 data points that now help drive proactive risk reduction.

By focusing on processes and a system to provide clear, positive health, function, and productivity outcomes, our successes continue to compound over time.

ENGAGEMENT—JASON HULME

The average number of visits per patient or the number of visits to discharge are metrics most medical clinics look at for the bottom line. It used to be, the more we saw a patient, the more money we made, but things are now more complicated. Clinicians are increasingly incentivized by insurance companies to see patients for fewer visits—the story goes, if you're a great clinician, they'll give you more money the less time you spend with your patients.

You can't argue with the logic that a superior clinician should help patients get better faster, but the business model of an insurance company is to reduce their costs, and the endpoint from an insurance perspective is almost never the endpoint from a resilience perspective.

To that end, the term "medical necessity" is a made-up term—courtesy of those same insurance companies—to dictate a scenario to not pay that doesn't really have the patient's best interest in mind.

In my clinic, we've always valued getting people out of pain and moving with integrity as effectively and efficiently as possible. The lifeblood of a clinic is referral business. Working within the confines of an insurance model, my assumption was always that getting people better, faster meant they'd be happier patients who'd refer more patients.

When I looked back at our data, I found that the patients who got out of pain the fastest weren't necessarily the ones who sent the most referrals. It became apparent there was a direct correlation that those who were with us the longest sent us the most referrals. That didn't mean the most visits, just the longest duration of care.

It seemed counterintuitive that getting people rapidly out of acute pain didn't set their world on fire to refer their friends and family. But we found that those who got to the point of not worrying about bending, twisting and rotating, or lifting or pulling were the folks who sent us the most business. We came to realize it's not a race to discharge; it's a race to resilience. The more activity we can promote, the more robust people become, and the greater their resilience to pursue the things that bring them joy and bring them closer to those they love, and to their communities.

You can absolutely get someone better in five visits, but what's better? The pain? Their movement? I tell every patient, "You're going to feel 'better' pretty fast, and that's great. But we really want to not need to see you back here for the next two years…and between now and then, for you to send us 10 people."

MONITORING RESILIENCE

Maybe people feel amazing within four visits, but the conversation is that I can't discharge them until I know they aren't just better, but that they're well. That means in two weeks, I want them back for a resiliency visit where we make sure their screens are good and we take them through a workout. Hopefully, they crush it while they're here; we give them a high-five and schedule them to come back with an extra one to two weeks added each time to the point where we're following up every 12 to 16 weeks.

It can be a little scary for some clinicians because when the patient comes back in six weeks, they have to face the facts. Did they actually internalize true resiliency and life-changing behaviors or did they slide back to a sedentary lifestyle and regress? If that happens, we didn't really move the needle because they weren't able to sustain themselves.

Being invested in not just the health, but also the wellness of your patients means you can only measure your success on how well you prepare them to navigate future challenges.

Some clinicians will be afraid those patients will never come back or believe their patients would never agree to pay out-of-pocket for a visit like that. At some point, my patients all end up paying cash for wellness visits because I explain the value upfront. They end up being lifetime patients not because they need me, *but because they trust me.* When we have that relationship and an injury comes up, they're quick to come to the clinic and we can resolve things much faster versus being reactionary later after things get bad.

Instead of looking solely at how quickly you can get patients out of pain, try looking at the show-up rate for those patients on their two- or six-week resiliency visits. Patients continuing to come in as you open the windows of time and allow them to take control will give you the best indicator of the value you're providing. If people aren't getting better, they're going to find someone else to help them.

My success rate is measured by those people who continue to show up because I empowered positive lifestyle or fitness changes they can use to keep themselves out of pain.

TACTIC—Monitor Your "Show Up Rate" (Phil Plisky)

I think the best business metric to track, one I learned from a private practice owner, was what he called "the arrival rates" or "the show-up rate." That single number predicted the financial bottom line more than anything else. Some people look at the cancellation rate metric, but to spin it in the positive, he found that an arrival rate of over 93% impacted the financial bottom line more than other metrics.

Obviously, life will get in the way of client and patient consistency, but by monitoring that number on a weekly, monthly, and quarterly basis, any deviation from around 93% meant further analysis was needed. That global number could be an indicator for him to assess his processes and hopefully identify the trends or causes before they became systemic.

> *Right out of the gate, I tell every team and athlete I work with, "We have two goals, and the second one is improving your performance. My first goal is to keep you healthy and on the field."*
> **—Eric D'Agati**

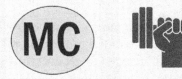

COMPLIANCE AND BUY-IN—MIKE CONTRERAS

If I had to break down how I've been successful, it's that I've been a firefighter for 30 years…and many of the people I work with are either also firefighters or utility workers who are similar. Firefighters need a certain amount of ego to cut a hole in a roof above a blazing fire in the same way a utility worker will climb a pole with 16,000 volts going through it. It takes one to know one; without sharing that experience, gaining their trust and confidence isn't easily done.

In my business, poor ankle mobility gives me as much information on the people who are at risk of injury as any dysfunction of the other patterns of the movement screen. For utility workers, the amount of strength, balance, and coordination required to climb and hang off of a pole on a one-inch spike and a rope is impressive. Full ankle mobility is the one thing almost every line worker needs.

Utility workers are on their feet all day, stuck in work boots, with tight calf muscles. Those three elements add up to locked ankles. That mobility restriction can impact every movement they engage in at work or at home. Due to the repetitive demands of the job, the only way to make a significant change is to make mobilization a component of that repetitive process.

I knew that to make an appreciable impact, the solution had to be so easy there was almost no excuse *not* to do it. Telling people with a physical job that they needed to carve out time to do a mobility routine before or after a grueling day of work was going nowhere. Short and frequent was going to be the best option, so we asked the crews to do a quick reset of calf stretching whenever they got out of the truck and to perform some cross-body reaching before climbing a pole. From those two simple actions, we measured drastic improvements in the resilience of the workers over three years of data. In the best year we had, we saw compliance from 78% of the 3,000 employees we screened. For context, if you can get anything over 50% compliance, most companies will pay you to come back every year.

MINIMAL EFFECTIVE DOSE

I could've dreamed up a much more extensive program to try to solve a lot more issues. But I knew 20% of the movement picture probably made up 80% of the problems, so I needed to get everyone invested and bought into addressing that 20%.

I didn't get that level of buy-in and compliance because everyone thought I was smart. I understood these guys—I was only asking them to do a couple easy things when they got in and out of a truck. But I realized if I were in their shoes, I probably wouldn't do it either. Because we shared a common mentality, I got them engaged by asking myself, "What's their *why*?"

Utility workers make a very good living doing their work, but their bodies end up broken. They have money and families, but their bodies are beat up. Even though they may look like a roughneck group, they're dads, brothers, and sons like everybody else. I know what it's like to be tired and sore, and then have to go back on shift.

Finding a plan that people would be willing to do consistently necessitated finding a minimum daily dose. We developed programs for 10 different companies that range from 10 minutes, to 20 minutes, to 30 minutes. I'm not convinced that 30 is better than 20, or that 20 with certain caveats is better than 10.

A lot depends on people's movement scores and the responsiveness of their nervous systems…and their consistency. But if I can convince them that 10 minutes of moving around means the difference between being able to enjoy their free time or play with their kids, it creates a much clearer return on the investment.

The screens and your programming don't exist in a vacuum—they offer an opportunity for awareness, education, and helping people connect the dots between movement and lifestyle. If we want to know whether we're making an impact on behaviors, we should monitor and track compliance with the lifestyle programming advice we dispense in the same way we do any other metric.

Screening is just a tool; people care less about the tool than how using the information will help make them feel better. It doesn't matter what the tool is saying if you can't translate the findings into something meaningful for your patients, clients, or athletes.

Tracking the willingness of people we work with to internalize our recommendations and change their behaviors is valuable because it acts as an informal measurement of how well we're connecting the value of our work to their lifestyles.

> There will never be 100% compliance, but there's always an opportunity to work on improving our delivery of education alongside our interventions.
>
> When we focus on ensuring that everyone understands what they're seeing or feeling in the context of the impact to the quality of their lives, we naturally see that compliance and buy-in increase. We magnify the benefits and durability of our work.

Impairments—Physical Limitations—Disability

Impaired body structures or physical limitations to performing an activity won't always drive people the same as losing the ability to participate or fulfill the roles in their lives.

If you have a bad knee that makes it hard to squat down, you'll find alternatives or work-arounds for a long time. But if you can't squat to be the catcher for your kid's baseball practice or you can't play the role of coach, athlete, or parent, you'll work a lot harder to find a solution to get you back there.

Risk factors are more than general projections. On a personal level, each creates and compounds limitations on our physical lives. Over time, we make conscious and unconscious choices to have a smaller physical life. One day, those limited physical experiences can reach a point of no return.

Find the opportunities to uncover those meaningful connections between a problem and the things people care about, and present your skills and abilities within that context.

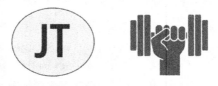

COMPLIANCE AND BUY-IN—JON TORINE

In athletics, the standard measure of a good or bad strength and performance team is typically the number of games or time lost to injury over a season. Coaches love when their athletes are getting faster or stronger, but the number one ability is availability. Keeping players in the game is the top priority for any team.

When I worked for the Indianapolis Colts, I literally lost sleep over that number. Part of the stress was knowing the number would ultimately be used to gauge my value to the organization, and part of my anxiety was because it's an inherently messy metric because it also captures things outside of your control.

In a game like football, injuries will occur, but the expectation is that an effective training program should minimize the incidence of certain injuries—like strains or overuse injuries. The expectation is that a well-performing rehab and performance team should be able to minimize the risk of those types of injuries and accelerate the recovery of those athletes who do inevitably get hurt.

While the coaching staff or organization may be measuring a strength coach's effectiveness primarily on that number, many strength coaches and trainers fall into the trap of trying to protect themselves by focusing their decisions and actions on improving that number at all costs.

They might agree to push an athlete back onto the field before ready, or they may take an overly conservative approach to training in the hope of avoiding too much added stress. They fixate on whatever it takes to keep that number as low as possible rather than focusing on all the other metrics telling them how effective they are.

However, the time or number of games missed isn't a measurement that tells us what to do. No, it's simply an indicator of the quality of the work we provide.

People often ask how to get a team or clients to buy into the Movement System approach. My response is to quit worrying about convincing someone to buy into your approach and just put it in action with everyone's best interests in mind.

We held players out after an injury longer than most other NFL teams because we had clear benchmarks in our return-to-play system. Our biggest concern was less on the initial injury a player sustained and more on the incidence of reinjury because each successive injury becomes more severe, and each period of recovery gets longer.

While the outside world and the media crushed us over how long we held guys out, the numbers at the end of the season showed that we had some of the lowest overall time or games lost in the league. We didn't make our decisions based on lowering that number to make ourselves look good—we based our decisions on putting the athlete's health first to meet the requirements needed to safely return and be productive on the field.

BEING TRANSPARENT WITH STANDARDS

We were consistent in testing and communicating to every player what their dysfunctional patterns indicated and why that put them on a path that looked different from the rest of their teammates in the weightroom or training room. We were letting the data we were collecting set our standard operating procedure, and once the players could appreciate our consistency in the standards and expectations, we started to see them take ownership of their scores and movement.

They asked to be rescreened, either because they felt better or worse, or they were sick of doing correctives instead of training with the rest of their teammates. At those points, we didn't need to do an exhaustive screen—we could do a quick screen that allowed us to progress a program quickly or justify why we needed to hold steady with the plan. In many cases, we began to see players checking themselves and making exercise decisions partly on their own because we had clear guidelines and options laid out based on how they were feeling and what the testing showed.

Rather than demanding codependency or a rigid system, we empowered the athletes to self-monitor and know if everything was good, off they went; otherwise, they knew what they had to do. We didn't start that way, but over time we created that culture and fostered a relationship of trust in each other because we were consistent in our message and process.

Movement and screening movement became a component of our player scouting assessment, our strength and conditioning program, and our return-to-play program with the medical team. I cared about monitoring and tracking players' movement scores just as much as their running times or weightroom numbers, but I cared more about their understanding of when their movement wasn't where it should be, and what steps they needed to take to recapture it.

By teaching this, we empowered them to take ownership when we weren't there. It allowed them to critically appraise their preparation before games and even their off-season programming because everyone was using the same measuring stick.

There's only so much control you can have over reducing or managing injuries, but you can absolutely control the systems and standards you establish. Set some standards for the outcomes you're hoping to achieve in health, function, or capacity, and then direct your focus toward how effectively your processes help clients and patients achieve and maintain positive change. Then you can see if the outcomes like production on the field, time lost to injury, or the recurrence of injuries change as well.

An effective system should tell you when you're the one negatively impacting the outcome at the potential risk of your ego. The screens were just one component within our larger system of feedback, but I have no doubt that the impact of my time with the Colts had less to do with how good I was at preventing injuries and improving performance and had almost everything to do with putting the athlete's success before my own and being transparent in constantly questioning and refining our processes and systems.

TACTIC—Rescreen at Natural Breaks in Activity
(Jon Torine)

The perfect time to rescreen movement is with a phase change in a training program. If you're a strength coach or a trainer with a periodized or tiered training plan, hopefully you have some kind of a deload or recovery week going into the next phase or shift in training. While you're turning down the degree of stress that week, you have the chance to see with a little more clarity what happened in those last four to six weeks of training.

To confirm your training program is working, movement should have a place alongside your metrics of strength, power, or speed. If your testing shows someone is running slower or strength hasn't budged, you'll be hunting for the reasons. There may be valid reasons for why someone doesn't make progress, but you should be prepared to acknowledge when it's something you're doing that's the culprit.

This is where that movement data point can sometimes act like the canary in the coalmine, warning that negative changes to function may be impacting capacity. Wouldn't you be interested in being the first to know if the whole team's shoulder mobility was regressing before they started showing up in the training room with pain? And wouldn't it be cool if you're the first to know so you could be the one to fix it?

Combining regular movement screens during those natural breaks or transitions in a training program along with informal screens for each athlete throughout the season is key. You have the opportunity to constantly question your program and check how well it's working for you...or against you.

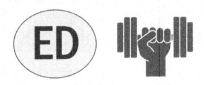

READINESS—ERIC D'AGATI

Make no mistake, instilling compliance and the behavior of self-management for people is hard. Not only do you have to provide a meaningful experience for them to understand why they need to make a change, you need to provide the tools and education so they understand what to do and how to check progress for themselves.

If we want to empower independence in any endeavor, we can't really accomplish that without providing people with a way to measure their own progress and ability. That's part of the reason telling someone what's wrong and what needs to be done doesn't often translate into action to make better lifestyle and activity decisions.

Think about a typical annual physical exam at the doctor's office. In a battery of tests, your blood pressure is taken, heart rate checked, and maybe your blood is drawn and analyzed. Despite the fact that those data points can change drastically from day to day and even hour to hour, a long-term plan is put in place. A medication is prescribed when one or more of those numbers are amiss, and the next visit to assess the merit of that plan is six months or a year in the future.

Some of those measures can't be easily self-assessed without professional help, but blood pressure or heart rate is something anyone can be taught to measure and understand at a basic level. With the explosion of technology for monitoring and tracking things like heart rate or activity level, there's almost no excuse not to educate and empower people to check these values on their own to gauge whether their choices and behaviors are working.

Movement is no different.

Every time you screen, you're capturing a snapshot of movement at that point in time. Physical therapists, chiropractors, and athletic trainers do this all the time—they check the range of motion of an injured joint or body part before and after a treatment session to measure if a change occurred. We understand the expression of movement can change rapidly and regularly, but too many times we base all of our decisions for a long-term training or treatment plan on an initial movement score.

If we believe that movement is an important signal of the equilibrium of health, function, fitness, and production, we should agree that regular measurement of movement should be a priority. But if we don't value that information enough to consistently collect it, why should we expect our clients to?

SCREEN EARLY, SCREEN OFTEN

Probably the most common question we hear in the FMS and FCS certification courses is, "How often do you re-administer the screens?" The somewhat unsatisfying answer is: Screen as often as it provides value to your decision-making.

Often a trainer or coach performs an initial intake FMS and maybe an FCS, puts the client on a corrective exercise and training program, and one of two things happens:

1. They progress to higher-level training and never retest that client until a problem arises.

2. They set regular time intervals to perform a rescreen, taking the client through the entire process, documenting the results, and addressing whatever they find.

You probably agree the first approach isn't as effective as the second. Testing once and then retesting only when something goes amiss is certainly more efficient from a time perspective, but it's purely reactive. It's like checking your blood pressure only once you start having chest pains. What you may save in an extra few minutes of occasional screening, you'll spend 10 times over trying to correct a problem that has grown to the point of creating obvious dysfunction or pain.

The second approach requires a more concerted effort to remain consistent, but regular screening means that even though you may not catch anything, you'll catch those percolating problems before they hit a full boil.

If your fitness client scored 1s on the active straight leg raise and the lunge pattern, you should be checking those patterns each session until they hit at least a 2.

Then, periodically checking in on those one or two patterns may be enough to ensure the positive adaptations are holding unless your eyes tell you it may be time for a full appraisal.

If someone initially demonstrates 1s on three, four, or five patterns, it will be far more valuable to consistently perform a full rescreen than waiting until you begin to see movement or production plateau or decline. But that still doesn't answer the question of, "How often should I rescreen?"

I've found it effective, at a minimum, to perform complete retesting at natural breaks. For athletes, it's at the start of preseason, some point in-season, and during the off-season. For the average fitness client, that might be when returning to training after a vacation or business trip. For any of those individuals, rescreening movement is critical when returning to activity after an injury or illness. A lot can happen to movement between natural breaks, but collecting that information and taking action even a couple of times a year is better than today's norm.

We should view the concept of acute and chronic movement adaptability in the same way we view tissue adaptability. Tissue can change rapidly, such as from a traumatic injury, and also chronically, as the product of hours and days and years of progressive training or, conversely, as the result of chronic inactivity or postural changes.

Movement can also change from the repeated expression of patterns and behaviors, but it can also change profoundly from acute, non-injurious events. I've seen football players who scored great on the FMS get the wind knocked out of them on a kick-off return, and the next day the ripples of altered function show up with breathing and shoulder mobility. Those changes can arise and persist from a less-than-one-second event. I want to know if two cross-country plane flights or two rounds of golf negatively affected my client's movement just like I want to know if a game or event affected my athletes.

Example Readiness Screen:

Top Tier of SFMA
Cervical flexion/extension/rotation, upper extremity reaching,
multi-segmental rotation/flexion/extension,
single-leg stance, overhead squat

Breathing Screen
Seated breath hold

Motor Control Screen
Lower extremity reach, upper extremity reach

**See Appendix page 353 for an overview of the SFMA.

TACTIC—Screen the Basics Every Time

If you do nothing else, screen breathing and basic mobility every time you work with a client or athlete—particularly mobility in the feet and ankles. Those key components set the stage for a productive training session, so why wouldn't you want to make sure the system is primed for success every time?

Better yet, teach your clients and patients how to screen and quickly correct those areas themselves. Detrimental changes can happen rapidly and result in a cascade of consequences if not caught quickly, so help them be that first line of defense.

SCREENING FOR READINESS TO TRAIN

If you work with athletes or those in a competitive environment, time is limited and risk is high; being able to quickly change course when indicated is key. You may only be able to formally screen an entire team of players three or four times a year to catch large variations through a season, but more actionable data requires more consistent, informal screening throughout the year.

The purpose of the movement screening is to get a baseline and see if there are modifications to make to your program. Even though a screen should take less than 12 minutes, it can be cumbersome or excessive for most professionals to implement if you only have 30 or 40 minutes in the session.

If I screened someone once and then the person played 36 holes of golf, took a red-eye flight, got in a fight with the spouse, and fought traffic before arriving at the gym, a lot of things could change not just in movement, but in the bigger picture of the nervous system. The training program was written based on where the client may have been a week ago, but if I don't know where things stand today, this person might not be ready for what was planned. The best corrective intervention today might actually be stopping the workout altogether.

In the words of strength coach Joe DeFranco, "You need a long-term plan, not a long-term program."

The long-term effectiveness of a training plan and the long-term success of people reaching their goals comes from a flexible approach instead of being a slave to a program. Proceeding with a training session based on what's written on a piece of paper over what you can see with your eyes or measure with tests is probably the number one reason people end up hurt from training. The "all out all the time" mentality needs to go unless you want to be the best referral source for your local medical professional.

Between formal screenings, don't assume all is well. Every day, the world is undoing your work. Once a baseline level of function is established where you're confident in a client or athlete's ability to tolerate training, on any given training day you need to efficiently determine the ability to absorb the stress.

A quick snapshot of how people are moving and their state of readiness lets you know if you can push the envelope in that session or if you need to modify or scrap Plan A in favor of Plan B.

That's where leveraging a daily readiness screen can indicate when things are looking good and it's safe to accelerate, and when to dial it back on the days that the feedback tells us things are off. Rather than performing a full FMS screen, in five minutes you could do something like the top-tier movements of the SFMA, a 30–40 second breathing screen, and a motor control screen to detect early signs of trouble.

You might choose to add other measurements like heart rate variability or another readiness metric and at the very least, you'll have a better collection of objective physical data to use alongside the subjective input of the person.

I view that quick screen as providing immediate feedback that:

- Everything looks good and feels good—I can proceed as planned.
- There's something I'm not comfortable with—whether that's a dysfunctional movement or pain—that I can break out and try to address with correctives.
    - If everything improves after the correctives, I can proceed with the plan after having taken that slight detour.
        - If I find single-leg balance is off, I can look at the lunge pattern. If a toe touch is limited, I can look at the leg raise. If mobility at the neck, spine, or shoulder is limited, I can work to restore that freedom of motion before putting weight on the client's back or pushing things overhead.
    - If I don't see improvement, today's plan needs to be adjusted or scrapped because nothing good will come from hammering a square peg into a round hole.

This is the green, yellow, red-light system in action. This may seem excessive, but if you come prepared with an idea of what a green, yellow, or red exercise or workout could look like that day, you have three paths to follow that may require a short diversion, but never risk your long-term success.

It can be deployed when delivering a treatment or training session or as a quick assessment before games and warm-ups just to make sure all systems are a go. Recognize when the data is telling you to protect, to proceed with caution, or to proceed as planned.

Measuring readiness and teaching people how to measure that readiness themselves allows you to build a flexible but resilient structure to your operation. Instead of just asking people how they feel before training or participating in a sport, you have an opportunity to meet athletes where they are that day through a little objective data.

Using that simple, real-time feedback loop doesn't require breaking out testing kits or doing elaborate formal testing, and it can give you additional context to say, "Today we need to be willing to bend so we don't break."

Think about it this way: During a sports season, how likely are you to cause a significant improvement in an athlete's performance or ability on a night-to-night or week-to-week basis? Are your actions more likely to produce a positive or negative impact? When you realize the risk-to-reward ratio is more dependent on risk reduction, you'll act accordingly.
—Jon Torine

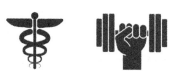

PUTTING MEASUREMENT INTO PRACTICE

Having confidence in the data and the indicators you collect and follow is the first step in learning to operate with a more holistic, data-driven mindset. There's no single metric that's the "best" or the most valuable relative to the others because all are inextricably linked. Changes in one metric can impact others, and those impacts might not be felt or seen in the short term. Fixating on a single measurement as the indicator of your effectiveness can leave you blind to the future effects on the health and resilience of your business.

The long-term success of a training program, professional practice, or business operation is less a reflection of the mapped-out plan, and more a reflection of the processes behind the decision-making. Even the most masterfully crafted training program or business model can fall apart because you can't predict where or when variables may insert themselves.

When you know the outcome you want to achieve and can convert your process into a series of questions with binary answers, the path becomes straighter because your decisions are more directed.

THE FMS DECISION TREE

Seeing it in print may make it seem complicated, but it's a simple branching logic tree. When you start from the top, the progression tells you when to stop or proceed.

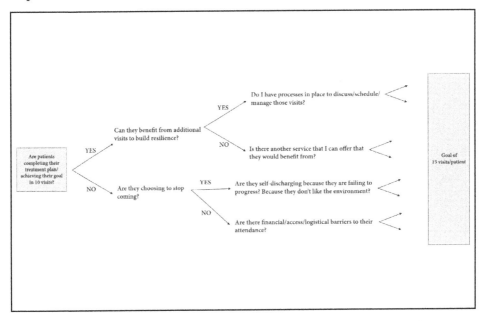

If your process isn't asking these questions, you may be able to skip steps, but you also run the risk of having to backtrack multiple times to discover where you left the path. Starting that process from the top allows you to build a database of relevant information for better decision-making as those decisions become more complex.

You're doing the equivalent of the pilot's checking and confirming of flipped switches and turned knobs before takeoff—following a standard operating procedure to support the complicated decisions to be made once the plane is in the air.

As you put together the questions to ask to develop your process, think about the types of information you're able to collect along the way.

The data point may be the same as the outcome—say, improving the number of visits per patient from 10 to 15. Rather than trying to come up with the perfect plan to get there, think about the questions between those two numbers. What are the assumptions you can test? What are the metrics that will produce the answers to inform your actions, and what's the minimum value of each metric you're willing to tolerate as the threshold to answer "Yes" and move forward?

Physical Data	Organizational Data
Pain Behavior (including SFMA)	Show-up Rate
Range of Motion	Compliance Rate with Visits and Overall Plan
Isolated Strength Testing	
Balance Testing (YBT or MCS)	Number of Visits per Client
Functional Testing (including FMS)	Number of Referral Sources and Referrals per Month
Capacity Testing (including FCS)	Revenue per Visit, per Client
Skill and Performance Testing	Games Lost to Injury
Time to Recovery and Return to Play	

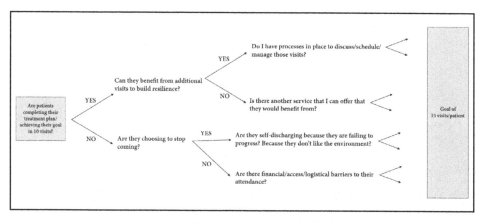

https://qrco.de/bcasLp

Working through a process like this should illuminate the assumptions that lack supporting data. When you encounter unknowns, you need to gather the information that will let you make the most informed decision.

We can't stress enough that the exact tactics or tools you choose are secondary to the strategic process you have in place to show you the way. The most successful professionals understand the margins when their data tells them to limit their exposure to the risk and when to take advantage of an opportunity to grow and adapt.

Recognizing those guardrails will keep you on the right path as you fill in the process with the best tools and tactics that produce measurable change.

OPPORTUNITIES FOR CHANGE

- ▶ Understand where you are and where you want to be as an outcome.
- ▶ Find opportunities to visually present your process to aid in your decision-making.
- ▶ Question your assumptions.
- ▶ Collect information from a variety of sources (patients and clients, your business, yourself) to verify or discredit those assumptions.
  - ▶ The more data, the clearer the picture. The more frequent the data collection, the more responsive and adaptive you can be—but you just need enough information to reduce risk and move forward.
- ▶ Set minimum benchmarks or checkpoints to guide your decision-making (if this = _____, then I _____).
- ▶ Fight to remain objective—remove yourself (your ego, assumptions, and opinions) from the decision-making as much as possible.
- ▶ Find opportunities (planned and impromptu) for full reassessments of your data or quick readiness screens to confirm you're staying on track.

CHAPTER EIGHTEEN

BUILD YOUR COMMUNITY, CHANGE YOUR CULTURE

- ▶ Is there a need in your community that's not being filled by another professional?
- ▶ What's your unique role in your local ecosystem of professionals?
- ▶ Have you cultivated relationships and resources with other practitioners in your market?
- ▶ What good is a community if you have nothing to share with it?

One of my core beliefs is that providing the greatest value in a health and fitness business isn't about selling supplements, gadgets, or apparel, or offering more services to capture more revenue. Instead, it's about building and strengthening your network.

That doesn't always align with many professionals' view of the field. The ways in which professionals are marketed makes us believe the competition is always looking for an advantage to take us down. That has fostered an environment where professions spend more time trying to protect their sphere of influence and trying to limit the scope of what someone else is allowed to do instead of fostering collaboration and an exchange of skills and information.

Our shared goal should be to be of service to our patients, clients, and athletes. My intent in developing the functional screens was to find a common connection in movement so we could all speak and understand the same language… and appreciate the value of each person's contribution toward that goal.

The growing network of movement professionals sharing their knowledge and methods around the world is something I'm incredibly proud of, but I've never asked anyone to be an evangelist for FMS. The success of those who adopted the Systems is a product of keeping good records and giving everyone the opportunity to benefit from their skills and knowledge.

Rather than asking, "What's in it for me," they looked around their communities and asked, "Is there a need I can address? Or is there someone doing it better whom I can learn from?" You'll own the market in your zip code when you understand where you can demonstrate value and where you can share and expand your expertise.

Approach building a community or network like a CEO would approach cultivating a board of advisors. Can you find the people in your community to provide skills and strengths complementary to your own, and also allow you to elevate your weaknesses? Can you find other trainers, coaches, or clinicians who value what you offer and with whom you want to work?

Be picky about those you choose to do business with—and hopefully they'll feel the same. Your reputations will be tied together, which is why finding people who share an understanding and appreciation for movement and the Systems can be so effective. Even though you all may be in different businesses or engaging with movement in different ways, common communication and the same quality control processes can align you in pursuit of a shared goal.

TACTIC—Expand Your Network

You can use *functionalmovement.com* to find like-minded professionals in your area who are already part of the FMS tribe, but finding those who already share a common language of movement should only be the start.

The greatest opportunity to learn and continue to expand your base of knowledge is by finding other qualified professionals in your immediate area who have complementary skills and offerings, but may not have been exposed to the Movement Systems.

Send an email. Introduce yourself in person. Grab a cup of coffee or a beer to sit down and learn their unique perspectives.

Not every attempt will result in a lasting friendship or referral source, but every attempt presents the opportunity to challenge your perceptions and systems. You might even create a ripple effect for people you'll never meet who will benefit from a new perspective on movement that you shared with an open-minded peer.

We work hard at finding people who speak our movement language because if we refer someone to a trainer or sports coach or they send us a new patient, we all have the confidence to say, "Here's the limitation we need to work on."

If you're a clinician discharging a patient to a fitness professional, you can feel more comfortable letting someone with a 1 on the push-up sneak out of your office because that's often a legitimate strength deficit and not a dysfunction, and you may not have time in the clinical picture to fix it. If you're a trainer or coach with an injured client or athlete, you can refer for treatment knowing the problem you uncovered will be addressed appropriately so you can do your work. Having the confidence, openness, and transparency in communicating the same strategy with every professional you refer to means everyone moves in the same direction as we take action.

LEVEL UP YOUR PEERS

Unfortunately, there may not be another professional in your community with experience using the Movement Systems. As you become more systematic and confident in your process and results, you'll also feel more comfortable educating your community. Support those people who are trying to use the FMS, and invest in helping level up your community. You have the opportunity to be a leader. The culture and systems you've built internally can create a massive impact if you liberate them beyond the walls of your gym or clinic.

For Dr. Hulme, this idea led him to question why there wasn't a systematic way for the athletic trainers in his region to know when to refer to medical professionals and when they could manage the treatment themselves. He identified a few coaches who'd been exposed to the FMS and YBT through different sports academies and approached them.

He started doing in-services for the athletic trainers in his county and doing group screenings on those teams where coaches already had some context on the screens. He found that many of those athletic trainers had already been through one of our training courses, but they weren't implementing the screens due to barriers they encountered in their work.

He started donating his and his staff's time to assist with coordinating team screenings, putting together the data into reports, and outlining ways to run group coaching and correctives. It became part of those teams' warm-ups and training programs—and certain teams flourished. It became a good thing in the community for everyone to be on the same page. It made the athletic trainers more effective in their role, reinforced the value of movement for the coaches, and positioned his practice as a resource for them all.

There are undoubtedly untapped opportunities in your local area where you can help elevate the skills of the professionals with whom you want to work, even if it's nothing more than forming a professional network for brainstorming ideas.

Actively sharing your unique experience and knowledge with your peers doesn't require additional money or staff, and it can spread like wildfire through your entire community.

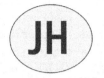

PROVIDE VALUE TO YOUR REFERRAL SOURCES
—JASON HULME

I can only imagine the amount of ink that's been spent explaining ways to get patients, clients, or athletes through your doors. When starting a business from scratch, some 90% of the effort goes into finding people to work with and finding the right connections who will send those people to you. Marketing is a profession unto itself!

There are plenty of tactics to deploy in driving new business, but the long-term stability of an operation is built on the strength of your referral strategy—a referral is the strongest form of marketing you can have. A referral will beat out the fanciest advertisement almost every time because people are generally unwilling to risk their reputation with a personal connection if they don't believe there's value in the recommendation.

When you're new to an area or lack the history or success stories to distinguish your value from the rest of the market, instead of just asking for someone's business, you need to establish a value.

When I first started my clinic and was marketing to medical providers, I believed that when primary care physicians saw musculoskeletal cases in the clinic, they were befuddled and hated working with them because they didn't have a way to treat them. I thought they'd look at me and say, "I've got five people to send you per day—thank you so much for being here." That couldn't have been further from the truth.

They thought they had things covered. For many musculoskeletal conditions, doctors work off an algorithm of their own, which is to first provide a muscle relaxant or anti-inflammatory medication. If that doesn't work, they go to a steroid dose pack. If that doesn't work, either get an X-ray or MRI, or go straight to an orthopedist or therapy. End of algorithm.

If you're a chiropractor or manual therapist, where do you fit into that equation? If you're a physical therapist, how are you differentiating yourself from the rest of the market?

The only way to be successful is to insert yourself into the narrative and become part of the algorithm.

When others in my geographic area said, "Don't bother talking to Dr. X, Y, or Z. They have physical therapy at their clinic; they're never going to refer to you." That, to me, was a small-minded approach. We got a foot in the door by saying, "We look at this with a holistic approach to full-body movement. We want the cases you've already said are nonsurgical, those you've sent to your in-house PT but who came back because they weren't progressing. Those are the patients we want."

We had a specific ask when approaching the doctors, not realizing how frequently that was a problem. Then we built trust by sending those patients back with measurable improvement.

TEACH SOMEONE A MOVEMENT PERSPECTIVE

Having confidence in the ability of our clinicians and asking for the hardest patients got us in the door, but the most effective tactic in providing value was to teach the primary care providers one to three of the movements in the SFMA.

We asked them about the most common musculoskeletal cases they saw in the clinic, which was most often low back pain, headaches, or neck pain. Before we jumped into a solution, we first asked them to help us understand how they looked at those cases from the pharmaceutical side so we could understand the different management aspects—what worked and what didn't work.

We asked them to educate us, and then we got to educate them. We suggested, "If a patient comes in with neck pain, ask them to extend their chin to the ceiling. We found from our internal data that if the chin and forehead aren't within 10 degrees of the horizon and they have pain or just can't do it, we can help dramatically." We inserted ourselves into the treatment narrative by giving them one quick test they could use to realize, "That's limited. You're the perfect person to go to Jason's office. This is his specialty."

All it takes is giving them one or two simple movements or a breakout, explaining what dysfunction can look like and all the other areas it can affect when present. It takes just one patient you can send back better, and that doctor will start to get on board with the functional model. You can create that initial loop for them to think, "If I see _____, that patient would benefit from going to _____."

A great side effect was that some of the doctors wanted to engage more deeply to understand how they could take a more active role in addressing functional problems. By helping them to better identify dysfunction within their exams, we ended up with more patients than we knew what to do with because we'd established a clear value in multiple ways.

And those doctors who were skeptical? They're getting marketed to every day of the week from different providers. Using the same narrative with a different slant helped us become a better connection.

I let them know I wasn't trying to step on their business or their existing relationships with providers. I showed them the same one or two tests and asked them to use the same test for challenging patients, send them to therapy, bring them back into the clinic, and retest.

I said I'd be back in a few weeks and would just be curious if they measured a change. If they saw a change, awesome—that meant folks they were working with were getting results. If there was no change (and I can't tell you how often they realized those patients came back exactly the same)—that's where I could show how I was different.

You can provide a better feedback mechanism with one or two simple and clear objective measures that help people cut through the subjective pieces that can cloud outcomes and also tease out the practitioners getting results. When we started to video record patients through their SFMA assessments and reassessments and took the videos to their referring providers, they were shocked by some of the outcomes we were getting.

When speaking to other providers, you ultimately have to *show* your value, not "tell" them. Everyone tells their referral sources their patients are getting better or they try to articulate a fancy or unique technique they're using. But being able to show a doctor one of the patients moving better and smiling is much more powerful than the best sales pitch you can dream up.

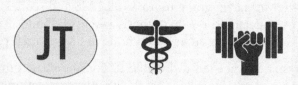

TRANSLATE DIFFICULT CONVERSATIONS—JON TORINE

When I was with the Colts, we performed formal movement screenings along with physical exams early in the off-season. We once signed a player from another team, a guy our doctor had cleared to practice after his physical exam. After our movement screening and other physical testing, we didn't like what we saw in his movement. At that point, we'd been doing the screens for a couple years, and what we saw with this player wasn't adding up. I went to our coaching staff and said, "Don't put this guy on the field. I think he's going to get hurt. Here's what our testing showed—here's what we know and what we don't know." Unfortunately, my message arrived a little late, and very early in practice, he got hurt.

Our team doctor came to me after practice when he heard the concern I'd expressed to the coaches and said, "I passed this guy on his physical exam, but you said he was going to get hurt. How did you know that?" I'd known this doctor for years. We had a great professional relationship, but I'd never fully explained the FMS and the testing we were doing. We didn't have a crystal ball, but had collected a lot of numbers to support our decisions and boost our confidence. I explained how we'd been implementing the screens into our work and why the results we saw pointed to an injury risk.

I asked him, "What made you pass him on his physical?" I'd never seen a true orthopedic medical exam and, at that point, I didn't realize how limited and "parts" driven it was. Passing the athlete largely relied on moving his arms and legs around, doing some manual muscle testing, and asking him to jump on one leg. Because the player said it didn't hurt and time was tight, the doctor gave him the thumbs up to practice right away…and that was it.

It wasn't an excuse—it's just a way of life in the NFL where getting players on the field is priority one. He immediately said, "If you have a better way of looking at this, I'm all for it."

Our team doctor had the perspective that if we had a better tool that could help before a guy went on the field or had a physical, he wanted us to be that first line. He didn't ask or need to know what a 1, 2, or 3 meant—he was never going to do a full FMS and score a player. He just needed to understand our hypothesis when we found dysfunction with this tool we were using so he could hone in on potential problems.

To do that, we needed to be able to communicate our language into terms he could use. He asked that if we noticed something, we write it up and get the message to him before the physical. It was rudimentary—simply saying we suspected a lower back or ankle to be the cause of dysfunctional movement. When the player was in front of the doctor, he could start from a better clinical model and be more targeted toward what he may not have otherwise looked at as closely.

Over time, he learned to appreciate the screens on a deeper level. We were able to work more effectively as a team from that first opportunity to translate the FMS for another professional. From there, the screen became part of the program—how we looked at players before we put them on the field; how we looked at free agents and rookies before bringing them onboard, and how we designed our team's training programs. Instead of being separate from the medical team, the strength and conditioning team became a vital part of it.

Align on a Plan with Other Professionals

There aren't many environments that are as outcome-driven as professional sports. Anything that can be seen as a competitive advantage or offers immediate benefits can take hold pretty quickly. I've done a lot of work training high school athletes, and it's largely the same story at the amateur level, although the impulse for adopting certain tools can be a little muted if the incentive isn't immediately clear.

In one case, I had an athlete who'd been cleared to train following a shoulder surgery. As I screened him, it was apparent he still had pain and poor movement, which meant I had to have a difficult conversation with him. He wasn't ready for me as a trainer, and I wouldn't train him until he was pain-free.

As I explained my reasoning, I discovered the kid stopped attending physical therapy after his therapist cleared him to train. That meant I had to talk to the therapist so I could understand his process because the athlete in front of me was still showing residual signs of surgery.

I called the therapist and said, "I just screened this athlete, and I think he needs more time with you. Even though you cleared him, I don't think he's ready."

I had to have the second difficult conversation with the parents about why his training was on pause. But…we sent him back to PT.

In a couple weeks, before he finished with therapy again, I spoke with the therapist and let him know I'd screen this athlete when I saw him again, and if he wasn't ready the second time, I'd send him back to therapy. This created a dialogue between us because he was familiar with the FMS, but had never thought of it as a part of his discharge process.

Once we established that connection where we were speaking the same language, everything worked out and that PT became a guy I referred people to, and he referred people to me as well.

Many people would look at that as calling out a PT and telling him how to do his job, when all I did was call and say the kid was still in pain. If I see pain with the simple movements of the FMS, I'd rather that person work with a medical professional instead of me—a strength coach with no medical background.

Putting both of our egos aside and working as professionals benefited everyone, and the Systems allowed me to work with a professional I didn't initially know because we found a common strategy.

When you can teach someone how to read the language of movement and help translate it into a particular role or skill, you're reinforcing the links between the layers of movement and fostering a stronger bond in your professional network.

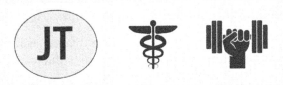

CONNECT WITH COACHES—JON TORINE

The greatest challenge in translating the screens into sports or skill training is that coaches and professionals in that world look at most things through the lens of an athletic test. The FMS doesn't look like an athletic test. The FCS has athletic movements, but it's easy for the pieces of the motor control screens or the loaded carry to confuse coaches or scouts when the best athletes don't always have the best scores.

We know those athletes with the best athletic measures don't always stay healthy or develop into the highest performers on the field, and yet the metrics that still get the most attention are who can lift the most, jump the highest, or run the fastest. Without a tool to reconcile those weightroom and on-the-field observations, many athletes are written off as lacking intangibles or not being coachable, when in reality, they may not currently be able to express their full athletic potential.

Basic physical literacy is the underpinning of those athletic movements. Having good shoulder mobility or control doesn't make someone an athlete who can throw or pitch well, but if that person can't demonstrate those qualities, the throwing and pitching potential will never be fully realized. We still need to teach the specific skills of pitching, but teaching works best when the person on the other end is there to receive that instruction.

Instead of coming to a coach and saying, "I'm here to fix your athletes," we're saying, "Here's what we can add to your repertoire," thereby acknowledging the tools and tactics that allowed them to succeed.

In football, about half the time, coaches are yelling at players to get their hips down to achieve a lower stance. If the cueing or coaching or yelling isn't working and the athletes are giving their best efforts, either there's a problem with the teaching or the athletes physically can't do what's being asked.

What if they can't get into a deeper squat because of a restricted ankle or a dysfunctional hip? What if a wide receiver can't rotate to catch a ball or change direction well when running a route because the spine and hips can't respond in harmony?

Basically, coaches scream about what athletes can't do or question their intelligence or commitment because they don't have a tool to identify when the problem lies in the fundamental ability to achieve a posture or execute a movement.

When I visit teams and universities, I spend most of the day bringing different staff together around a common system of screening, just as I did with our Colts team physician. I ask the coaches to let the performance staff work with a struggling athlete for a few minutes a day—not promising to fix a problem, but allowing them the chance to identify a possible movement limitation and remove barriers to success.

When the performance staff can identify the struggling athletes whose barrier to learning a sports skill is actually dysfunctional movement, and can then demonstrate a visible improvement in how an athlete moves and responds to coaching, it takes a lot less convincing the coaching staff when it comes time to implement a larger movement-focused strategy.

TACTIC—Volunteer Your Experience (Mike Contreras)

Whether it's connecting with players and coaches, firefighters, soldiers, or tactical athletes, our business begins with relationship-building. Very few people turn down free. Opportunities will always be available to volunteer and provide repetitions to learn as long as you can demonstrate a benefit.

Getting outside your clinic or facility to present education, workouts, or self-care services is necessary to break into competitive or athletic environments, but you first need to break through the culture. Meeting people on their level and embedding yourself into the culture of athletics or of a firehouse provides a better perspective of what they need to do and the challenges in their way.

However you can, seek out the environments or groups where you hope to make an impact and engage with the physical culture you find. Before you try to implement some grand design or new strategy, you have to develop the trust that comes from a good will offering of your help and support.

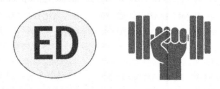

CONNECT WITH COACHES—ERIC D'AGATI

When I first began consulting with pro sports teams, I wanted to be non-threatening because the teams didn't have anyone on staff looking at movement from the angle of the FMS. I wasn't there to be the athletic trainer or the strength coach—I was there to look at movement and help the two communicate with one another.

They wanted to keep players healthy and make people stronger and faster, with just enough cross-collaboration to keep things moving smoothly. My role was to help figure out a clean system linking their efforts where they might not have the time or ability to do it on their own.

When I had the opportunity to consult with the New York Giants football team, I didn't tell anyone what to do—I just asked that the staff of both the training room and the weightroom try to apply the same grading and appraisal of the movement system to see if we could all agree on the "whys" behind a player who couldn't squat or one who pulled a hamstring.

Even though they were approaching players from opposite ends of the movement spectrum, they could more easily meet in the middle and see opportunities. That almost immediately created a better working relationship because they recognized the unrealized potential in better handling the athletes transitioning between rehab and training.

Today, most professional sports rehab teams have adopted a more movement-focused approach to injury prevention, but even still, more injuries are being viewed through the lens of load management rather than restoring functional movement.

Coaches and players believe they can keep the tread on the tire longer if they don't take the car out of the garage as much, without considering that if the wheels are imbalanced, they'll wear out faster either way.

Link Your Findings to Production + Performance

Many relationships I've forged in sports developed from fostering a connection of the Systems back to athletic performance. I'd watch coaches working with athletes I'd trained and would look for those moments when they struggled getting a concept across to a player.

For example, a pitcher was struggling trying to get his body over his front leg. I suspected dysfunction was impacting the movement; during a break, I spoke with the coach off to the side and said, "I don't think he has the ability to do that."

Once I explained my reasoning, the spotlight was on me to do something about it...or risk losing credibility with this coach. Screening a single movement pattern—but specifically the active straight leg raise—showed how the athlete lacked the control to feel how to properly hinge his hips.

I ran a couple of quick correctives to get him to understand how to better hinge his hips, and magically, he could do what the coach was asking. It wasn't about showing the coach how to coach, but how to recognize when the coaching might be falling on deaf ears. I was showing him a new tool he could use to do something about it.

As a trainer or strength coach trying to develop relationships with sports or skill instructors and coaches, your goal should be to provide a client who's a malleable ball of clay, ready to apply the coaching they receive. You need to help other professionals avoid wasting their or their athletes' time getting good at bad reps. Taking 200 repetitions a day is only beneficial if it's reinforcing a good fundamental skill. If not, athletes are just getting tired, and worse, perfecting a bad pattern.

The Movement Systems also allow you to become more critical when you see skill coaches in action. You'll recognize those who are just running drills with no real emphasis on the teaching aspect versus those actively tailoring the approach based on what they see.

Effectively teaching a skill is accomplished the same way as effectively retraining a movement pattern: by scaling the difficulty and complexity of the task to find the threshold for success. Providing those coaches and instructors with the tools to recognize when a barrier to success is a conceptual roadblock, a mobility limitation, a lack of stability or control, poor patterning, or a limited capacity can make you a valuable resource and a trusted referral.

TACTIC—Networking Works

> Even if you're professionally hyper-focused on a single level of physical growth and adaptation, it's shortsighted not to recognize that using a team approach is often in the best interest of your client. This will reflect positively on you as the coordinator of these resources.
>
> Depending on your skill set, have at least one health professional to call on for the clients who present with pain or health concerns, one wellness professional to address risk factors and act as the gatekeeper to fitness, and one fitness professional, performance professional, or skill coach for those clients whose goals lie in higher dimensions.

THERE'S STRENGTH IN A TRIBE

The world would have you believe everyone is your competition in pursuit of success because it considers making the most money as the desired result. I've worked with enough professionals to know those who thrive aren't those treating every other therapist, chiropractor, trainer, or coach as an enemy, or those trying to squeeze every last dollar out of their clients. Those who succeed all understand the power of the tribe and building and sharing a culture that's collaborative, integrated, and dynamic in serving the needs of a community.

If you can provide for the needs of your client base by building and strengthening your network, you can grow into something larger, more stable, and more diversified than anything you could have constructed on your own.

OPPORTUNITIES FOR CHANGE

- Find those open-minded, like-minded professionals in your community.
- Foster a collaborative relationship by providing them value and, in turn, gaining a resource for your clients.
- Believe that being of service and leveling-up your network and community fosters long-term growth for you and your peers.
- Create opportunities to learn and grow together.

CHAPTER NINETEEN

BUILD YOUR TEAM

- ▶ What are the values you look for when choosing someone to add to your team?
- ▶ What would it take for your team to make the same decisions you would?

To grow personally and professionally, you need to find other open-minded and curious people. Finding and collaborating with those in your community is essential to help your business grow, but as you see those referrals and your appointment slots filling, you'll inevitably bump up against the next emotional and physical hang-up: You need someone to lean on if you want to continue to grow.

We all have different thresholds for the volume of work we can tolerate, but successful business owners hit that point when they start daydreaming about the vacation they want to take or the kid or family they want to see. When you're operating a business while wearing all the hats of promoter, administrator, and practitioner, any time spent away from your business means "everyone" is on holiday.

Hiring someone to handle administrative duties is one thing, but you'll also need to find another practitioner to provide treatment or training to spread the workload. It's an exciting time when you hit that phase of growth, but most people add the first one or two members of their team out of necessity (or desperation). They hire based on skills or the role they need to fill because when they're busy, they just need the help.

When your goal is to build a sustainable business, strategies and processes also need to factor into both finding the right people, as well as supporting their growth and development.

That's hard to do without good skills and leadership, but it's even harder to recruit and hire the right talent without systems that ask the right questions and provide the right feedback to make sure the person you hire isn't just skills on a page. You want someone who can grow along with the business.

IDENTIFY YOUR PEOPLE

Looking for the right people to expand your team is similar to looking for those professionals to collaborate with in your community. Who would be the most valuable resource to support you and your clients? Who can support your business and can continue to grow and develop into more? What are the traits and qualities you value in those with whom you'll literally surround yourself?

Finding the answers to those questions is dictated largely by your personal preferences or needs. Rather than letting your instincts or first interaction guide your decisions, write out the qualities or traits you consider non-negotiable. If you're the average of the five people you spend the most time with, you need to recruit a staff who'll consistently push the collective average higher.

Luckily, people with intrinsic value to a team often have the same traits.

- They provide a unique or complementary perspective.
- They leave their egos at the door.
- They have a sense of humor.
- They're low maintenance.
- They're highly respectful.

The team members at Functional Movement Systems don't have to be experts or bring the best resumes. As long as they bring a good attitude, making sure they get the right training is easy because enthusiastic people become educated people.

Identifying the qualities you value is your first filter. Don't automatically disqualify people if their technical skills aren't at the highest levels or if they lack a full grasp of your systems or approach. Most skills can be taught and improved upon, but good luck teaching an adult to be more respectful or have a sense of humor. Knowing which qualities are non-negotiable is probably the most important element—there's no easier way to sabotage your business than adding someone that poisons the delicate chemistry of the culture you've built.

When hiring new employees for his Sports and Fitness Performance training facility, Coach Frank Dolan looks for six basic traits.

- **Personal Responsibility**—Enjoying complete freedom to choose your response to outside circumstances and to improve your life through things you can influence

- **Growth Mindset**—Having belief that everyone can change and grow through knowledge, application, and experience, and that setbacks and failures aren't only part of the process, but are necessary to get better

- **Olympic Mentality**—Being dedicated in your preparation to something that gives your life meaning and purpose, something that demands an all-out effort and the fullest expression of your talents and values

- **Focus on Quality**—Taking a professional approach to what you do by always doing your absolute best—focus on the little things that make a big difference

- **Care**—Taking the time to really understand what people want, believe they can do it, challenge them to be the best they can be, and have their backs through the entire process

- **Positivity**—Leading with optimism and enthusiasm, having faith and belief that things will work out for the best and infusing energy and fun into everything you do

Although each trait could mean different things to different people, it would be hard to argue against hiring for people who are willing to learn and grow, caring about helping other people, and meeting others with optimism and enthusiasm. If you can find those attributes, you should be able to teach them a decision-making process or the technical skills needed to be successful.

The specific skills you're looking for may evolve as the needs of your business change over time, but the traits, much like your principles, should be non-negotiable. Building a successful team requires more than just finding professionals with the right mix of traits and personalities that gel.

Success is a product of those compatible people coming together around a shared vision, a shared purpose, and a systematic process toward a shared goal.

Don't let the degrees, certifications, or experience get in the way of finding those who are genuinely interested and motivated by challenges and working as part of a team.

If you want your team members to demonstrate your core values, put those values into practice and invest your time going deeper to help your staff members thrive. When you bring those people into an environment of fluid, open communication and collaboration, you set the stage for rapid expansion and growth.

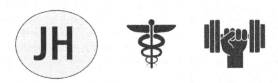

INVEST INTERNALLY—JASON HULME

The professionals we hire to join our team are already self-motivated to learn and improve themselves, but we dedicate time to training as a team because we can only be as effective or efficient as the weakest link.

Every Monday, we have a two-hour full staff meeting to review the active patients in our practice and discuss the challenges we and they are facing. Every Wednesday from nine to noon we close the clinic for staff training. The staff is paid as normal, but for five dedicated hours each week, we're auditing our abilities and asking:

- How is this patient progressing? What does the patient need more of?
- What techniques and tactics are working?
- Where does someone need more support or a little more guidance on what action to take?
- What can we each be doing better to support the work of our other team members?

For those five hours a week, we all teach and we all learn. If we have new staff, we're testing them or having the team teach new areas techniques or areas they have been investigating to maintain seamless continuity of care. It's interactive and makes us all better. When we go back to work, we're fired up the rest of the day.

Thinking of that time as five hours of lost revenue is shortsighted. Patients and clients are falling away—firing you, going somewhere else, or barely hanging on—and you won't even know it's happening if you're not giving yourself time to pay attention.

Most people get stuck when they become the bottleneck in the growth of their business. That approach to diagnosis and getting people better and out the door quicker will get you more referrals, but when the floodgates are open, that system will get tested if you're the only one who understands it. If patients or clients only want to see *you* because you hold some "secret recipe" no one else on your team possesses, you'll never maximize your business because you won't be able to maximize the value of the rest of your team.

The kiss of death comes when your referral sources call and say, "We only want our clients to see you." When patients show up and feel like they're receiving substandard care because they aren't being seen by the "best" clinician, you're heading down a challenging road. It can feel good to be viewed as the guru of your practice, but it should serve as a warning that something isn't interchangeable between you and your staff.

That level of synergy doesn't happen organically. It takes time, effort, and leadership to formally train and bring a team together around a standardized process. If you've done the work to hire open-minded, curious people, putting those processes in place shouldn't limit each team member's autonomy in how they practice; it should help elevate the standard of everyone's ability.

A good system is intended to provide feedback first, and it can create an incubator of ideas and tactics for people motivated to learn from the feedback. When a team culture emerges where everyone owns their roles and responsibilities and patients receive the same standard of care no matter who they work with, we see a shift take place. Rather than feeling like they aren't getting to work with the "best" person in the clinic, patients actually thrive because they feel like they have an entire squad of people behind them.

Only with a good team around you, functioning together under standard operating procedures, can you confidently build a self-managing practice. If your goal is to build something that allows you to step away without risking the continuity of the entire operation, dedicate time and resources to promote the growth of your team before it stifles the growth of your business.

Investing in your team early and often is one of the best investments you can make.

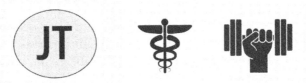

CREATE A TRUE TEAM APPROACH—JON TORINE

The Colts had a medical management team that consisted of strength and conditioning, athletic training, rehab and sports medicine staff, as well as our team doctors, head coach, our president, and a couple other personnel. In our meetings, we piled into a big conference room, and if people couldn't be there, they were on via a speaker phone on the table. We assembled that team because we understood breakdowns in communication is the biggest barrier to success in most organizations.

The intent of constructing that team was partly to allow us all to do our jobs more effectively, but really, it was a directive from our coaches and leadership at the top to ask, "How do we not silo this information on behalf of the players?"

When we gathered people whose principles and values were aligned committed to transparency, it created the opportunity for open conversation and disagreements that helped align us.

The word "alignment" is interesting because creating alignment doesn't mean "agreement." Alignment doesn't mean we agree on a particular method to accomplish a goal or that we leverage someone to get our way. Alignment means committing to the same problem, the same outcomes, and the same measures of success, and supporting each other in that process.

When you're aligned around a system, the message and the methods within that system can change every minute. Most of us fight over methods because we're emotionally or intellectually tied to what we do, but that's the wrong approach.

There should always be the opportunity to use your method. If the feedback from the system shows it works, we should all know more about it. If your method doesn't work, was this an isolated case where it didn't fit, or does the feedback suggest it's time to throw it out?

Health	Wellness	Fitness	Production

| Medical Staff | Rehab Staff | Performance Staff | Coaching Staff |

Can everyone align on the greatest bottleneck/barrier/metric at the center of the problem?

Can everyone value and measure it?

Who is most able to address it?

Once a week on Monday nights, we went around that conference room to review the status of every injured player on the roster. The conversation usually proceeded along these lines:

Athletic Training and Rehab:
Where is he in his recovery? How much time do you need?

Team Doctors:
What are you thinking? Rehab says he'll be out three weeks; the medical team says two weeks, and the training staff says two weeks. Let's set expectations on a plan.

Strength and Conditioning
What can this guy be doing in the meantime to be ready to return?

Coaches and Personnel:
What adjustments do we have to do in regard to the roster?

If there was a surgeon or someone outside the organization who worked with the player, we'd get those people on speakerphone and collect their input as well. In confusing cases, we'd work to determine the experts we could call to get a clearer answer.

That meeting might go 10 minutes or it could be two hours—the expectation was it would take as long as necessary to align on a path forward to put the players, and ultimately the team, in the best position to succeed. It's a simple concept to implement, but it's not always easy to sustain. It requires everyone to put ego aside and open themselves up to feedback and debate.

WELCOME FEEDBACK

To add another layer of accountability, we made the meeting open to anybody—especially the players. If a player wanted to hear us discuss his situation and his status for the week, he was welcome to attend.

Working at that level of transparency and openness with your athletes is both terrifying and liberating. Do they have a difference of opinion? Do they want to hear what the doctor or the front office is saying about them? Do they understand what their recovery will look like, and what they need to do this week and next?

It was an open-door policy in the truest sense because if everyone in that room believed an athlete was ready and he didn't think he was—or vice versa—how could we align on the best course forward?

Again, alignment doesn't mean agreement.

I watched a high-level executive and one of our star players get into a shouting match in the training room because the player felt he was ready to play and the decision had been made to hold him out of an upcoming game. When the culture of a team is to put someone's long-term health and well-being above the outcome of a game, it might create conflict in the moment, but how do you think players respond when they understand it's to protect them from themselves?

As a matter of fact, I used to gauge when my athletes were ready by how angry they got at being held out. When players didn't put up a fight or half-heartedly argued they wanted to play, I knew they didn't really feel ready to return. When they looked like they wanted to strangle me, I knew they felt ready and capable to hit the field again.

Do you think athletes are more or less likely to lay it on the line for you when they know your interest lies in their success versus your own? The culture from the top down through the coaches and staff to the athlete with the Colts was: Don't take longer than you need, but definitely don't take shorter than you need.

Anyone who's dealt with an injury knows the physical and mental grind it can take to get back to activity. When you rush players back and they get reinjured, it can be devastating individually and for the team.

There were no raises for getting guys back early and there were no punishments if it took a little longer—that's the wrong kind of motivation to get people to do their jobs well.

The intellectual prowess of the people I worked with during my time with the Indianapolis Colts was staggering, but the success of the organization was less about having the smartest people in the building as much as it was about that level of collaboration. Our organizational mandate demanded transparency and accountability. So much of the success of that organization was directly tied to the strategy of placing each athlete as the central focus and creating formal and informal opportunities to communicate and exchange ideas.

> "The number one way to discriminate is to treat everyone the same, because they don't all need or deserve to be treated the same. They need to be treated in a way that puts them on a progressive path forward."
> —*John Wooden*

The 4x4 demonstrates this sentiment perfectly because each box contains the behaviors and tactics to solve that individual's limitation.

AVOID BEING THE BOTTLENECK

Building your team of trusted professionals sets the stage to scale your operation, but there's a balancing act that needs to occur at this stage in the growth of a business. On the one hand, allowing everyone to find their own way in the system will end in more frustration and miscommunication than synergy. On the other hand, trying to individually maintain too tight of control on part of the process can mean the bottleneck to growth might be you.

The greatest challenge in applying systems across entire businesses or teams is implementing them before they're fully fleshed out or understood by the person doing the implementation. If you haven't worked out the kinks on your own, keeping everyone on the same wavelength will be that much harder when you can't control the process for each and every person.

When we originally formulated the processes that followed the movement screens and assessments, I didn't know how to deliver them across an entire practice. Rather than making a sweeping change or attempting to teach everyone a process that wasn't fully formed, I took it upon myself to put in the work by performing twice as many evaluations as anyone else in the clinic. I took on the extra evaluations and paperwork so I could test our models in a petri dish. By the time I was 35, I'd probably done two to three times the number of musculoskeletal exams of any clinician my age.

I was doing the initial two or three treatments, testing out my process. When cases were going the way I expected, I could hand them over to one of my colleagues to follow my plan of care. That approach exposed me to more outcomes in a shorter period than most other people because I was giving my stamp of approval on what needed to be done. My assistants loved to catch me being wrong.

My ego had to go out the window because the expectation I set was that I should be the first to find out when I'd misjudged a situation. It fostered a bit of a competitive spirit and it kept me honest while putting pressure on myself and the team. If the clinic or patients weren't doing well, it was because of me—and I could change *me* more easily than changing everyone else.

I had confidence in the skills and abilities of my clinicians and assistants to follow through; their initial value was to vet my strategies without worrying about the assessment piece of the puzzle. I didn't need to be there on graduation day. I just needed to set the expectation for what that outcome should look like and check in to reevaluate when needed. I wanted to know my failures, and I wanted the outliers, the malingerers, and the "problem" patients in my treatment room—I wanted to see when I needed to leave the system, or when the system would fix the problem.

When I had enough confidence in the data and the feedback I was personally seeing, I taught the assessment process to everyone on the team, feeling confident in adding layers of feedback in the clinic. Those lessons learned in isolation ensured that our combined efforts didn't create more noise or confusion. If there's one defining characteristic of the leadership I've tried to practice, it's continuing to refine my communication toward greater accountability.

The Movement System calibrated all of us in the same direction to the point it almost didn't matter who touched a patient because we were all using the same filters to stay on track toward the same outcome.

BUILD A CULTURE AROUND THE SYSTEM

If your goal is to scale and grow your business while being unwilling to compromise on quality, you need to think about how to deploy these systems with the ultimate goal of removing yourself from the process. You'll always struggle to focus your attention on the decisions that go into growing your business if you can't loosen your grip on the day-to-day management of everyone coming through your doors.

It's ego that compels us to see every client and give our stamp of approval or disapproval to feel connected and responsible for the final result. If you want to make a bigger impact in your community and grow to be more than a single treating clinician or personal trainer, you'll have to cast your ego aside and focus on how to elevate the effectiveness of everyone around you. In a true team environment backed by enough integrated training, even though everyone may not have the same number of repetitions or insights, they'll have everything needed to carry on without you.

You need to recognize where the value of your time lies. That realization, unfortunately, often comes through hardship. In the case of clinicians, many are seeing the direction of the profession shift toward medical insurers reducing payments and adopting a flat-fee, outcome-based model. The idea is to incentivize those professionals who get better results, rather than those who spend the most time with their patients.

In that scenario, whether we spend one minute or an hour with a patient, you'll see the same amount of money. Project that out with the number of visits you're currently doing and you could see more than 40% of your income evaporate in a year. I don't care what business you're in, if you discover your income will decrease by 40%, you'd better dedicate your time optimizing your internal processes to correct that imbalance or you'll go out of business.

The solution would usually come through better efficiencies—shrinking the time spent per patient or reducing the amount of time the "skilled" employees need to spend with each person, allowing them to see more people or focus on higher value activities. Ask a patient how it feels to have the treatment time cut in half, and sadly, they're more likely to blame the practitioner in front of them than the insurer paying the bills. Maximizing productivity and the revenue return on your time is always critical, but we can't forget that productivity is an equation: *Productivity = (total output) / (total input)*.

You can boost productivity by reducing inputs (time spent with patients) while also trying to maintain or increase the output (number of patients seen), but that becomes a harder equation to solve if we also consider quality. Not so different from "move well, before you move often," trying to squeeze more out of any system only increases the likelihood the quality of the output will suffer, especially if the processes aren't there to ensure consistent quality in the first place.

The barrier to productivity is that every process has a rate-limiting step—essentially the slowest step—that impacts how quickly the entire sequence of steps can be completed. A fast-food restaurant is limited by how long it takes to prepare edible food; bodily reactions are limited by the available enzymes or catalysts and how long they take to work. If you compromise the number of steps or try to shorten the duration of steps, the integrity of the process itself starts to break down.

INTEGRATE THE TEAM INTO THE PROCESS... OR THE PROCESS INTO THE TEAM

The beauty of a team environment is that rather than squeezing more out of fewer or shorter steps, we can find greater efficiency and productivity from shortening the gaps *between* the steps. Decreasing the time it takes to communicate, translate, and respond to information between members of the team, especially with handoffs, protects the quality of our product when everyone is in alignment with the system and actions it demands.

When each member of the team knows how to capture a consistent quantity and quality of information, everyone can learn to see patients through a similar set of eyes. Learning the principles that define what that information means allows people to understand how to speak and act in their own unique way that still aligns with the process of the group. It's like throwing a no-look pass in basketball because you trust your teammate is filling a specific role, but processing and responding to the information in the same way you are.

You need to guide your team along the same path you took in mastering the delivery and interpretation of the screens to naturally create a more efficient and resilient business model. This will liberate you from less critical responsibilities.

> *"We offer three kinds of service...You can have it fast, good, or cheap—but you can only pick two.*
>
> *GOOD and CHEAP won't be FAST.*
>
> *FAST and GOOD won't be CHEAP.*
>
> *CHEAP and FAST won't be GOOD.*
>
> —*A sign behind my grandfather's desk*

Anyone from a high school volunteer to a retired groundskeeper can be taught how to take blood pressure and heart rates, measure range of motion, test reflexes, perform the top-tier of the SFMA, or score an FMS or FCS. It's the synthesis of that information that requires an advanced skill set and a deeper understanding of what it means.

Even those business metrics like show-up rate, the average number of visits and sessions, or referral rates can easily be taught to staff as indicators of the effectiveness of the system. If everyone in your gym or clinic understands the required battery of tests and information and they're all competent in collecting that data, everyone can make better decisions from the same reference points.

If you sit down with a new client with those basics already laid out by an assistant or a junior team member who performed screens and an intake, your time and energy can go into movement breakouts, diagnostic testing, or refining the most appropriate interventions. That either means you can be more productive with the same amount of time or accomplish what you need to in less time.

In both instances, your confidence should be much higher in delegating a plan to a staff member and then checking in as needed, knowing everyone appreciates the same gauges to monitor improvement.

A POTENTIAL WORKFLOW FOR AN INITIAL PATIENT VISIT

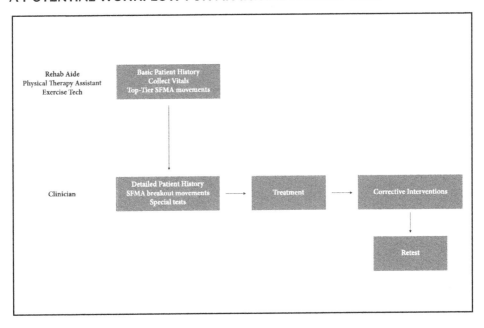

A POTENTIAL WORKFLOW FOR FOLLOW-UP PATIENT VISITS

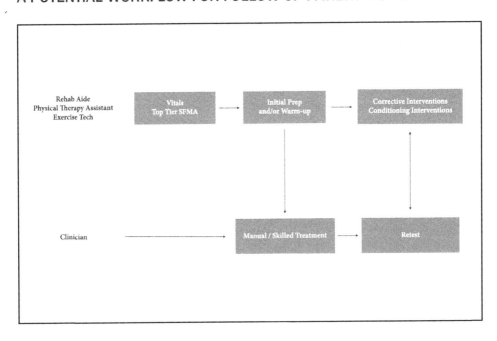

As the team becomes more fluent in the shared language of movement, gaps between the skills or roles of teammates starts to blur and merge into a frictionless experience where almost any team member can drop in and work with someone without skipping a beat. The level of skill of each practitioner should only dictate the breadth of the decision tree from which they operate. When the data indicates a need for a more advanced set of eyes, there should be no hesitancy or confusion over who needs to step in.

Building a team is an inherently challenging endeavor because it extends beyond finding motivated people with the right set of skills. That's one reason the most talented sports teams don't always win championships, and the companies with the most talented employees aren't always the most successful.

Creating a solid foundational structure of communication from which everyone can operate demands that you help each of your employees understand the systems in place and show them where their entry and exit points lie on the path.

This allows everyone to work at the edge of their abilities and expand their value and effectiveness in the team. If you hope to someday remove yourself from day-to-day operations to expand and scale your business, that collective effort must be focused and coordinated on building and reinforcing itself.

OPPORTUNITIES FOR CHANGE

- ▶ Identify those traits and qualities you want reflected in your team.
- ▶ Implement systems and processes to educate and train your team to install a culture of collaborative success.
- ▶ Share your knowledge at every opportunity—don't become a silo of information.
- ▶ Develop a plan and process to empower each team member to take ownership of their roles and allow those roles to grow with them.
- ▶ Systematically remove yourself from the process and see if what you constructed can stand on its own.

CHAPTER TWENTY

SCALE YOUR BUSINESS

- ▶ Where's the best area to invest your resources to help grow your business?
- ▶ Is there another way in which to deliver your services or skills to reach more people or have a greater impact?
- ▶ What does success look like for you?

The idea of stepping away from the day-to-day operation of your business can be pretty appealing. Being able to focus most of your attention on all the demands of opening a new facility or expanding your operation is what many of us want. But scaling your business shouldn't even enter your mind if you haven't handled the previous steps of tapping into your community, building and training a team, and you haven't established reliable processes and metrics to track your progress.

Maybe you've constructed a good team; you're getting great results, business is growing and you want to build even more momentum. Maybe you've already reached that point like a lot of business owners when you feel the need to dramatically grow your operation.

When people hit that inflection point of wanting to add new or different services or expanding their space or locations, it's rarely a resource problem that sabotages their progress—it's the lack of all of firmly established, foundational systems. You can't develop superior long-term athleticism on a weak and dysfunctional body, and you can't build a sustainably growing business on weak and dysfunctional teams and processes.

Think you're ready to test the resilience of the business you've constructed? First, imagine what would happen if you stepped away for a week or a month. If that immediately sent a shiver up your spine, you're probably like most owners, stuck in the day-to-day operation because there's no solid structure to hold onto.

Of course, some owners make the decision to stay in the trenches and don't want it to grow more than that. They want a good quality of life and to be a great resource for the community. Maybe they find fulfillment in different aspects of their lives. Implementing a process-focused approach can still improve the effectiveness and efficiency of their business, and make things a lot less stressful, but not everyone has the goal to radically expand their businesses.

However, for those of you who are the type of people whose motivation and fulfillment comes from wanting to broaden your influence or your profession, you'll need to fight to continue to grow, both personally and professionally. If you've become the bottleneck in the process of growth, you'll never move the needle of enacting change on a larger scale.

- How tight are your internal processes for recognizing and responding to problems?
- How well have you trained and embedded your team into those processes?
- How comfortable are those team members, loving the brand, the values, and the place where they work?

If those pieces aren't right, you're never going to be able to move out of the day-to-day, because you'll constantly be pulled back and hung up for a thousand reasons. You can't market enough to get enough clients. Or maybe you have plenty of patients, but your team culture is one where people feel others are making money off of their efforts and are unwilling to support each other. How smoothly or poorly your attempt to grow and scale goes is a direct reflection of everything you've put together up to that point.

Scaling successfully means you've probably maximized the resourcefulness of your operation. The question becomes where to invest your precious resources to compound your success. That may mean more people, more space, more offerings, or some combination of the three, but as with every other step on the path, you can use the lens of your principles to inform those decisions with respect to the natural processes of growth and adaptation.

INVEST YOUR RESOURCES

Nowhere is the balance of resources and resourcefulness clearer than in the basic construction of a health and wellness operation. You can't have enough space or enough enthusiastic people, but both of those resources are costly. Chasing too much of either before you need them is a quick way to failure.

The constraints of a budget, no matter how large, will always force you to decide where to allocate your money—and your decisions matter. In the image-driven health and fitness field, too much of that budget often gets spent on the latest machines, tools, gadgets, or a commercial space in a trendy location. That might get people's attention, but it's a losing proposition because you'll need to continually keep up with the latest and greatest to differentiate yourself.

I've found the most success allocating my spending toward maximizing the quality of the members of the team and the amount of space dedicated to movement. Improving the quality of the resources protects the quality of the product. I hope I've convinced you of the value of investing in the growth and development of your team, but if your goal is to get people moving, the environment you build better be full of opportunities for movement.

Whenever I open a new clinic and walk a doctor through, I listen for, "Hey, where are your lines of equipment?" I want to hear that so I can say, "We don't get people sitting. We get people moving." I point out that half the equipment they're probably thinking of has a seat, but the only chairs or tables we have are for treatment, waiting, or resting. After the message sinks in, the response is almost always, "I never thought about it that way."

If someone is trying to convince me they're safe to return to exercise or training, I'm not going to base my career on how much weight they can move on a leg extension or a leg press machine. If I have parents wondering if their kid can compete in a sport, I want the space to be able to show them if the kid can't do a standing long jump.

Functional exercise is an unpopular concept because of the false notion that it's something dictated by specific pieces of equipment or exercises that often resemble a circus act. If you have a business dedicated to a functional approach to promoting health, wellness, fitness, or production, it should mean that no matter what tools or equipment you have, the environment is one that allows for the full expression and development of movement.

In our case, if you can cover the patterns of the neurodevelopmental progressions or the FMS, you can easily cover the activities of daily life and the lifelong maintenance of development movements.

What's Your Gauge for When the Clinic's Running Well?

Just as with the Systems, we need baselines for the efficiency and effectiveness of our daily operations. Some can be subjective; others need to be objective. We've got financial markers, patient or client compliance and improvement, employee happiness and advancement, overall mood...we need to weigh them all.

That said, in the best-running clinic I ever had, I'd often hear one refrain from patients who'd observed the workplace during their therapy sessions. They'd smile and say, "I wish I could work here."

These weren't PTs. They were folks from every segment of the population. But they knew enough to appreciate a well-oiled machine—especially one that made them feel and move better.

Approaching the space from a functional perspective serves two purposes. First, you can be more resourceful with your space, fitting more bodies into an area that isn't occupied by huge, immobile exercise machines. Second, it allows you to be more resourceful with your equipment budget, purchasing equipment pieces that serve multiple purposes. A good set of free weights, resistance bands, foam rolls, stall bars, a mat table, and some medicine balls provide roughly 100 times better return on investment than the latest exercise machine because they allow you to scale both functionally and financially.

MAXIMIZE YOUR SPACE AND YOUR STAFF

Building a strong team and optimizing the free square footage in which to work allows you to grow into your space until that inevitable point when you feel the pressure on the space. The only downside of a movement-focused approach is that if you're successful, at some point you'll have patients and clients literally running into each other while doing their work. The challenge then becomes finding that threshold number of bodies in the room that doesn't impact the quality of care.

Too many people make that jump early, believing that doubling the size of their footprint will double the revenue they can generate, only to find they hadn't maximized the opportunities available in the previous space. Remember, space is just as limited by the clock as it is by square footage. How creative can you be with time?

What feels like the pressure of too many patients or clients to handle can sometimes be the pressure of inefficiencies in how the team works as a unit. I can't stress enough how important it is to nail your internal processes early and to maximize the team and space you have now. You don't want to discover your system is broken when the stakes are higher after you've added more rent and salaries.

Investing resources in your team first and your space second allows you to grow in a more natural way. Giving everyone the tools and knowledge to take on expanded roles and responsibilities puts quality before quantity and protects you against failure to adapt.

I'm always trying to identify quality people and support the people with whom I work. I made sure that every one of my clinic employees eligible to sit for the strength and conditioning exam became certified in their first six months on the job; I wanted them to be able to engage more deeply in the clinic and also in the community. They were able to provide support and value for high school sports teams and create a bridge to the clinic.

I also love bringing in interns or students from the community or through local universities because it allows me to develop potential future employees for new opportunities I find.

There's a good chance that if I'm the favorite or most valuable affiliation experience for physical therapy students, I'll have the opportunity to hire them, or they may choose to hire me to continue to educate them in their careers. Focusing the bulk of my resource investment in people translates into better and more capable members and leaders of my practices, a deeper pool of potential employees and collaborators, and a huge professional network that offers access to even more resources.

There's always risk that comes with expanding or starting a new business. Providing specific guidance on what that looks or feels like is purely an academic exercise because there are so many factors that come into play when it comes time to expand. No two people will have the same financial or staffing resources when it feels like time to take that leap, and the availability of space and even personal factors can do more to dictate the threshold of risk a business owner is willing or able to cross.

You're the only one who can ultimately determine if that's the correct path to take. Learn what you do best and then structure your environment and invest your resources to support that service, putting quality before quantity.

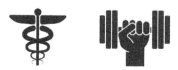

EXPAND YOUR OFFERINGS—
GRAY COOK AND MIKE DEIBLER

I already mentioned my preference for finding experts in their respective layers of movement to work with collaboratively. If I need to coach someone through an Olympic lift or a periodized training plan, I can do it, but I'd rather call in specialists to take the work I've already done and infuse it with what they do best. That approach helps keep me improving in what I do best, while learning just enough outside my specialty to advise intelligently and to know when to defer.

I've seen more success in this field by professionals recognizing what they do well and then figuring out new ways to deliver that value than successes by professionals who try to add more services to their menu of mediocre skills.

Today, I am most fascinated by new ways to offer our unique skills and services, and none more than the virtual delivery of health, fitness, or performance. If there's anything we've learned from the challenges of the COVID pandemic, it's that many people will continue to pursue fitness in the absence of gyms and training facilities and, with guidance, many of them prefer the convenience of working out or rehabbing at home.

Technologies are flooding the market, offering ever-more-advanced digital applications and virtually connected bikes, treadmills, and resistance machines for consumers to access physical therapy and personal training that's faster, cheaper, and more convenient than ever before. But without establishing risk and setting movement baselines, they're essentially just delivering the same old programs through a more convenient technology.

In the face of quarantines and mandatory shutdowns, most trainers, coaches, and health care professionals quickly pivoted to offering their services virtually just to stay financially afloat. Maintaining the same level of quality service and results while completely altering the nature of the work is hard enough, but competing with so many other options forced some business owners to come to terms with the fact that the quality of their offering was drastically diminished. Stripping away the atmosphere of a trendy facility, access to fancy equipment, or highly supervised treatment or coaching turned out to be less important to a lot of people than being able to engage with exercise on their own schedules.

The public shift toward training at home using the latest piece of exercise equipment certainly feels more pronounced than it was in the past. I doubt it will ever completely replace the connection and community that comes with working with others in person, but this moment in time has shown there's a demand for virtual health and fitness options. Plenty of people can be successful, engaging with their health, wellness, fitness, and production in a new way.

Now, there's offering your services virtually as a means to keep your business alive, and then there's offering those same services as a part (or the entirety) of your normal business model. From a financial resource standpoint, offering your services virtually is arguably the lowest cost option with potential benefits in the flexibility of where and how you deliver your service. Offering your services through a broader virtual or digital model offers access to a massive pool of potential clients online, but ask anyone with significant experience offering virtual training or treatment how great it is, and they might tell you to be careful what you wish for.

Mike Deibler of San Diego Premier Training is a great example of someone succeeding in the virtual training space. Mike works virtually with a wide range of clients and athletes from around the world, a segment of whom are training to compete in Spartan and obstacle course races. A significant portion of this book has been dedicated to communication and guiding your patients, clients, or athletes through a movement experience—much of Mike's success has come from recognizing that a virtual model demands an incredibly high level of communication and feedback.

No matter the client, he always asks himself, "Can we accomplish what this person needs virtually?" Making the shift to treating or training clients in this way can be overwhelming and more time-consuming than working with them in person—especially if you don't create guardrails and tighter feedback loops to stay on track.

If you've developed the strategies and processes to be successful working with your clients and patients in person, you can be successful transitioning into a virtual model as long as you're clear with the expectations and criteria for yourself and your clients from the beginning of the relationship.

IS THIS PERSON SET UP FOR SUCCESS?

This can be a hard judgment; even though we may want to offer this option to as many people as we can, it won't be for everybody. No one wants to turn down clients, but if people get hurt or don't get the results they want, it'll reflect on you.

Even though philosophically we should take the same approach whether working with someone virtually or in person, if the ability to troubleshoot and be expansive with the training is handicapped by working remotely, where can we shift our focus to address other barriers to success?

Here being even more diligent with your intake process sets the stage for everything else. Working with people online is probably a different experience for them too, and some may have never considered working online with a trainer or coach. More time spent on the frontend, finding out as much as possible about the clients and their lifestyles, will absolutely make you more effective on the backend as you lay out the process.

The top priority, as always, is to identify pain or significant problems with movement. Always follow up on that priority by identifying any additional risk factors. You may wonder how to do this remotely, but there's no insurmountable barrier to performing a movement screen remotely. The first book I wrote, *Athletic Body in Balance*, walked the reader through how to do a self-screen. It helped a lot of people get themselves on the appropriate corrective path with just a dowel, a doorway, and a piece of tape.

There's ideal—performing the screen or assessment in person—and then there's optimal, based on the situation. Don't let perfect be the enemy of good. If we can acknowledge there will naturally be some erosion of the quality of data, the responsibility is on us to capture enough data to chart a safe and effective path forward.

Plenty of practitioners have performed some version of the FMS or SFMA as part of a virtual evaluation and have been able to capture enough good information to make a decision without diving deep into the scoring or assessment.

Sometimes that really needs to be done live, and sometimes, with a little guidance, people can perform it independently and can film themselves doing it. The right method is whichever provides confidence in collecting acceptable information that helps drive your decision-making.

If a person's vital signs, movement scores, or lifestyle behaviors indicate deeper assessment or attention is needed than can be effectively delivered online, you'll feel confident in pointing them to a local medical or fitness professional. Struggling to solve problems remotely will frustrate all parties involved and will likely produce a result that doesn't make anyone happy.

But if we can help people establish even a little awareness around issues we feel confident in addressing, we can still make it easier for that person to continue down the right path.

WHAT ARE THE GOALS?

Looking at goals brings us back to whether the person is seeking independence or performance. A self-motivated client with good physical awareness may be independent enough to succeed with a guided program and interactions, but not every client will possess those qualities.

For all clients, we need to understand if they're safe to pursue activities and able to independently engage with those activities before we can focus on pushing the boundaries of their ability. We don't need to be with clients for every rep of their exercises, but if there are concerns about function, motivation, or there's another need for coaching in real-time, they may not be safe enough or independent enough to succeed with a solely virtual program.

Gathering good data is essential when working with clients remotely. Without awareness of potential barriers to success and the ability to address them, the likelihood of a positive outcome or experience goes down dramatically.

The better we can understand the gap between clients and their goals, the better we can project where challenges may arise. This will help in choosing the right combination of strategies to move someone toward independence and the best outcome.

The bulk of that answer comes from setting the best possible baseline and identifying the greatest opportunities on which to focus.

The FMS is a non-negotiable for Mike's screening. Even though it's not a perfect solution, he can walk a client through the screen using a broomstick, some string, and a couple chairs to at least identify those movement patterns that are clear 1s or 0s.

From there, any other testing is largely dictated by what tests can provide valuable, actionable data that are safe for clients to be instructed how to perform.

That might be components of the FCS, a timed 1.5-mile run, or strength measurements if he feels comfortable with someone performing strength testing with a partner. It's becoming easier to capture quality health and fitness data remotely, and there's no excuse to not be collecting good, valuable data.

The question becomes, "Can we gather enough information to tell us where this person is relative to the goal, and do we and the client possess the confidence, ability, and resources to pursue and achieve that goal in a semi-independent manner?"

Sometimes that answer is, "No." We need to be comfortable communicating that with the client's best interests in mind. Sometimes the answer is, "Maybe," and a blended in-person and remote approach may be beneficial to build toward independence.

But even when the answer is a clear, "Yes, this person can succeed with a fully remote relationship," the most effective strategies are still dictated by a client's independence and our ability to deliver the level of care and service needed to succeed.

TACTIC—Find a Local Certified Professional

If you really want to get a true FMS score before proceeding with an online client, see if there's someone local to your client who can perform a screen on your behalf. There's a worldwide network of professionals trained in delivering the movement screens, and we have plenty of stories of people personally screening clients for online trainers.

Having a conversation with a local resource demonstrates the commitment you have in your client's success, which far outweighs the perceived risk there may be in "losing" that client to someone else.

STRATEGIES FOR DELIVERING VIRTUAL CARE

Live Video Sessions	Pre-Recorded Video	Static Photos with Instructions
Opportunity: Easier to gather and provide feedback from direct observation Opportunity to tailor your verbal instruction to determine what's working Opportunity to demonstrate exercise from multiple angles for better comprehension	**Opportunity:** Clients can perform on their own schedule Clients can watch videos multiple times for reinforcement Allows them to work at their own pace Scalable solution (your schedule doesn't factor into the program)	**Opportunity:** Clients can perform on their own schedule and at their own pace Ability to print and use if internet access is a barrier Scalable solution (can sell as more generalized, templated programs)
Challenge: Only scalable to a certain degree (limited by schedules) Difficult to capture a 360-degree perspective of how someone is moving	**Challenge:** Less immediate feedback Verbal cueing or limited viewing angle of movement may limit comprehension	**Challenge:** Often a one-size-fits-all approach Doesn't allow for verbal instruction and cueing May be a barrier in interpretation of the written instruction Nuance of movement lost from static images

The best strategy typically demands more than just a single solution. The pros and cons of any single solution need to be weighed against the needs and abilities of the clients and the time and resources you're able to commit.

Regardless of what you both agree on as the best course of action, poor behaviors, habits, lifestyle, and movement may be standing in the way of their goals. Anyone can design and distribute an online training or rehab program, but supporting lifestyle changes creates a compound effect on other positive behaviors that promote independence. None of those demand your constant presence to make a positive impact, although they do require you to prioritize and monitor their effects.

Delivering the level of service required for success is important, but you also need to consider how to deliver the level of communication required to generate the critical feedback to keep you on track.

HOW WILL YOU COMMUNICATE?

In an environment where you're not able to capture immediate real-time feedback, how will you respond to your client's needs? How can you avoid text messages at midnight from clients in different time zones or the email updates that read like novels?

First, never assume clients understand what you're asking of them or that they'll exercise an appropriate level of caution when they encounter an exercise or instructions they don't completely grasp. You may not conceive of every question or scenario that might arise, but you need to consider how to communicate exactly *what* you want them to be doing, and also *how* and *why* they should be doing it.

When your manual or physical methods of working are taken away, you'll appreciate the heightened value of clear communication and effective coaching. During a live virtual session or via pre-recorded audio or video, you don't have the benefit of catching subtle signs of dysfunction or of providing a bit of corrective pressure on a body part. People will succeed to the degree you're able to deliver your message in the most accessible manner.

During the on-boarding process, clarity is key. Your interactions with remote clients will be less frequent than if they're physically present in your facility, and establishing clear expectations when you have the first conversation with a client can save your schedule and your sanity.

Setting transparent expectations of how the process will work and why they need more or less guidance or oversight builds a collaborative decision. There's nothing worse than losing a client who struggles through the first two or three workouts. You won't even know it, and by the time you do a check-in, you'll discover the person has opted out.

A good default would be to communicate in some fashion two to three times a week. That can come in the form of an email or a call, or a short text message to let them know you're there for support—anything that lets you measure compliance and motivation is critical here. Depending on the amount of time you're willing to commit or how well someone is responding, that could be a little more or a little less, but it's best to initially opt for more frequent communication.

Creating a process around how and when you communicate is key. We've seen practitioners schedule formal check-ins with clients on certain days of the week. These consist of a recap and goals for the following week, and include questions about obstacles, pain, or problems encountered. Setting specific days for clients to check in and days to follow up prevents the creep of emails and messages every free minute of the day, and allows you to more efficiently batch your correspondence time.

Tracking the information you collect during those formal sessions on a simple spreadsheet can help you spot trends or emerging barriers to improvement.

Client Tracking Log Example

Client Name	Check-In Date	Session Number	Goals	Progress Toward Goals	Questions	Obstacles	Pains

The better you get at capturing and interpreting this data, the easier communication becomes. More dependent clients require more frequent and immediate feedback, along with a broader communication strategy to keep them engaged. Supplementing live instruction of new phases or exercises with pre-recorded exercise videos or tutorials and more frequent check-ins become essential in the early stage of working with these clients.

As their independence grows, the need for real-time feedback loops may decrease and allow for less one-on-one time and more self-sufficiency in managing their programming. Those fully independent clients following a purely written or pre-recorded program might make good progress with nothing more than a weekly email or text and a monthly live check-in.

You'll always have to find the right balance of oversight and guidance, and until these clients demonstrate a good level of comprehension and awareness of the plan, always err on the side of caution. It takes more time remotely to trust that a client can do a movement safely. There's rarely a benefit to throwing a new or unique exercise into the mix if someone doesn't understand how it should feel or what it should produce.

> # TACTIC—Plan for the Frequently Asked Questions (Mike Deibler)
>
> Write down every question you get along with the answer because you'll likely see them again. Once you start to see the most common five or six emerge, do yourself a favor and create a FAQ document to save time in the future.

WHAT WILL YOU CHARGE?

So what's the value of your service when it's delivered virtually?

I don't need to tell you that every market is different and can tolerate only a certain price point. When you think about the price at which to offer this kind of service, or really any service, it's helpful to think of it in terms of how much time it'll take. Will you spend hours customizing a plan for each client and working with people one on one? Or will you work from templated plans with less frequent check-ins?

If you simply think in terms of the hourly investment per client, build a price off your normal rate. For the number of hours per month, charge accordingly, just as you would in person.

Charging that amount can feel uncomfortable for some professionals, but I believe that's because they feel this is an inferior product. If all you're doing is teaching exercises, you're right—you're providing something people can learn for free on the internet. Any amount you charge will be too much.

If you're putting in the same time and effort to deliver a comprehensive virtual experience as your in-person sessions, you should feel comfortable in the quality of the product you provide. If you're saving time by using templates, then maybe charge less, but if you're providing one-on-one treatment or training, a customized program, and even more of your time and availability than you would in person, your price should reflect the value you offer.

Designing two or three offerings based on the level of independence that someone wants and needs can help you deliver a "high-touch" individualized experience or a more automated and cost-effective option.

We all need to acknowledge that many people view the services of physical therapists, chiropractors, personal trainers, and even some coaches as a commodity. When you're a commodity, price and convenience are the main drivers behind the choices people make.

It's a saturated market for online training that consists of free options and templated, one-size-fits-all programs. Trying to compete in that market is a race to the bottom, and one that puts quantity over quality.

The market that's not saturated is the one with professionals who are setting themselves apart, taking the time to understand and be thoughtful about the approach they take in this new landscape. Before you start compromising on the price of your service, remember that there are more than enough people willing to suffer a little bit of inconvenience (whether time, commitment, or cost), as long as you refuse to compromise on the value you deliver.

The opportunity is there, if you're willing and able to take it.

OPPORTUNITIES FOR CHANGE

- Before offering new services or solutions, start with a process to determine if you are maximizing the resources you currently have.
- Don't expand into a new space until you can physically feel the pressure of your current environment, having already maximized its efficiency.
- Invest resources in your team first, and your space second.
- Give everyone on your team the tools and knowledge needed to take on expanded roles and responsibilities.
- Before adding more space, consider opportunities to deliver your services in a virtual or hybrid model.
- Determine what your time is worth to you, and ask if your effort matches the value you are providing.
- Make certain that your internal systems prioritize communication and feedback so that every patient/client/athlete you work with (whether in-person or virtually) is set up for success.

CHAPTER TWENTY-ONE

BE TRANSFORMATIONAL, NOT TRANSACTIONAL

- ▶ How do you distinguish between a manager and a leader?
- ▶ Who's affected the most by the professional decisions you make?
- ▶ What are you giving back to your profession?

For most people, the hardest transition in running a business isn't going from being an employee to being a boss. It's not going from hustling on your own to building and running a team. It's not even scaling up from a single clinic or gym to multiple locations.

The hardest transition is moving from being a manager to being a leader.

Those terms aren't interchangeable. A good manager is technically sound and tactically viable. This person is able to understand and can communicate the skills needed for success, and can adapt and respond to changing situations. As Eric D'Agati says, "Good coaches are so good at the technical, they become obsolete. But they're so good at the tactical that you can't live without them."

> *"If your actions inspire others to dream more, learn more, do more and become more, you are a leader."*
> —**John Quincy Adams**

When you're able to educate and communicate effectively, your technical impact allows your team to continue to operate at a high level even when you're not around. The tactical piece makes you indispensable because not everyone is willing to seek feedback and learn to find the right mix of tools or methods for success. A great coach whose technical knowledge has been ingrained in the athletes could miss practice for a week…and everyone on the team would still perform well. But if they aren't on the sideline on game day, the loss of the tactical abilities will be significantly felt.

The difference between a manager and a leader is that a manager pushes from behind and a leader guides from the front. A good leader possesses the technical and tactical skills required to be successful, but more importantly, a leader is willing to be accountable for the failures and is radically transparent in the analysis of what went wrong and how to fix it.

In sports, when people move from being an assistant coach to head coach, they quickly realize it's easier to make suggestions than decisions—particularly when those decisions need to be broadly applied.

Assuming the role of a leader means there's now not only a lot more on the line, but the buck stops with you. You're not just holding people to a performance standard, you are setting the standard. Any failure of the team to meet that mark should be an opportunity to investigate what you could have personally done better.

TACTIC—Empower Your Team (Frank Dolan)

I created a budget in my business for what I call "strategy sessions." I told my trainers that at any point throughout someone's training, they should feel empowered to schedule a 30-minute meeting with the client or athlete if they felt it was needed.

If they felt someone's goals had changed or they needed reinforcement or support in changing behaviors or nutrition, they had autonomy in setting up that time to talk and I would pay them extra for that time.

There's no extra cost to the client. I wanted to incentivize the team to be thoughtful. From a client's standpoint, that's value that goes well above and beyond what's expected. From a trainer's perspective, it's an opportunity to have a deeper, more meaningful conversation than what happens during a training session, and it helps us get better outcomes.

I want to help everyone who works for me develop their skills and abilities, and my business has benefited from their transformations.

OVERCOMING A TRANSACTIONAL MINDSET

The willingness to assume that level of responsibility, accountability, and risk in pursuing new ideas isn't something we all possess. Failure, criticism, and being wrong are all real consequences of leading from the front, and the fear of the criticism that comes with trying something different than the standard often stops people in their tracks. The rest of the world is holding onto tradition or protecting their positions until the general consensus gives them confirmation and permission to change because the lens through which they view change is transactional. "How can X get us more money, clients, or attention? What do I have to give up to try X?"

That's why "hacks" have become an industry unto themselves—a marketplace promising shortcuts to rewards with little risk in a fraction of the time. You can sometimes hack your way to immediate short-term gains, but hacks lack sustainability. They provide a solution with the promise of a result, without the necessary step of understanding what you're doing…or not doing. If everything is viewed as a transaction, it inevitably leads to a place of putting yourself before your clients and patients because the question you're asking is, "What's *my* risk to reward?"

You can succeed with that transactional mindset. Waiting for external confirmation or shortcutting the process may even reduce the risk of failure. Unfortunately, it also limits your ability to take advantage of larger opportunities. New concepts on the leading edge of any field rarely come out of evidence. New ideas come out of those who go first and take a laboratory approach to a different way of thinking or looking at a problem to solve.

Those are people who have an idea, spend years—or maybe it's 10,000 hours—creating a consistent value and critically vetting everything with, "Is this significantly better? Can doing X better allow me to be more objective, resourceful, or effective?"

The motivation isn't how to gain more of X, but how you can add more value to the service you provide. You can take advantage of the gap in the value of the services you're able to provide relative to your competition long before everyone else catches on and follows your lead. That's moving from a transactional mindset to a transformational mindset.

Reinvesting in your success compounds itself, allowing you and your business to grow steadily and sustainably compared to those who overvalue the importance of short-term gains.

A leader looks to change the parts of tradition that need to change and adds to the parts of tradition that still work. That doesn't mean all leaders are innovators or even early adopters of a new concept or technology, but they all strive to remain objective and radically transparent as they continually push the boundaries of their work and teams.

A leader's value is directly tied to the actions taken in service of the development of the individual, the community, the team, or the organization. That dedication may ultimately be rewarded in the form of more money, attention, or accolades, but that's purely a happy side effect of a true leader being in it for transformation, not transaction.

HOW TO ADOPT A TRANSFORMATIONAL MINDSET...

- ▶ Use natural obstacles to test strategy and build character. Don't try to buy your way or hack your way out of a problem, because you'll see it again and again.

- ▶ Demonstrate that leadership is a responsibility, not a title—earn it or lose it.

- ▶ Foster grit and intrinsic value while developing skill—no one likes the talented asshole.

- ▶ Celebrate individual achievement, but never over service of the team. When even the franchise player realizes there's no "I" in team, the organization gets better.

- ▶ Remove entitlement at every opportunity. Do your job; own your stats—only your mom believes your excuses.

- ▶ Use failure to teach and unify—failure is inevitable, so embrace and own the lessons it brings.

- ▶ Reinvent culture through objective transparency and systematic non-failure and refresh it continuously.

- ▶ Look upstream and start identifying and taking action on risk. Trying to find new ways to fix the same old problems in front of you only gives your competition time to find better solutions before you do.

CHAPTER TWENTY-TWO

FIND YOUR PATH

I volunteer to teach physical education once a week at my children's elementary school. The class sometimes doesn't look like what most people would expect. We have kids jump off the first row of bleachers and try to stick a landing. Then we have them do it with a beanbag on their heads…and then continue to add complexity and demand. Or we might have them balancing on half-foam rolls or walking on balance beams. There are no lesson plans. No "exercises."

The last 10 minutes of the class, we talk about who did well, who wants to do better, and what we can do about it. We're imposing an obstacle without an answer.

They learn to pattern each other. They watch each other and learn, and my job is to scale it—to put them at the edge of their ability and let them figure out these physical obstacles and work through their movement problems. They find themselves in an uncomfortable situation that demands developing mental toughness and learning intuitively through experience.

We can't have someone sitting on the bleachers, waiting while everyone else participates. We can work with an individual child within the group, with everyone doing the same thing but scaled to foster motor learning and that adaptive response in developing movement. From there, it's just a matter of letting them play and explore and be children—and allow those activities to naturally grow and expand their physical ability and resilience.

I mention that story not because I think you should volunteer to teach a gym class for 10-year-olds, but because it captures the essence of everything we should strive for in our work. Every one of us is in the business of physical education. It's something we've lost as a culture and is the root cause of so many of the challenges and problems that patients, clients, and athletes bring to us to solve.

> *"There comes a point where we need to stop just pulling people out of the river. We need to go upstream and find out why they're falling in."*
> —**Desmond Tutu**

If we're to have any hope of making a big enough impact to change the trajectory of our physical culture, we all need to do our parts in reestablishing each layer of movement back at the source. That's not solved by prescribing sets and reps or corrective interventions—it's solved by fundamentally changing how we deliver and empower physical awareness to those we work with, and how we provide them with the tools to navigate their physical lives. Not everyone will take you up on the offer to hold that space, but that doesn't mean you shouldn't always strive to teach people how to live within their own bodies.

It's always easier to see what could be added—more supplements, more forms of exercise, more tools, more certifications. People think of "survival of the fittest" in terms where those with the most strength, money, time, or resources are able to rise. But nature and history have shown us the strongest, the smartest, or those with the most resources don't always stick around the longest.

Being rich in resources may provide more protection during challenging times, but long-term success still boils down to who can respond and adapt more readily to a constantly evolving environment. In almost every example, it's those who are the most resourceful, getting by with less, who ultimately survive and thrive.

Grit and determination are necessary elements for sustained growth and development personally and professionally. If there's one area we can all benefit from the application of those qualities, it's in pursuit of greater resourcefulness first, and resources second. Taking this mindset into your interactions with patients and clients, your approach to treatment and training, your business dealings, and your life in general may hold back rapid growth, but it ensures that your roots are set firmly in the soil before you start adding branches to your trunk.

MOVING FORWARD IN THE MOVEMENT BUSINESS

I hope this book gave you a new perspective on building a holistic approach to how you work with your clients and how you operate your business. I believe our work with Functional Movement Systems succeeded in establishing some of the common language on what quality human movement should objectively look like. If nothing else, it exposed that nagging problem that's negatively impacting the health and fitness of our modern society—that many of us are simply applying variations of the same solutions that fail to address what's most often a movement problem.

Differentiating yourself in what has become an incredibly important and increasingly crowded field means offering value and an approach to service that goes beyond the standard of care.

Our goal was always to create something effective and consistent to support our own work and our own clients, but in teaching others, we've been able to assess whether our systems and tools provided the same value over a larger scale in the hands of others. Over time, the processes have been repeated, expanded, refined, and modified—always supported by the data collected and run through the same filters to prevent our egos or motivations from getting in the way of progress.

The 4x4 matrix presented in these pages is our latest attempt to refine our work into a more complete system of decision-making strategies we hope will inform your practice and provide value to you and your clients in the same way as the Functional Movement Systems.

Just say no to dogma. Whatever screens or assessments you use, you should always have a why and a process that allows you to objectively test and assess your perception and behavior. There's no "one" way and there's no "right" way, but if we're all holding our work up to the same measuring stick, we can begin to agree on what looks like a "better" way.

Don't let someone else's data (ours included) dictate your path. Always engage with anything new in a critical way. Choose your course, pick the measurement tools, and filter them through a system to see what the data has to say about the impact of your choices.

		Physical Adaptation			
		Awareness	Protection	Correction	Development
Physical Growth	Production	?	-	+	=
	Fitness	?	-	+	=
	Wellness	?	-	+	=
	Health	?	-	+	=

Look again at that 4x4:

- In which layer of movement does your greatest professional impact lie?
- Which row or rows offer new opportunities to expand your value or expertise?
- What's the value or tactical expertise you can impart to your patient, client, or athlete to promote independence within each column of adaptation?
- What are you doing to fill each of those boxes for yourself and others?

The answers to these questions (and all those that came before) will be as unique as each person with whom you work. But each of us can find the same clarity and direction in our individual actions by filtering our inputs and outputs through the same systematic process

We all must embrace the opportunity and the responsibility to help others cultivate their own physical growth and adaptation in a natural, systematic, and sustainable way.

We all must be committed to guiding and empowering others towards independence on that journey.

We all must hold ourselves to the highest standards of accountability and transparency—grounded in objectivity, without ego, and always in service to our patients, clients, athletes, peers, and communities.

If we can all stand together on that foundation and work toward the same destination, I have no doubt that each of us will find the best tools, tactics, strategies, and support to make the journey uniquely our own.

APPENDICES

SYSTEM OVERVIEW

RISKS TO MUSCULOSKELETAL HEALTH

RED/YELLOW/GREEN LIGHT EXERCISES

STANDARD OPERATING PROCEDURE OF MOVEMENT

EXAMPLE PATIENT PROGRESS NOTE

RECOMMENDED READING

AN OVERVIEW OF THE FUNCTIONAL MOVEMENT SYSTEMS

SFMA: SELECTIVE FUNCTIONAL MOVEMENT ASSESSMENT

The Selective Functional Movement Assessment (SFMA) is a clinical assessment for those experiencing pain. It's a movement-based diagnostic system that systematically finds the cause of pain—not just the source—by having healthcare professionals break down dysfunctional movement patterns in a structured, repeatable assessment.

When you head to the hospital for shooting arm pain, the immediate course of action is to check your heart, not your arm. The symptoms down your arm are a result of a problem elsewhere in the body. Similarly, the SFMA focuses on underlying dysfunctional movement to find the cause of pain. This concept is better known as regional interdependence—how seemingly unrelated problems are actually driving the dysfunction. The SFMA fills the clinical need to assess for stability and/or motor control dysfunctions, as well as mobility dysfunctions.

The SFMA is the first organized system that takes into account altered motor control, the inability to coordinate proper movements. This system allows us to identify the correct problems—mobility versus motor control—to best equip clinicians for a successful outcome. The SFMA uses the neurodevelopmental perspective, the way we learn to move as infants, to create a system to reteach our brains how to communicate with our bodies to reprogram motor control.

Although we encourage all fitness and health professionals to learn the SFMA Level 1, the actual certification is reserved for allied healthcare professionals. Following Level 1, SFMA Level 2 teaches healthcare professionals how to use the SFMA findings to guide their interventions emphasizing our "3 Rs" approach of Reset, Reinforce, and Redevelop to immediately integrate mobility techniques and motor control reprogramming tools into clinical practice.

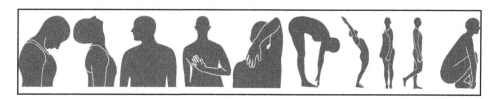

FMS: FUNCTIONAL MOVEMENT SCREEN

The Functional Movement Screen is a standardized movement-pattern filter to gauge how someone, no matter the age, is moving in everyday life. It takes into account both mobility and stability and equips the professional with information to make programming decisions with precision and purpose. This information enables us to quickly screen movement to identify the biggest opportunities for those with whom we're working.

The FMS identifies movement patterns the individual moves well in, those patterns that can be developed or loaded for fitness. It also identifies patterns that aren't ideal and need to be protected and corrected. This distinction removes guesswork and doubt. At the end of an FMS, you'll have a baseline and valuable information to create a program specific to the individual to foster an environment to meet the goals and keep the person healthy.

We encourage all fitness and healthcare professionals to learn the FMS, as it offers a better understanding of the true relationship movement patterns play in our health, fitness, and production goals. FMS Level 2 establishes a foundation for your programming—the smooth transition from movement dysfunction to competency fostered by creating customized exercise selection while simultaneously limiting the factors that inhibit progress.

The FMS is a critical piece of any standard operating procedure to determine if your clients are safe to follow a path of fitness and production, or whether they need to resolve pain or dysfunction to ensure success in their physical journeys. This is where we exit an injury or musculoskeletal health problem and enter a new strategy of performance or independence in physical life.

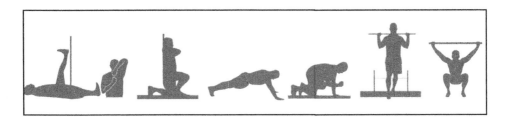

YBT: Y BALANCE TEST

Asymmetries in function are a major factor in increased injury risk. The Y Balance Test (YBT) is the tool we use to quantify a person's motor control and functional symmetry. YBT allows us to "quarter" the body—left versus right and upper versus lower—to test how the core and each of the extremities function under bodyweight loads.

The Y Balance Test was developed through years of research of injury prevention and identification of motor control changes that occur after injury. It provides a map that identifies roadblocks to a person's functional performance both in the rehabilitation and performance worlds.

The YBT course is available to all healthcare and fitness professionals. Learning and implementing this testing tool can offer clear, measurable benchmarks to ensure the fundamental quality of movement is intact.

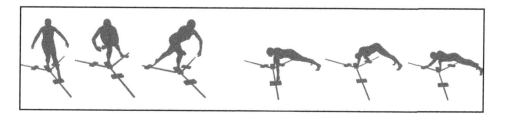

FCS: FUNDAMENTAL CAPACITY SCREEN

The Fundamental Capacity Screen (FCS) is an innovative approach to general fitness testing that dissects the fundamental fitness issues hindering those you train from reaching their true potential. The FCS was designed to test four key components of athletic capacity and identify issues affecting the ability to:

- Control balance
- Maintain posture under load
- Produce power
- Store and reuse energy

FCS education is a resource for any professional whose focus touches these four key components of fitness. Appreciating why and how to test these and providing corrective and conditioning strategies for athletes and active individuals can restore a level of quality to training and conditioning movement.

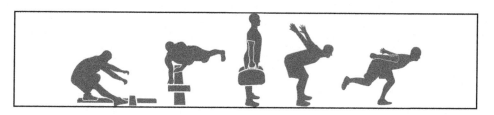

FBS: FUNCTIONAL BREATHING SCREEN

The Functional Breathing Screen is a novel screen built around the "EAARS" model of breathing function, designed for both the fitness and healthcare provider to capture the presence of functional and dysfunctional breathing patterns. Functional breathing is:

- ► Efficient,
- ► Adaptive,
- ► Appropriate,
- ► Responsive, and
- ► Supportive of health.

Recent research has shown us that breathing dysfunction is multi-dimensional in nature and includes three primary categories or dimensions of dysfunction: the biochemical dimension, the biomechanical dimension, and the psychophysiological, symptomatic dimension. The presence of dysfunctional breathing affects overall health and musculoskeletal system performance. It contributes to many symptoms and functional disturbances, including those affecting the musculoskeletal system. It can contribute to decreased pain thresholds, impaired motor control and balance, and subsequent movement dysfunction with each of these impairments adversely affecting performance in fitness and rehabilitation.

Functional Movement System's breathing curriculum introduces the screen and several related tools to assess and test for breathing dysfunction alongside a breathing retraining approach. Grounded in the same neurodevelopmental progression as our other corrective strategies, the approach to restoring natural breathing pattern is valuable in both fitness and rehabilitation settings.

RISKS TO MUSCULOSKELETAL HEALTH

My interest in risk factors is driven by the same curiosity about movement that led to the development of the Functional Movement Screen.

In those early days, I didn't set out to add something new to training or rehabilitation. I was just a young, frustrated PT confused by lots of missing pieces. In the 1990s, medicine was overlooking serious musculoskeletal issues because there was no movement component to a general physical exam.

Enter the FMS. It does what it does well, but as I've often said, if all it does is identify the 20 percent or so of people previously cleared for activity who have pain with movement, it serves a great purpose. (It can and does this and much more.)

But it's 2021 and though we've steadily grown, the FMS is still unlikely to be used in your general practitioner's office. Movement still isn't part of a physical exam that deems a person "well."

So here we are in the 2020s. Half of all American adults have a musculoskeletal health condition and it's the most commonly reported medical condition for adults aged 18–64. If you don't think those numbers are crazy, what if I told you that annual musculoskeletal health spending exceeds spending on national defense?

… And movement is still not part of a physical exam.

Current research on risk factors for musculoskeletal injury reinforces just how much we're missing in healthcare… and how that hands us the responsibility.

I like to break this data into six categories: Pain, Body Composition, Medical History, Balance, Movement and Activity Level. Here's how I think of each category:

Pain:[1,2] This one is simple. Does the individual report pain on a questionnaire or with movement or with any movement assessment, test, or screen?

Body Composition:[8-11] Here's another simple one. A BMI of 25 or more is a significant musculoskeletal risk multiplier. You can calculate this, but questions can still help.

Medical or Behavior History:[1-4] This can put up the usual red flags, but it's worth noting that a previous time-loss injury is considered a musculoskeletal health risk factor. This is where a more robust client or patient questionnaire can yield great information. It's up to you to word the questions to elicit the most objective answer you can get, but don't just think "previous surgery" because this is also about lifestyle and behavior. Think sleep (hours per night), hydration (glasses of water per day), and more as you try to uncover the history and lifestyle that can be affecting other risk categories.

Balance:[2,5] Low scores and asymmetries on quartering balance tests are risk factors for musculoskeletal health.

Movement:[6-7] General movement dysfunction and asymmetry, as well as muscle strength asymmetry, are considered risk factors.

Activity Level:[9] This is another simple one: Reduced physical activity puts an individual at risk for musculoskeletal health issues.

All of these categories are in your realm of care, but you should already be focused on three in particular.

Which three? The only three that are actionable today: Pain, Balance, and Movement. These three have effective and efficient feedback loops.

These three also happen to have objective tests associated with them, making my response to melding musculoskeletal health with general health simple. First, let's broaden our view to include what we've labeled as health risks such as high BMI and low cardiovascular fitness, as risk factors for musculoskeletal health as well. Then, take action where you can by using the Functional Movement Screen and the Y Balance Test when exiting rehabilitation and before changing activity levels.

Now let's get back to that algorithm. The discussion of the categories is obviously general—in this setting it has to be. But the guidance from the research isn't general. These musculoskeletal health risk factors have quite specific measures. Functional Movement Systems is currently working on an algorithm that considers all of these risk factors through movement self-screens based on the FMS and YBT with extensive health questionnaires covering sleep, nutrition, and physical activity. Organizing and weighing this information and providing appropriate guidance focuses attention on the weakest links to reduce risk and build health, wellness, and fitness.

1 Teyhen, D. S. et al. What Risk Factors Are Associated With Musculoskeletal Injury in US Army Rangers? A Prospective Prognostic Study. Clin. Orthop. Relat. Res. 473, 2948–2958 (2015).

2 Teyhen, D. S. et al. Identification of Risk Factors Prospectively Associated With Musculoskeletal Injury in a Warrior Athlete Population. Sports Health 1941738120902991 (2020).

3 van Meer, B. L. et al. Which determinants predict tibiofemoral and patellofemoral osteoarthritis after anterior cruciate ligament injury? A systematic review. Br. J. Sports Med. 49, 975–983 (2015).

4 Toohey, L. A., Drew, M. K., Cook, J. L., Finch, C. F. & Gaida, J. E. Is subsequent lower limb injury associated with previous injury? A systematic review and meta-analysis. Br. J. Sports Med. 51, 1670–1678 (2017).

5 Plisky, P. J., Rauh, M. J., Kaminski, T. W. & Underwood, F. B. Star Excursion Balance Test as a predictor of lower extremity injury in high school basketball players. J. Orthop. Sports Phys. Ther. 36, 911–919 (2006).

6 Busch, A. M., Clifton, D. R. & Onate, J. A. Relationship of Movement Screens with Past Shoulder or Elbow Surgeries in Collegiate Baseball Players. Int. J. Sports Phys. Ther. 13, 1008–1014 (2018).

7 Kiesel, K. B., Butler, R. J. & Plisky, P. J. Prediction of injury by limited and asymmetrical fundamental movement patterns in american football players. J. Sport Rehabil. 23, 88–94 (2014).

8 Bastick, A. N., Runhaar, J., Belo, J. N. & Bierma-Zeinstra, S. M. A. Prognostic factors for progression of clinical osteoarthritis of the knee: a systematic review of observational studies. Arthritis Res. Ther. 17, 152 (2015).

9 Chapple, C. M., Nicholson, H., Baxter, G. D. & Abbott, J. H. Patient characteristics that predict progression of knee osteoarthritis: a systematic review of prognostic studies. Arthritis Care Res. 63, 1115–1125 (2011).

10 Nicholls, A. S. et al. Change in body mass index during middle age affects risk of total knee arthroplasty due to osteoarthritis: a 19-year prospective study of 1003 women. Knee 19, 316–319 (2012).

11 Reyes, C., Leyland, K. M., Peat, G. & Cooper, C. Association between overweight and obesity and risk of clinically diagnosed knee, hip, and hand osteoarthritis: a population-based cohort study. Arthritis (2016).

RED, YELLOW, AND GREEN LIGHT EXERCISES

The exercises listed below are certainly not "complete," but should provide guidance on how to approach the application of exercise with dysfunctional movement patterns.

Many of these exercises (and more) can be found in the exercise video library on *functionalmovement.com*.

	Red Light (Protect)	Yellow Light (Develop with Caution)	Green Light (Correct and Develop)
Active Straight Leg Raise	Hip-Hinging (Deadlift Movement) Running Jumping	Step-Ups Lunges Split-Stance Exercises	Tall- and Half-Kneeling Chops and Lifts Upper Body Training Core Work
Shoulder Mobility	Overhead Pressing Overhead Pulling Handstand Position Work	Horizontal Pressing and Rowing Partial Turkish Get-Up Rack-Position Carries	Deadlifts Kettlebell Swings Farmer's Walk and Carries
Ankle Mobility	Lunges Split-Stance Exercises Running and Jumping	Deadlift Kettlebell Swing Single-Leg Deadlift	Half-Turkish Get-Up Half-Kneeling Chop/Lift Upper Body Work
Rotary Stability	Asymmetrically Loaded Exercise (Single-Arm Snatch, Kettlebell Swing)	Partial Turkish Get-Up Half-Kneeling Chop, Press, or Lift Deadlift and Squat (Symmetrically Loaded)	Floor Press Symmetrically Loaded Upper Body Work
Trunk Stability Push-up	Pressing (Standing) Kettlebell Swings Ballistic Drills	Deadlifts Squatting Push-Ups	Step-Ups Split-Stance Exercises Single-Leg Deadlift
Inline Lunge	Lunges Split-Stance Exercise Running and Jumping	Deadlift Kettlebell Swing Single-Leg Deadlift	Half-Turkish Get-Up Half-Kneeling Chop/Lift Upper Body Work
Hurdle Step	Single-Leg Exercise Running Carries	Deadlifts Squats (Symmetrically Loaded)	Half-Turkish Get-Up Half-Kneeling Chop/Lift Suitcase Deadlift
Deep Squat	Squat Variations	Single-Leg Squat Split-Stance Lunge Running	Turkish Get-Up Deadlift, Single-Leg Deadlift Tall- and Half-Kneeling Chop and Lift

	Red Light (Protect)	**Yellow Light (Develop with Caution)**	**Green Light (Correct and Develop)**
Movement Control	Overhead Pressing Running Jumping	Single-Leg Training Horizontal Pressing	Bear Crawls (Upper Body) Half-Kneeling Throws Balance Beam
	High-Impact and Heavy-Weighted *Balance* Stress		
Postural Control	Running Jumping Ballistic Moves	Half-Kneeling Single-Arm Kettlebell Press Turkish Get-Up	Six-Point Carries Kettlebell Hold and Turn Half-Kneel Kettlebell Halos *And All Movement Control Green Light Exercises*
	High-Impact and Heavy-Weighted *Spine* Stress		
Explosive Control	Running Jumping Ballistic Moves	Medicine Ball Throws Jump Rope	Indian Club Swing Rope Wave Progression *And All Movement and Postural Control Green Light Exercises*
	High-Impact and Heavy-Weighted *High-Intensity* Stress		
Impact Control	Running Jumping Bounding	Jump Rope (Single-Leg and Advanced Techniques)	Indian Club Slam Jump Rope, Basic *And All Movement, Postural, and Explosive Control Green Light Exercises*
	High-Impact and Heavy-Weighted Acceleration, Deceleration, Direction-Change Stress		

STANDARD OPERATING PROCEDURE OF MOVEMENT

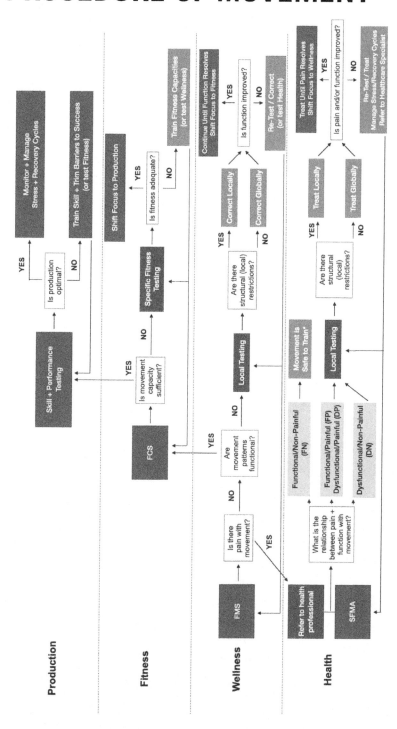

EXAMPLE PATIENT PROGRESS NOTE

Dear Dr. Brown, Thank you for referring Janet Johnson to our clinic for evaluation and treatment of low back pain. We have seen her for six visits and she has expressed a 30% reduction in pain. Her movement patterns and daily function reflect that same 30-40% improvement.

A simple pain scale

The SFMA and MCS are my movement tools for patterns

I'm still concerned about a balance issue as she attempts to stand on her left leg only and I feel it is the primary contributor to her original complaint of low back pain. We have identified two key impairments in her left lower extremity that are largely responsible for her left-sided balance issues. They are: a 45% strength deficit in left hip extension and a 20% restriction in left ankle mobility. See attached function and impairment sheet.

This statement connects function and symptoms in a logical and reasonable way

This statement relates general function to specific impairment measurements

I anticipate that she will need three to four more visits in physical therapy, but I would like to space the visits to once per week. This should allow us to monitor her reduction in pain and full return of function. If you have any questions or concerns about this note, please feel free to contact us.

Demonstrate a plan towards resolution and independence

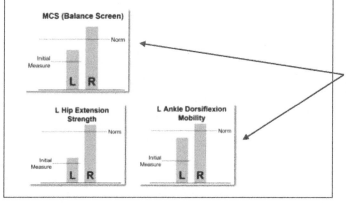

I borrowed the idea for bar graphs from JTech ROM and strength reports

RECOMMENDED READING

This book makes specific reference to many works from diverse disciplines. Countless other authors who weren't referenced have greatly influenced my thought processes, both generally and concerning movement. Here are a few of the most impactful, followed by my greatest takeaways.

The Talent Code: Greatness Isn't Born. It's Grown. Here's How
Daniel Coyle

Talent is Overrated:
What Really Separates World-Class Performers from Everybody Else
Geoff Colvin

    Practice deliberately. Fail fast with feedback.

Principles
Ray Dalio

    Radical transparency and algorithmic thinking aren't just assets in financial models.

Range: Why Generalists Triumph in a Specialized World
David Epstein

    Beware of sacrifices for specialization. Know the benefits of generalization.

The Checklist Manifesto
Atul Gawande

    Standard operating procedure doesn't undermine professionalism; it's its hallmark.

Linchpin: Are You Indispensable?
Seth Godin

    Use your creativity to become indispensable.

Upstream: How to Solve Problems Before They Happen
Dan Heath

    Don't let someone else find your upstream problem.

A Hunter-Gatherer's Guide to the 21st Century:
Evolution and the Challenges of Modern Life
Heather Heying and Bret Weinstein

> We've forgotten that form and function are intrinsically linked.

The Obstacle Is the Way
Ryan Holiday

> Challenge your resourcefulness with fixed resources. Obstacles will always be there.

Moneyball:
The Art of Winning an Unfair Game
Michael Lewis

> Permission to change perspective. The correct way to challenge fixed mindsets is to be statistically armed.

Risk: A User's Guide
Stanley A. McChrystal

> Threats x Vulnerabilities = Risks
> Do you know what and how to measure?

In Defense of Food:
An Eater's Manifesto
Michael Pollan

> Transfer the concept of "whole food" to "whole movement."

Start with Why
Simon Sinek

> Distill your WHY, HOW, and WHAT statements. You won't get it right the first time, so practice.

Leaders Eat Last
Simon Sinek

> Communication and accountability starts at the top.

Extreme Ownership:
How U.S. Navy SEALs Lead and Win
Jocko Willink

> Own and articulate your principles in action and word.

CONTRIBUTOR BIOS

ERIC D'AGATI

As the founder of ONE Human Performance, Eric consults with many top sports teams and organizations, including the New York Giants and the New York Islanders. Eric's education includes a degree in Exercise Physiology from William Paterson University and post-professional certifications from numerous organizations, including the NSCA. He has lectured at diverse universities and clinics, including the Mayo Clinic, NJSIAA, Frank Glazier & MegaClinics football coaches clinics, and dozens of speed and conditioning camps. He's also been a guest SAQ Trainer at Nike Football Training Camps. Eric is the former Strength & Conditioning Coordinator for NY/NJ Juggernaut Professional Fast-pitch Softball, is the inventor of the Performance Progression Pyramid training system, creator of 5 Tool Training, strength training for baseball and softball, and is the founder of Strong Kids, an after-school fitness program for children.

JON TORINE

Jon spent 17 years as a strength and conditioning coach in the NFL, where he handled all facets of the strength and conditioning programs and was part of the medical management team. In addition to S&C, his duties included team nutrition and hydration, team circadian rhythm management, building an intern program, assistance with college and free agent evaluations, and working closely with the rehabilitation and physical therapy staff in return-to-play efforts. During this time, he used the Functional Movement Screen to help guide his training decisions. His experience using the FMS in a high-level group situation is broad, and his expertise in working with elite athletes is notable.

JASON HULME

Jason excels in working with people suffering from pain and athletes at all levels at his chiropractic clinic, Active Spine and Joint Center in Hendersonville, TN. He supports his Nashville running community, including serving three years as the Hendersonville Half-Marathon Medical Director. In 2017, Dr. Hulme was appointed by Governor Haslam to the Tennessee Board of Chiropractic Examiners. Only two years into his leadership on the examining board, the Federation of Chiropractic Licensing Boards appointed him committee chair of the Certified Chiropractic Clinical Assistant (CCCA) program.

Jason was recognized by the Tennessee Chiropractic Association as the 2020 Chiropractor of the Year for his outstanding achievement in his decade of practice. He's a sought-after national speaker known for his ability to share his knowledge effectively in a way that inspires others.

MIKE CONTRERAS

Mike has been a firefighter for over 30 years. During that time, he's held various positions, including Firefighter, Firefighter/Paramedic, Fire Captain, Fire Academy Coordinator, Battalion Chief, and is currently a Division Chief. Mike is an NSCA Certified Strength and Conditioning Specialist (CSCS) and an NWCG Safety Officer. He has worked with fire departments, the US military, police departments, and large utility companies to implement a movement-based solution to reduce the risk of illness, injury, and worker's compensation costs.

Mike's extensive experience and education have led him to develop the FMS Health and Safety (FMS HS) program. His unique ability lies in taking a complex subject and providing a simple solution. The FMS HS system focuses on human performance, risk identification, and mitigation, which can be utilized in the everyday workplace and customized to fit any environment.

MIKE DEIBLER

Mike is a personal trainer certified with ACE, NSCA (CSCS), and CFSC. His history as a former All-American high jumper with a background in exercise science has helped him develop extensive knowledge in performance and fitness coaching. He owns San Diego Premier Training in San Diego, CA, and has a long career as an educator in the fitness field. He's the Director of Education for Exercise ETC, a continuing education company for fitness professionals, and is an adjunct faculty member at Miramar College. Mike has also been featured in articles from multiple publications, including *Men's Health, Women's Health, Health and Fitness Magazine,* and *Shape*.

FRANK DOLAN

Frank is the owner and operator of Sports and Fitness Performance Training Centers (NY) and has been a sports performance coach since 2001. During that time, he's trained youth, high school, college, and professional athletes from the ranks of MLB, the NBA, and the NHL. In 2014, he was named to the Nike Training Network, and has consulted for Nike Global Training, Nike NYC, and Equinox Fitness Clubs. Frank is currently an adjunct professor at Hofstra University and Suffolk County Community College on Long Island, where he lives with his wife and two boys.

INDEX

4x4 movement matrix
introduction to 78
using the 3 Rs in 163

A

adopting a transformational mindset 344
algorithmic thinking, principle of 15
American health, current state of 37
assisted vs active vs reactive 174
facilitation techniques for 205
Athletic Body in Balance, self-screening 333
awareness
capturing for your clients 161
using play to develop 249

B

battling ropes as a corrective 211
biases, professional affinity toward 25
Boyle, Mike
chef vs line cook analogy 29
joint-by-joint approach, the 166
bracing to provide stability 172
breathing
changes in during rolling 172
control begins with 199
techniques of 200
building your team
be transformational, not transactional 342
creating a team approach 316
finding the right people 312
foundation building 311
integrating the team into the process 322
investing internally 314
strategy sessions for empowerment 342
traits to look for when hiring 312
business measurements
determining importance of 267
organizational data 293
business network
building of 295, 298
volunteering your experience 305
business scaling, *see scale your business*

C

charts and graphs, list of
4x4 grid, questions of 255
4x4 matrix and production 238
building a stable foundation 44
client tracking example 338
confidence-reality ratio in screening 124
confidence vs competence 32
corrective 4x4 matrix, the 203
depth of expertise 88
depth of expertise, opportunities of 90
depth of expertise, risks of 94
finding the bottleneck in the staff 317
FMS decision tree, the 292
graphic showing FN/FP/DP/DN 148
growth, opportunities for 33
identify risk first (FMS/SFMA) 136–137
joint-by-joint approach, model of 166
movement, posture, explosion, impact 210, 229
movement, SOP of 363
patient progress note, example of 365
potential workflow for patient visits 324
quantifying the layers of movement 138
risk factors and odds of future injury 67
RNT, feed the mistake 206
screens pyramids 237
Venn diagram of SFMA/FMS/FCS 213
clients, understanding the needs of 121
clinical metrics 276
clinical outcomes, measurement of 269
Colvin, Geoff, *Talent is Overrated* 101
comfort vs discomfort 40
communication
clincian to doctors 271
establishing trust 158
increasing value with 159
language of movement, the 159
value of and need for 155
with non-FMS coaches 304, 306
with non-FMS medical professionals 301
competency, capacity, skill continuum 223
competency vs capacity 44

371

compliance and buy-in
   firefighters and utliity workers 279
   professional athletes 282
confidence vs competence 32
Contreras, Mike
   contributor bio 370
   screening firefighters, utility workers 115
   sidebar: compliance and buy-in 279
   sidebar: institutional outcomes 272
   tactic: volunteer your experience 305
correcting movement, process of 216
   standard operating procedures for 194
corrective 4x4 matrix
   measuring movement competency 206
   SFMA, tool for decision-making 203
corrective exercise
   assignment of home exercise 197
   frustration of 218
   role of 191
   vs sustainable activity 248
Cosgrove, Alwyn, customer quote 155
COVID pandemic, business lessons of 331
Coyle, Daniel, *The Talent Code* 101
create systems, principle three 72

D

D'Agati, Eric
   contributor bio 369
   good coaches, defining 341
   initial goals, determining 278
   key questions for clients 126
   level of effort for training value 128
   sidebar: connect with coaches 306
   sidebar: readiness 286
Dalio, Ray, transparency, algorithmic 15
DeFranco, Joe, long-term plan quote 289
Deibler, Mike
   contributor bio 370
   tactic: plan for frequent questions 339
   ways to expand business 331–332
developmental sequence, the 55, 57
   measurement of 9
Dolan, Frank
   contributor bio 370
   tactic: empower your team 342
   traits to look for in hiring 312
Dunning Kruger Effect, the 32

dysfunction
   different than pain 149
   patterns, using the SFMA for 152
   vs deficiency 193

E

exercise as an additive reinforcement 48
expectations, setting of 177
experiences, creation of for clients 161
explosive control, progression of 217
explosive control vs impact control 211
extrinsic vs intrinsic cues 175

F

failure vs non-failure 68
feedback
   accountability partners for 113
   building your system for 112
   tests, screens, assessments 107
   welcoming of 318
Ferriss, Tim, *The Four-Hour Body* 242
firefighters, screening of 272–273
first move well, then move often 54
fitness
   making fitness into competition 39
   measurement of 50
   sacrificing function for 185
foot and ankle, prioritizing mobility of 167
foundational mobility and control 216
function as an entry point, definition of 52
Functional Breathing Screen, details of 356
functional movement patterns 216
functional movement progression 238
Functional Movement Screen
   as the entry point in your system 135
   as used with the SFMA 151
   common mistakes with 76
   decision tree of 292
   details of 354
   development of 58
   early problems in application 74
   establishing a baseline 73
   finding pain during 147
   introduction to 11
   patterns, importance of 198
   scoring system overview 138
   uses for 117

Functional Movement Systems
  auditing system of 7
  non-negotiables of 102
  standard operating procedures of 79
function vs structure 43
Fundamental Capacity Screen
  introduction of 11
  measuring minimums for capacity 208
  rescreening of 215
  uses for 118, 212
  when to move to 137
fundamental movement patterns 216

G

goals
  helping your clients develop 126
  how will clients know when reached? 127
  underestimating pressures of 99
Gray's whiteboard talks, list of
  breathing and corrective exercise 200
  exercise and activity 231
  function and form 37
  how to focus on the weakest link 259
  mobility, starting with 169
  moving with ease 146
  physical obstacles and education 345
  solving obstacles from the ground up 173
  standard operating procedures 78
  systematically reducing your options 293
  valuing physical currency 84
  wellness exploits the overlaps 213

H

healthcare, movement model in 92
Hulme, Jason
  contributor bio 369
  identifying referral options 297
  mindfulness/pain journal 151
  non-negotiables list 100
  quote: diagnosis drives the boat 150
  sidebar: clinicial outcomes 269
  sidebar: engagement 276
  sidebar: invest internally 314
  sidebar: value for referral sources 298
  split, point of challenge with 105
  splits in building a business 265
  tactic: hold your prognosis 130
  tactic: promote self-selected fitness 244

human performance, development of 15

I

impact control, progression of 217
independence vs performance 241
injuries
  asking your clients about 129
  movement screening and 142
institutional outcomes, examples of 272
intake form, suggestions for 132
intrinsic vs extrinsic cues 175

J

John, Dan, keep the goal the goal 141
joint-by-joint approach 166
journal, mindfulness/pain 151
judging the value of training 128

K

Kiesel, Kyle, military personnel research 65
Kraus-Weber study 38

L

layers
  health, fitness, or performance 42
  health, wellness, fitness, or production 49
Le Corre, Erwan, MovNat, creator of 245
Lee, Bruce, strategies and tactics of 28
  be like water quote 99
Lewis, Michael, *Moneyball:*
  The Art of Winning an Unfair Game 7
lifestyle survey, need for and method 122
lights system, the
  example exercises of 188, 361
  example strategy of 225
  introduction to 187
  when to implement 290

M

mentorship vs apprenticeship 13
minimums, management of 101
mobility and stability, joint-by-joint 166
mobility, strategies for 168
Motor Control Screen, overview of 210
motor milestones, discussion of 55
motor patterns, correction of 212

motor/postural control
    confirmation of 170
    reinforcing mobility gains for 196
movement
    capacity vs competency 62
    components of 34
    global patterns of 25
    language and development of 56
    layers and definitions of 49
    natural development of 47
    problems, starting with why 26
    screening, rules for 61
    standard operating procedure of 363
movement behavior
    form or function, driven by 9
    implementation of screen at discharge 93
    movement control, progression of 217
movement hierarchy
    explosive control vs impact control 211
    movement layers, functional measures 63
movement matrix, 4x4
    introduction to 78
    use of the 3 Rs in 163
movement principles
    description of 24
    principle one 54
    principle two 63
    principle three 72
    movement screening, scoring of 139
    see also, Functional Movement Systems
multi-segmental flexion pattern
    interventions to correct, examples of 207

N

non-negotiables
    identifying yours 99
    Jason Hulme's list 100

O

opportunities in business
    enhancing others' skills 90
    for fitness professionals 95
    for medical professionals 93
    identifying your non-negotiables 99
    recognition of 87

opportunities for change
    building your team 325
    choosing what to work on 219
    creating community 309
    dysfunctional movement 180
    dysfunctional vs painful movement 143
    evaluation of your process 239
    expanding your business 340
    for your clients 132
    implementation of the screens 118
    independence vs performance 250
    introduction of 103
    in your professional practice 108
    measuring your systems 294
    protecting your clients 190
    when dealing with pain 153
    your communication with clients 160

P

pain
    as the signal, not the problem 150
    considerations of in your business 145
    discovered during screening 140
    how to watch for during screening 147
    identification of 136
    mindfulness/pain journal 151
    painful patterns, training of 148
    vs dysfunction, difference between 149
patient progress notes, example of 365
patient visits, potential workflows for 324
patterns
    dysfunctional, using the SFMA for 152
    lights system and 226
    of the SFMA and FMS 202
    recognition, the skill of 106
    screens and assessments of 216
    starting from 61
    use of for elimination 165
    vs postures, description of 57
performance vs independence 241
Perry, Mike, client non-negotiables 101
physical adaptation
    layer of 80
    looking for opportunities in 84
physical awareness, creation of 70
physical data, measurements of 293

physical growth
   layer of 80
   looking for opportunities 84
play, practice, train, difference between 245
Plisky, Phil
   military personnel research 65
   monitoring your show-up rate 278
postural control, carry screen for 217
postures, examples of 171
President's Council on Youth Fitness 38
production
   improvement of 224
   retraining skill and performance for 235
   vs performance, definitions of 51
professional growth
   determining your path 91
   generalist, route of 89
   questions to ask yourself 83
   specialization, considerations of 88
proprioception, external load for 174
protect, correct, develop
   movement principle two 63
   reinforce the change 181

Q

questions to ask your clients 126–129
quotes, list of
   Albert Einstein 24
   Alwyn Cosgrove 155
   Archilochus 103
   Arie de Geus 35
   Bruce Lee 28
   Dan John 141
   Desmond Tutu 346
   Earl Cook's desk sign 323
   Eric D'Agati 278, 341
   General Sun Tzu 25
   Harrington Emerson 23
   Harry S. Truman 18
   Jason Hulme 150
   Jocko Willink 79
   Joe DeFranco 289
   John Quincy Adams 341
   John Wooden 19, 319
   Jon Torine 291
   Mark Twain 72
   Richard Feynman 12
   Tony Dungy 264

R

radical transparency, principle of 15
reactive neuromuscular training
   definition of 174
   facilitation techniques of 205
readiness screen, example of 288
reconditioning capacity 228
red, yellow, green lights, *see lights system*
referral sources, providing value for 298
reflexive control and stability 201
reinforce the change 181
reset, reinforce, redevelop, the 3 Rs
   examples of 182–183
   test, action, retest, delivery, table of 192
   when to move between the layers 222
resilience, monitoring of 277
retesting, rescreening
   at natural breaks in activity 285
   did the correction stick? 186
   timing of 287
   to gain buy-in 177
risk
   factors for musculoskeletal injury 357
   identifying movement risks 65, 184
   management of 65–66
   questions to ask at the entry point 53
   removing negatives 67, 183
rolling, integrity of 172
Rose, Dr. Greg, corrective matrix 204

S

scale your business
   expand your offerings 331
   investing your resources 328
   maximize space and staff 330
   new technology options 332
   virtual training in, *see virtual training*
   what are your baselines? 329
   what does success look like to you? 327
scoring screens, clear priorities 140
screening groups
   goals and process of 232
   planning for 114
screens
   as a guide 138
   comparison across groups 76
   don't practice the test 165

screens, *continued*
   evaluating client perception of 123
   FMS, FCS, YBT, performance testing 236
   for competitive athletes 289
   linking the threads together 164
   mastering before implementation 109
   movement screening 60
   providing context for your clients 141
   use the full screens, not parts 111
   vs assessments 60

SFMA
   as used with the FMS 151
   categorizing patterns of 147
   details of 353
   dysfunction and pain, correction of 195
   finding pain during 147
   introduction of 11
   Jason Hulme's use of 269
   patterns of, simple to complex 195
   the 3 Rs approach 162
   uses for 117
   when pain is identified in the FMS 136

self-appraisal and awareness
   questions to build upon 14
   stages of 32

self-awareness, lack of as a risk factor 125

self-limiting exercises
   description and examples of 230–231

show-up-rate, monitoring of 278

sidebars, list of
   assigning home exercise correctives 197
   correcting behaviors 208
   dissecting layers of movement 81
   dysfunction vs deficiency 193
   empowering people 169
   failure vs non-failure, commentary on 68
   fire service testing overview 273
   gauging a well-run clinic 329
   impairments, limitations, disability 281
   integrity, compromise of 189
   movement system case study 237
   non-negotiables for clients, list of 101
   postures vs patterns 57
   practicing the tests 165
   readiness screen, example of 288
   sacrificing strategy for tactics 114
   screening the top-tier (SFMA) 117
   screens vs assessments 60

sidebars, list of *continued*
   standard operating procedures 78
   sustained success, secrets of 152
   symptoms vs signs 146
   tactical filters, layers of 256
   three biggest mistakes of the screens 141
   understanding where your skills end 91
   wants vs needs 51

signs vs symptoms 146
specialization, discussion of 88

split, a point of complexity
   challenges to business 105

stability
   building from the ground up 203
   reintegrating patterns with 201
   static vs dynamic 171
   strategies for 173

standard operating procedures 363

strategy vs tactics
   in the professional environment 27
   sacrifices of 114
   strategy tests and reinforces tactics 28

stress and recovery, explanation of 127
structure vs function 43
symmetry, prioritization of 204
sympathetic system, potential triggers 131

T

tables, list of
   4x4 grid, evaluating your own 260
   4x4 matrix, development 223
   adding elements to correct and restore 71
   assisted, active, reactive training 174
   discovering opportunities, fitness 95
   discovering opportunities, medical 93
   dysfunctional vs deficient 193
   examples of the lights exercises 188
   facilitation techniques 205
   identified movement risk factors 65
   information needed, actions of 82
   layer of movement, FMS definitions 49
   levels of movement, rating of 41
   light system strategy 225
   light system strategy, expanded 226
   minimal acceptable qualities 228
   mobility strategies 168
   modifiable movement risk factors 184

tables, list of *continued*
  movement layers, functional measures 63
  multi-segmental flexion 207
  opportunities for physical adaptation 84
  patterns and postures, SFMA/FMS 202
  physical adaptation vs growth 347
  physical data vs organizational data 293
  physical growth, adaptation, actions 80
  postures, static vs dynamic stability 171
  production, fitness, wellness, health 254
  red, yellow, green lights, controls of 362
  red, yellow, green light exercises 361
  removing elements to reduce risk 68
  risk factors, odds and relative risk 66
  self-limiting exercises, examples of 231
  strategies for delivering virtual care 336
  testing to confirm each layer 42
  the 3 Rs, correction element 194
  the 3 Rs, expanded 182
  the 3 Rs, protection element 183
  the 3Rs, redevelopment 222
  the 3 Rs, reinforcement element 192
  the 3 Rs, test, action, retest, delivery 162
  the 3 Rs, use of in the 4x4 matrix 163
  what does your testing tell you? 53
tactic sidebars, list of
  be flexible when training groups 234
  capture function with capacity 215
  confirm the integrity of rolling 172
  confirm that your corrective stuck 186
  deliver the same action differently 174
  don't label a person's movement 227
  efficiently maintain function 232
  empower your team 342
  everything is educational 271
  expand your network 296
  find a local certified professional 335
  find and fix the foundation first 268
  hold your prognosis 130
  invest time in breathing 200
  monitor your show-up rate 278
  networking works 308
  plan for the frequent questions 339
  prioritize mobility, foot and ankle 167
  prioritize symmetry 204
  promote self-selected fitness 244
  random practice 212

tactic sidebars, list of *continued*
  rescreen at natural breaks in activity 285
  screen the basics every time 289
  screen the "good" side first 124
  use play to develop awareness 249
  video feedback 158
  volunteer your experience 305
team building, *see building your team*
testing and retesting to gain buy-in 176
the 3 Rs, *see also tables list*
  reset, reinforce, redevelop 162
  use of in the 4x4 matrix 163
Torine, Jon
  comment about standards 184
  contributor bio 369
  risk-to-reward ratio 291
  sidebar: compliance and buy-in 282
  sidebar: connect with coaches 304
  sidebar: create a team approach 316
  sidebar: translate conversations 301
  tactic: rescreen at natural breaks 285
  Tony Dungy quote 264
tracking your clients successes, failures 160
training and exercise, client history 128
training groups, need for flexibility 234
Tsatsouline, Pavel, kettlebell expert 245

U

utility workers, functional needs of 279

V

video in business
  use of in virtual training 336
  use of with your clients 158
virtual training
  building an online FAQ 339
  charging for 339
  client tracking example 338
  communication options 337
  evaluating potential for success 333
  expanding your business to include 332
  getting a local FMS score 335
  goal setting for 334
  intake process of 333
  stragegies for 336

W

wants vs needs 51
weak link
  correctives for 191
  explanation of 179
workflow, fitting the screens into 109

Y

Y Balance Test
  details of 354
  introduction to 11
  Motor Control Screen and 210

DEDICATION

A pair of constants were with me throughout the process of this book, two life experiences I never thought I'd have to consider:

The first, that I'd write a business book. I have my partners to thank for this because they made me become a better businessman.

The second was that I'd become a father again in my late 40s. Well, my Zena is 10 years old as of this writing. Her development has been another welcome opportunity to witness the miracle of movement growth and healthy adaptation.

So, Z—This one's for you and all your great moves!

GC

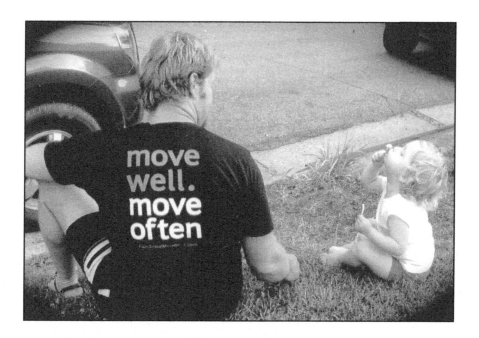

Made in the USA
Coppell, TX
29 September 2022